Emergency Psychiatry

Emergency Psychiatry

edited by

Juan E. Mezzich, M.D., Ph.D.

Ben Zimmer, M.D.

Western Psychiatric Institute and Clinic
University of Pittsburgh

International Universities Press, Inc.
Madison, Connecticut

Library of Congress Cataloging in Publication Data

Emergency psychiatry / edited by Juan E. Mezzich, Ben Zimmer.
p. cm.
Includes bibliographies and indexes.
ISBN 0-8236-1647-9
1. Psychiatric emergencies. I. Mezzich, Juan E. II. Zimmer, Ben.
[DNLM: 1. Crisis Intervention. 2. Emergencies. 3. Mental Health Services. WM 401 E531]
RC480.6.E443 1990
616.89'0025–dc19
DNLM/DLC
for Library of Congress 88-13599
CIP

Manufactured in the United States of America

Contents

Contributors

Jose M. Albornoz-Ruiz
T. A. Ban
Ellen Bassuk
P. N. Burvill
Erwin A. Carner
F. Cashman
Gerald A. Coffman
William R. Dubin
M. R. Eastwood
Karen J. Evanczuk
Irl Extein
Beverly J. Fauman
Michael A. Fauman
M. E. Garralda
Samuel Gerson
R. D. Goldney
W. Guy
N. Gregory Hamilton
Melissa Klein
S. K. Littmann
Reba J. Mathias
Juan E. Mezzich
John Monahan
Kevin M. O'Keeffe
Richard A. Perlmutter
Charles J. Rabiner
Sidney H. Schnoll
Andrew E. Slaby
Larry L. Smith
S. Stiasny
Laurence R. Tancredi
G. Voineskos
Howard M. Waxman
Kenneth J. Weiss
W. H. Wilson

University of Pittsburgh Invited Commentators

David Brent, M.D., Assistant Professor of Child Psychiatry, Child Psychiatric Treatment Service, Department of Psychiatry, Western Psychiatric Institute and Clinic

Cleon Cornes, M.D., Associate Professor of Psychiatry, Director, Depression Prevention Clinic, Western Psychiatric Institute and Clinic

Karen Evanczuk, M.S.N., Nursing Clinical Manager, Diagnostic and Evaluation Center, Western Psychiatric Institute and Clinic

Jeffrey L. Geller, M.D., M.P.H., Assistant Professor of Psychiatry, Law and Psychiatry Program, Western Psychiatric Institute and Clinic

Lynn H. Hackett, M.D., Assistant Professor of Psychiatry, Medical Director, Geriatric Psychiatry Inpatient Unit, Western Psychiatric Institute and Clinic

Peter B. Henderson, M.D., Professor of Child Psychiatry, Director, Residency Training in General and Child Psychiatry, Western Psychiatric Institute and Clinic

Shirley Hill, Ph.D., Associate Professor of Psychiatry and Psychology, Director, Substance Abuse Treatment and Alcohol Research Program, Western Psychiatric Institute and Clinic

Jonathan M. Himmelhoch, M.D., Professor of Psychiatry, Director, Research Affective Disorders Clinic, Western Psychiatric Institute and Clinic

George A. Huber, J.D., Assistant Professor of Psychiatry, Administrator, Western Psychiatric Institute and Clinic

Stanley D. Imber, Ph.D., Professor of Psychiatry and Psychology, Director, Treatment of Depression Collaborative Research Program, Western Psychiatric Institute and Clinic

David J. Kupfer, M.D., Professor and Chairman, Department of Psychiatry, Director of Research, Western Psychiatric Institute and Clinic

Robert S. Marin, M.D., Assistant Professor of Psychiatry, Geriatric Psychiatric Module, Western Psychiatric Institute and Clinic

Joaquim Puig-Antich, M.D., Professor of Psychiatry, Chief, Child and Adolescent Psychiatry, Western Psychiatric Insitute and Clinic

Charles F. Reynolds III, M.D., Associate Professor of Psychiatry & Neurology, Director, Sleep Evaluation Center, Western Psychiatric Institute and Clinic

Loren Roth, M.D., M.P.H., Professor and Vice-Chairman, Department of Psychiatry, Chief, Adult Clinical Services, Director, Law & Psychiatry Program, Western Psychiatric Institute and Clinic

Shawn C. Shea, M.D., Assistant Professor of Psychiatry, Medical Director, Diagnostic and Evaluation Center, Western Psychiatric Institute and Clinic

Paul Soloff, M.D., Associate Professor of Psychiatry, Head, Mood Disorders Inpatient Unit, Western Psychiatric Institute and Clinic

Meyer Sonis, M.D., Professor of Child Psychiatry, Program Director, Office of Education and Regional Programming, Western Psychiatric Institute and Clinic

Duane Spiker, M.D., Professor of Psychiatry, Western Psychiatric Institute and Clinic

Ronald D. Stewart, M.D., F.A.C.E.P., Associate Professor of Surgery, Assistant Professor of Anesthesiology and Critical Care, Director and President, Center for Emergency Medicine of Western Pennsylvania

Paula Trzepacz, M.D, Assistant Professor of Psychiatry, Medical Director, Psychiatric Consultation/Liaison Service, Western Psychiatric Institute and Clinic

Jack A. Wolford, M.D., Professor of Psychiatry, Western Psychiatric Institute and Clinic

Foreword

David J. Kupfer, M.D.

Although psychiatric emergencies constitute an extremely important level of activity in the practice of our specialty, academic discussions of emergency psychiatry traditionally deal with this critical issue, if not as an afterthought, in a perfunctory manner toward the end of most textbooks of psychiatry. Rarely is the topic of emergency psychiatry a focus for grand rounds; even less frequently do most departments of psychiatry invite a visiting lecturer because of his or her expertise in this area. A manual of psychiatric therapeutics is probably the forum that comes closest to dealing with emergency psychiatry "up front"; but, here again, most authors opt for reviewing the application of various treatment regimens rather than tackling what I consider to be the most important issue—the assessment of individuals in a state of psychiatric crisis.

It is fitting that increased attention be given to psychiatric emergencies since it has been suggested that over the last 40 to 50 years, the increase in public sector use (Voineskos and Lowy, 1985) of psychiatric emergency rooms has been greater than the rise in use of any other hospital facilities. In the Western Psychiatric Institute and Clinic of the University of Pittsburgh, for example, the number of emergency visits per year reached 5,670 in 1988. Some of this increased utilization can be traced to the public policy decision to deinstitutionalize a large number of patients with chronic psychiatric illnesses from the state hospitals in which they had long been cared for, to less restrictive community treatment. The need to provide crisis intervention for these individuals during periods of exacerbation of their illness and the continuing effort to avoid long-term rehospitalization has increased the pressure on staff to develop sophisticated diagnostic and evaluation procedures under the umbrella of a walk-in emergency room. And given the legal ramifications of court-ordered evaluations, it would appear that psychiatric emergency rooms will have to be used more in the future than they ever have been in the history of the profession. The increase in psychiatric emergency visits attributable to these developments and more has sharpened the need to educate medical students, residents, and faculty about decision making in a psychiatric crisis.

This book of readings, compiled and edited by Drs. Mezzich and Zimmer, stands alone as a unique source of papers and annotations focused on the major issues in emergency psychiatry. The book moves from the general to the more specific, dealing first with broad assessment, forensic, and educational issues to establish a basis for the topics that will follow. It then goes on to review a variety of behavioral emergencies, including the two issues that, together, are the keystone of psychiatric emergency room situations—suicide and violence. The evaluation of the patient who poses a danger to himself or to others and the management of the crisis such an individual poses has probably led to more writings in emergency psychiatry than almost any other topic. The readings drawn together for this book acknowledge that psychiatric emergencies know no age barriers; a child or adolescent or an elderly individual is as likely as a middle-aged adult to present with a psychiatric emergency. This book pays particular attention to the special problems of those patients at age's extremes. It also acknowledges another influence that has contributed to the flooding of psychiatric emergency rooms—the general increase in alcoholism, illicit use of all types of drugs, and the more life-threatening combination of alcohol *and* drugs. Overdue attention is devoted to the patients we have come to see all too frequently in both psychiatric and general emergency rooms, the "chronic crisis" patients who use the emergency rooms in lieu of a regular and stable schedule of follow-up care. Finally, attention is given to a situation psychiatrists may deal with less often as a crisis than do their general medical colleagues—death and dying.

The management and disposition of patients posing a psychiatric emergency raises a number of important issues that are dealt with in this volume: how to select the appropriate intervention strategies, be they pharmacologic or nonpharmacologic; when to hospitalize, when to release, and when to seek further consultation; and how to plan a setting in which to handle psychiatric emergencies, including discussion of innovative models that have been used successfully.

This book develops for the reader in step-by-step fashion a method for the assessment and management of psychiatric emergencies. It provides sufficient information concerning the emergency handling of specific types of behaviors to be used as a textbook of psychiatry. Perhaps most importantly, however, this volume gives the clinician a direct opportunity to read substantially more on the surprisingly neglected topic of emergency psychiatry than has been put between two covers to date.

References

Voineskos, G., & Lowry, F. (1985). Psychiatric emergencies. In: *A Method of Psychiatry*, eds. S. E. Greben, V. M. Rakoff, & G. Voineskos. Philadelphia: Lea & Febiger.

Acknowledgments

It is a pleasure to express appreciation for the help and stimulation received from all those people who made this book possible. Our colleagues at the Diagnostic and Evaluation Center of the Western Psychiatric Institute and Clinic, University of Pittsburgh, have nurtured this project in many ways. They include faculty psychiatrists, nurse clinicians, psychiatric, emergency medicine and family practice residents, psychology interns, medical, social work, and nursing students, and with particular distinction, Shawn Shea, M.D. and Karen Evanczuk, R.N., M.S.N., Ph.D. who over the past several years have worked closely with us. Ihsan Salloum, M.D., while studying emergency psychiatry helped us scholarly with a thorough review of the basic literature, in the computerized aspects of which Ms. Barbara Epstein, Ms. Ester Saghafi and Ms. Patricia Reavis were of invaluable aid. We are indebted to David Kupfer, M.D., Chairman of the Department of Psychiatry of the University of Pittsburgh, for writing the Foreword reflecting on his continuous support for our academic work, and to the distinguished members of the faculty who graciously prepared the commentaries which substantially enrich this reader. Special thanks are owed to Ms. Carol Gettings, who went several steps beyond her administrative assistant duties to edit, type, and assemble the manuscript with her unique touch of care and elegance. Margaret Emery, Ph.D., and the staff of International Universities Press greatly facilitated our work with their advice and sustained enthusiasm. To our families, we wish to express our sincere gratitude for their generative stimulation and invigorating support.

We would also like to thank the following journals, who allowed us to reprint the original articles:

American Journal of Psychiatry, 135:198–201 (1978); 137:1513–1517 (1980)

Annals of Emergency Medicine, 10:481–484 (1981)

Archives' of General Psychiatry, 41:1001–1004 (1984)

Australian and New Zealand Journal of Psychiatry, 14:1–15 (1980)

Canadian Medical Association Journal, 120:421–425 (1979)

Child Psychiatry, 24:261–267 (1983)

Community Mental Health Review, 2:4–13 (1977)

Hospital and Community Psychiatry, 32:687–698 (1981)

Hospital Medicine, 19:116–155 (1983)

International Journal of Psychiatry in Medicine, 10:189–204 (1980–1981)

Journal of the American College of Emergency Physicians, 6:315–323 (1977); 8:275–279 (1979)

Journal of the American Geriatric Society, 32:343–349 (1984)

Journal of Operational Psychiatry, 12:21–23 (1981)

Maryland State Medical Journal, 21:53–60 (1972)

Psychiatric Journal of the University of Ottawa, 9:36–41 (1984)

Psychiatric Quarterly, 54:190–197 (1982); 54:33–37 (1982)

Psychiatric Annals, 12:799–806 (1982)

Introduction

Juan E. Mezzich, M.D., Ph.D. and Ben Zimmer, M.D.

The word "emergency," from the medieval Latin *emergentia,* refers to a sudden, urgent, unforeseen occurrence requiring immediate action, while the word "psychiatry" denotes the science and art of diagnosing and treating mental disorders. On these etymological grounds, as well as reflecting current usage, emergency psychiatry can be defined as the field involved with the evaluation and care of urgent behavioral disturbances. The latter implies a call to immediate action. This, of course, does not mean that emergency care involves or requires superficial clinical skills. In fact, it demands sophisticated diagnostic, management, and dispositional competence plus high efficiency, as decision making here must take place under time constraints. Furthermore, the setting of emergency care (a psychiatric evaluation clinic or a general hospital emergency department) is typically one of the most important if not the principal gate for entrance to care at a health facility, emphasizing the crucial and widely reaching institutional role of such a unit, including its centrality for a well-implemented clinical information system.

Two critical elements of competent emergency care must be mentioned at this point, as they reflect its complexity and scope. One is *systematic assessment,* the main role of which is to provide the bases for sound emergency management, hospitalization, and referrals. Furthermore, it furnishes data for the evaluation and planning of clinical services as well as for clinical and epidemiological research. It involves the delineation of key psychopathological syndromes such as organic mental conditions, affective disorders, substance abuse, and personality disorders as well as of other important clinical aspects such as dangerous behaviors, concomitant physical disorders, occupational and interpersonal functioning, and social supports. Pertinent to these endeavors is the use of semistructured procedures that may increase rigor in data collection while allowing flexibility both in the conducting of the interview and in the integration of information obtained from various sources (the patient, accompanying persons, past clinical charts, referral documents, and so on).

The second critical element is the *consideration of systems issues for making management and disposition decisions.* One perspective here involves attention to various treatment levels and strategies to suit the patient's needs. This encompasses, first, psychotherapeutic interventions such as that reflected in the therapeutic tone of the initial evaluative interview, dealing with an explosive family situation on the spot, and initiating a series of crisis intervention appointments. Also pertinent here is the use of psychopharmacological agents such as neuroleptics for psychotic and agitated patients, antiparkinsonian agents for extrapyramidal reactions, benzodiazepines for impending delirium tremens, and thiamin for the Wernicke's encephalopathy of some alcoholics. Admission and referral options include hospitalization programs of various orientations and lengths of stay, partial hospitalization, and outpatient programs with various psychotherapeutic, pharmacological, and sociotherapeutic emphases. A parallel perspective involves attention to different spheres of influence and social systems such as the patient's family and its particular developmental stage, problems, and concerns; social networks that may need to be mobilized; and the legal system that often interfaces, synergistically or conflictually, with the clinical care system regarding patients presenting dangerous behaviors. Also important here is the consideration of ethnic issues. They involve not only variations in the way psychopathology presents itself, but also potential discrepancies between clinician and patient in the way they conceptualize illness and cure that may hinder patient compliance and implementation of care.

A READER ON EMERGENCY PSYCHIATRY

The basic purpose of this book is to present stimulating and pluralistic views for understanding the critical patterns and issues of emergency psychiatry.

The book first reviews general concepts and methodological issues, then describes the most important forms of behavioral emergency, and finally takes up key strategies for intervention and service organization.

I. General Issues

This section introduces us to broad conceptual and methodological considerations in emergency psychiatry. Its purpose is to furnish a framework for understanding the field as a whole, examining its larger questions, and setting the stage for the discussion of specific behavioral emergencies and therapeutic strategies.

The first chapter presents a penetrating and synthetic review of critical issues in emergency psychiatry as perceived by an eminent clinician and scholar, Dr. Slaby. The emphasis he places on a biopsychosocial approach for understanding the patient and for planning treatment and management is particularly cogent. The commentary that follows touches on the human sensitivity required for emergency work and on the special concerns of primary care professionals in outreach and rural settings. Legal and forensic considerations are the subject of the second chapter in which the author, Dr. Tancredi, a psychiatrist and a lawyer, analyzes the clinician's responsibilities for providing quality care while maintaining sensitivity to the patient's rights. The discussant, a lawyer with extensive clinical administrative experience, focuses on the duty to protect as well as to treat. The unique role of the emergency department in the acquisition of key psychiatric skills, such as integration of information, patient interviewing, and the effective use of various care settings and social supports, is discussed by Drs. Oliver and Rabiner in chapter 3. In the comments that follow, a highly experienced residency director elaborates on the need for a truly educational experience to include not only exposure to a meaningful reality but also competent and timely faculty feedback. The final chapter of this section, by Dr. Mezzich, reflects on the decisive importance of systematic assessment for adequate clinical care. It presents a semistructured approach to psychiatric evaluation, which involves the use of all sources of information available, standardization of the areas and items to be covered, flexibility in the conducting of interviews, and a multiaxial diagnostic formulation. The role of semistructured procedures in emergency care and in the teaching of interviewing is discussed further in the ensuing comments.

II. Specific Behavioral Emergencies

Part II deals with the various forms that behavioral emergency can take: the ways in which they present, their underlying mechanisms and associated factors, and the particular management problems they pose. The topics covered include some highly pressing psychopathological syndromes; two foremost emergencies—dangerousness to self and others; urgencies at both extremes of the life cycle; and the special challenges presented by the frequent requester of immediate care, and by death in the emergency department.

Nosological matters are discussed first, in chapter 5, in terms of the elucidation of an organic basis in behavioral disturbances, with particular attention paid to delirium, its differential diagnosis and assessment procedures. In chapter 6, Dr. Schnoll examines substance use disorders regarding life-threatening overdoses, and the enduring demands on the clinician posed by alcohol and drug abusers. The major forms of psychosis are reviewed in chapter 7, with an emphasis on the need for specificity in diagnostic assessment in order to facilitate management in general and treatment with psychopharmacological agents in particular. The most dramatic of the neuroses (i.e., hysteria), is examined in chapter 8 with respect to its presentation in emergency settings and the environmental problems it generates. Regarding lifelong maladaptive patterns, the case of borderline personality pathology is considered in chapter 9, including self-destructive elements, manipulativeness, and attempts to split the clinical staff. In all of these cases, the need to inscribe emergency management within the perspective of longitudinal care is emphasized.

Self-dangerousness is reviewed in chapter 10, in particular with regard to its changing trends (e.g., increasing suicide rates in female), the difficulties and available guidelines for assessing suicidal risk, and its exacting management through intensive work by multidisciplinary teams. With respect to dangerousness aimed at others, a brighter outlook is presented in chapters 11 and 12 for its prediction within the framework of emergency commitment proceedings, and suggestions are offered for the safe assessment and management of violent patients in the emergency department.

Life-cycle emergencies are presented next in chapters 13 and 14, and include, first, the patterns of symptomatology and family and social factors in emergency referrals to child psychiatric clinics. The case of the geriatric patient is then considered and the need for comprehensive evaluative approaches. Warnings are expressed about dichotomizing patients as either "medical" or "psychiatric," when in fact, many patients present a combination of these problems.

Finally, the special demands posed by the frequent visitor to the emergency department are considered in chapter 15, including the feelings of anger and frustration often aroused by these patients and the need for identifying and maintaining a primary treatment facility for consistent longitudinal care. In chapter 16 the phenomenon of death in the hurried and impersonal environment of the emergency setting is discussed, and the need to care and console in these situations.

III. Management and Disposition Issues

The third portion of the reader is concerned with approaches to care in emergency psychiatry. This encompasses consideration of broad therapeutic strategies, decision-making processes, and organizational issues.

In chapter 17, the principles and implementation of crisis theory are reviewed, with additional comments offered about adapting crisis concepts to the needs of practicing clinicians and empirically assessing their therapeutic impact. The role of psychopharmacology in the emergency department is discussed in chapter 18, focusing attention on the use of neuroleptics for severely agitated, violent, and psychotic patients as well as of sedative hypnotics for anxiety attacks. Invited comments point out that effective information gathering using all sources available is critical to emergency management.

The relevance to hospitalization decisions of various aspects of the clinical condition, as articulated in an expanded *Diagnostic and Statistical Manual of Mental Disorders* (DSM-III) multiaxial formulation, is considered in chapter 19. Among all psychopathological conditions, the presence of psychosis, regardless of type, appears to be most strongly associated with inpatient admission. However, among all axes of the diagnostic formulation, the highest correlation was found for impairment in adaptive functioning. Discussed next, in chapter 20, is the complex role of the psychiatrist as consultant in a general emergency department. Such role encompasses medical, social, and emotional factors in a way that attempts to be both scientifically grounded and humanistic in attitude. The commentary emphasizes the operation of multilevel systems in this environment, with pressures originating from the patient, his family, hospital administrators, and the consultant himself.

The final chapter, on care delivery systems, examines patterns of emergency service use and the scope of patients' needs, on both of which strategic planning for efficient management of clinical problems should be based. Highly relevant to this process is the routine collection of information on patients seen, as this may be valuable for the planning not only of emergency services but also of the various clinical programs to which patients are referred. Additionally pertinent here are the grounding of the definition of an emergency more on the patient's perception of urgency than on severity of pathology, and the need for multidisciplinary professional coverage to ensure adequate attention to the diversity and plurality of problems presented in an emergency setting.

STRUCTURAL ELEMENTS

The reader was built around a set of topics dealing with key conceptual and methodological questions, specific behavioral emergencies, and management and disposition matters. A selection of published articles covering these topics are the backbone of the book. To complement them and enhance their critical reading, a set of editors' comments appear at the beginning of each section and invited comments by

University of Pittsburgh faculty follow each chapter, which also has an annotated bibliography.

Emergency psychiatry has been for some time a key area of clinical service and is now becoming important also for scholarly consideration and research. In regard to patient care, it demands high psychiatric skills, particularly involving interviewing which is both sensitive and informationally thorough, and making efficient management and disposition decisions. The latter should pay appropriate attention to all forms of treatment and various interfacing systems such as the local hospital administration, health and social agencies, and the legal system. In this regard, the emergency department constitutes an important site for professional training. In fact it is uniquely suited for the acquisition of some of the most critical psychiatric skills.

For services planning and evaluation as well as for clinical and epidemiological research, the emergency department also plays an important role, especially when it constitutes a principal entry to the health system and is connected to a well-implemented clinical information system.

I

GENERAL ISSUES

Part I addresses questions such as the following: What are the cornerstones of psychiatric work in emergency settings? What kinds of theoretical models and clinician attitudes are most conducive to effective emergency care? How do quality of care and sensitivity to patients' rights combine as responsibilities of the treating clinician? How do the duty to treat and the duty to protect interface in emergency care? What does the emergency department offer as a training site for such central professional skills as interviewing, efficient decision making, consultation with other professionals, and coordinated use of various treatment programs and facilities? What are the particular assessment requirements for sound emergency care and what is the role of semistructured procedures in such endeavors?

1

Emergency Psychiatry: An Update

Andrew E. Slaby, M.D., Ph.D., M.P.H.

Nowhere in psychiatric care is greater or more diversified expertise required than in the delivery of emergency services. When a patient presents in crisis, the clinician needs skill in rapid, focused interviewing, in the differential diagnosis of behavioral disorders, and in understanding how the patient's case history and cultural background, which help determine the symptoms of even the most biologically induced disorders, may be used by a therapist in managing the patient (Slaby, Lieb, and Tancredi, 1981).

The human organism threatened by an external stressor or by internal physiologic decompensation defends itself holistically to prevent destruction of the personality's integrity. Emergency psychiatric clinicians must determine the degree to which a number of psychological, sociological, biological, and existential factors have altered an individual's functioning. The clinician then works to develop a biopsychosocial management plan to rapidly restore the patient's functioning and, ideally, bring about some growth as a result of the crisis (Goldberg and Slaby, 1981). The goal of emergency psychiatry is not

This chapter was first published in *Hospital and Community Psychiatry* (1981), 32:687–698, and it is reprinted by permission.

merely the amelioration of anxiety and depression and the return to baseline functioning but also growth, so that the individual will be more of a person.

To achieve these goals, emergency clinicians need a variety of therapeutic skills and a knowledge of the medical management of acute psychiatric dysfunction. They must have sufficient knowledge of systems dynamics to enable them to work well as a member of a team and to deal effectively with other medical services and community agencies. Consultation skills and sensitivity to systems issues are imperative so that patient flow and referral run smoothly, given limited funds, evolving legal sanctions, institutional boundaries, psychopathology of patients' families, and the fact that in crisis all of us involved in treatment may respond in self-defeating ways.

Emergency clinicians, more than other psychiatric clinicians, must be able to make decisions under stress and to change those decisions if they prove wrong. They must tolerate ambiguity and realize that often there is no one correct choice but, given a limited number of options, only a preferred choice. Finally, crisis clinicians must be aware of what they know and do not know and what resources are available to help them.

In this review, I will focus on recent advances in the delivery of emergency psychiatric services. This effort does not pretend to be comprehensive. Along with a review of some basic principles, it covers new developments in diagnostic psychiatry; treatment of drug toxic and withdrawal states; management of acutely psychotic, self-destructive, and violent patients; and staff burnout—the occupational hazard of emergency psychiatric clinicians.

DIAGNOSTIC PSYCHIATRY

The cornerstone in the delivery of emergency psychiatric care is diagnosis. Diagnosis must guide treatment decisions and has been demonstrated to be an important determinant of dispositions (Errera, Wyshak, and Jarecki, 1963; Schwartz and Errara, 1963; Tischler, 1966; Baxter, Chodorkoff, and Underhill, 1968; Shader, Binstock, Ohley, et al., 1969; Gross, Herbert, Knatterud, et al., 1969; Hanson and Babigian, 1974; Gerson and Bassuk, 1980; Slaby and Perry, 1980). Differential diagnosis of mood, thought, and behavior disorders is critical. For example, depressed mood, in addition to being a symptom of bipolar and unipolar affective illness, schizoaffective disorders, schizophreniform disorders, chronic schizophrenia, cyclothymic disorders, dysthymic disorders, borderline personality disorders, and some adjustment disorders, is also present in a large number of medical disorders (Slaby et al.,1981; Table 1.1). Similarly, the differential diagnosis for anxiety states and schizophrenia includes a number of medical and psychological conditions (Tables 1.2 and 1.3). Emergency clinicians must also be aware that while stress leads to alterations in behavior it does not, perforce, lead to psychological illness. Symptoms seen at a time of stress may be largely due to medical illness like migraine equivalents or hyperthyroidism precipitated by stress.

Some nonpsychiatric emergency clinicians believe that patients presenting in psychiatric crisis are sent to psychiatrists for disposition only after they are medically cleared. In most emergency rooms, medical clearance indicates that, based on a superficial physical examination, there are no gross indications of major organic illness. It does

Table 1.1
Medical Disorders Presenting with Depression

Addison's disease	Digitalis toxicity
Alcohol intoxication	Distal effects of cancer
Antihypertensive medication (such as methyldopa, propranolol, reserpine) toxicity	Disulfiram (Antabuse) intoxication
Arteriosclerosis	Encephalitis
Barbiturate intoxication	General paresis
Benzodiazepine intoxication	Hepatic failure
Carbon disulfide intoxication	Hepatitis
Carcinoma of pancreas	Hyperparathyroidism
Cerebral tuberculosis	Hyperthyroidism
Cerebrovascular syphilis	Hypoglycemia
Cessation of amphetamine or cocaine use	Hypokalemia
Cirrhosis of the liver	Hyponatremia
Corticosteroid toxicity	Hypothyroidism
Cushing's syndrome	Infectious mononucleosis
Degenerative diseases of the central nervous system (e.g., Alzheimer's disease, Huntington's chorea, Pick's disease)	Levodopa intoxication
Diabetes	Multiple sclerosis
	Occult malignancy
	Pernicious anemia
	Postviral infection syndrome
	Renal failure
	Subdural hematoma
	Thallium intoxication

From Slaby et al. (1981), reprinted with permission.

Table 1.2
Differential Diagnosis of Anxiety States

Adjustment disorder with anxious mood	Impending myocardial infarction
Agoraphobia	Insecticide (organophosphate) intoxication
Alcohol withdrawal	Internal hemorrhage
Amphetamine and similar sympathomimetic intoxication	Lead intoxication
Atropine psychosis	Mitral valve prolapse
Barbiturate and similar substance withdrawal	Normal anxiety
Bipolar affective illness	Obsessive-compulsive disorder
Borderline personality	Panic disorder
Caffeine intoxication	Paroxysmal atrial tachycardia and other cardiac arrhythmias
Cannabis intoxication	Phencyclidine intoxication
Cerebroarteriosclerosis	Pheochromocytoma
Cocaine intoxication	Phobic-anxiety depersonalization syndrome
Encephalitis	Postconcussion syndrome
Generalized anxiety disorder	Posttraumatic anxiety disorder
Glue sniffing	Pulmonary embolism
Hallucinogen intoxication	Schizophrenia
Homosexual panic	Simple phobia
Hypertension	Social phobia
Hyperthyroidism	Subacute bacterial endocarditis
Hyperventilation syndrome	Temporal lobe disease
Hypocalcemia	Temporal lobe epilepsy
Hypoglycemia	Unipolar affective illness
Hypokalemia	

From Slaby et al. (1981), reprinted with permission.

not indicate, however, that the alteration in mood, thought, or behavior is not an atypical form of a major or even life-threatening physical illness.

In a recent study of 658 consecutive psychiatric outpatients, 9.1 percent were found to have psychiatric symptoms caused by previously unrecognized medical illness (Hall, Popkin, Devaul, et al., 1978; Hall, Gardner, Stickney, et al., 1980). Other estimates are that unrecognized medical illness causes anywhere from 33 to 60 percent of psychiatric disorders (Maguire and Granville-Grossman, 1968; Johnson, 1968). In a study by Maguire and others, 33.5 percent of 200 consecutive inpatients (the majority of whom were admitted for profound depression or incapacitating psychosis) were found to have medical illnesses; 49 percent of that number had illnesses that previously were unknown to either the patient or his physician (Maguire and Granville-Gross-

Table 1.3
Differential Diagnosis of Schizophrenia

Addison's disease	Hypothyroidism
Adjustment reaction of adolescence	Idiosyncratic alcohol intoxication
Alcohol hallucinosis	Insecticide (organophosphate) intoxication
Alcohol paranoia	Isoniazid intoxication
Alcohol withdrawal	Lead intoxication
Amphetamine intoxication	Levodopa intoxication
Atropine psychosis	Manganese intoxication
Bacterial meningitis	Mercury intoxication
Barbiturate and similar substance withdrawal	Methyldopa (Aldomet) toxicity
Bipolar affective illness	Multiple sclerosis
Brief reactive psychosis	Niacin deficiency
Catatonic schizophrenia	Normal pressure hydrocephalus
Cerebral neoplasm	Paranoia
Cerebroarteriosclerosis	Paranoid schizophrenia
Cerebrovascular syphilis	Pernicious anemia
Chronic undifferentiated schizophrenia	Pheochromocytoma
Corticosteroid toxicity	Phencyclidine intoxication
Cushing's disease	Porphyria
Degenerative diseases of the central nervous system (e.g., Alzheimer's disease, Huntington's chorea, Pick's disease)	Pyridoxine deficiency
Digitalis toxicity	Schilder's disease
Disulfiram (Antabuse) intoxication	Schizoaffective disorders
General paresis	Schizophreniform disorders
Hyperparathyroidism	Systemic lupus erythematosus
Hyperthyroidism	Temporal lobe epilepsy
Hypoparathyroidism	Thallium intoxication
	Thiamine deficiency
	Tubercular meningitis
	Wilson's disease (hepatolenticular degeneration)

From Slaby et al. (1981), reprinted with permission.

man,1968). In another, more recent, study of 2,090 lower-socioeconomic outpatients, 43 percent had major medical illness, of whom 46 percent were undiagnosed by the referral source (Johnson, 1968). The patient's medical illness strongly affected his psychiatric state in 69 percent of those cases, and in 18 percent it appeared to be the sole cause of the psychiatric symptoms.

Unrecognized medical illness can contribute to the clinical presentation of patients with organic brain syndromes (Koranyi, 1979; Jarvik, Ruth, and Matsuyama, 1980). Tsuang and associates found significantly more deaths due to infectious and circulatory disease in a group of 200 schizophrenics, 100 manics, and 225 depressives compared with the general population in Iowa (Tsuang, Woolson, and Fleming, 1980). The absolute mortality for deaths due to neoplasm was not significantly different for the groups.

Neurosyphilis still causes 4,000 deaths a year in the United States, and recent statistics suggest that if every person in the country were tested for syphilis, approximately one million untreated cases would be found (Binder and Dickman, 1980). It is now thought that a significant number of patients with agoraphobia—once considered a predominantly psychological illness—may have mitral valve prolapse. A study of 25 agoraphobic women and 23 controls using an array of cardiac examination techniques found 11 agoraphobic patients, but only two control women, with mitral valve prolapse (Pariser, Pinta, and Jones, 1978; Kantor, Zitrin, and Zeldis, 1980). Organic brain syndromes have long been recognized as a complication of bacterial endocarditis; it is now known that they also may be an early feature of nonbacterial thrombotic endocarditis (MacKenzie and Popkin, 1980).

Specific psychiatric symptoms can be as complex in etiology as broader behavioral abnormalities like depression and psychosis. Delusions of parasitosis—a fixed mistaken belief that one is infected by parasites—can be caused by use of psychostimulants (particularly amphetamines, cocaine, and methylphenidate), temporal lobe epilepsy, schizophrenia, delirium tremens, and monosymptomatic hypochondriacal psychoses (Liebowitz, Nuetzel, Bowser, et al., 1978). The differential diagnosis for catatonia includes, in addition to classic catatonic schizophrenia and affective disorders, some 40 other organic conditions including bilateral chronic subdural hematomas, periodic catatonia, disulfiram therapy, focal lesions in the brain (as in the basal ganglia, limbic system, temporal lobes, and diencephalon), aspirin intoxication, ACTH intoxication, neuroleptic use, and a number of other infectious and toxic and metabolic conditions (Gelenberg, 1976; Gelenberg and Mandel, 1977; Woods, 1980; Weddington, Marks, and Verghese, 1980; Goldberg and Slaby, 1981; Slaby, 1981).

Just as organic illness may appear as psychological illness, so too the emergency clinician may be confronted with psychological illness presenting as organic illness. When no apparent organic etiology is found for delirium, it is usually attributed to transient viral infection, a peculiar drug response, or another nonspecific condition. Profound affective illness may present as delirium (Bond, 1980) or dementia (Slaby and Wyatt, 1974; Demuth and Rand, 1980; Goldberg and Slaby, 1981; Slaby et al., 1981) or contribute significantly to the clinical picture.

Diagnostic assessment of psychiatric emergencies of medical and surgical inpatients may be particularly difficult, as a number of subtle psychological and physical factors may interact to create the patient's crisis. The acute psychological changes seen in patients following removal of cataracts (postcataractectomy syndrome) is due in no small part to anticholinergic intoxication (Summers and Reich, 1979). Factors contributing to postcardiotomy delirium can include the impact of the open-heart-surgery recovery room on a patient made vulnerable by disease and surgical trauma, the change in the postoperative cardiac index, postoperative infection, atelectasis, blood loss, pain, the effect of anesthetic agents or other medication, electrolyte imbalance, and a previous history of psychopathology exacerbated by surgical trauma (Heller, Kornfeld, Frank, et al., 1979; Slaby et al., 1981).

Hall reported that more than 90 percent of the medical illnesses undiagnosed in psychiatric patients can be found by psychiatric and physical examinations that include a neurological exam, a 34-panel automated blood analysis, complete blood count, urinalysis, electrocardiogram, and sleep-deprived EEG. He recommended the set as an initial evaluation battery, particularly for patients facing involuntary commitment to a mental hospital (Hall et al., 1980).

Current data suggest that computerized axial tomography (CT) has an overall accuracy rate of 90 to 98 percent in detecting brain abnormalities. Skull x-rays are only about 50 percent accurate. Computerized tomography identifies significant nonacute diseases such as cerebral atrophy, porencephaly, and old infarcts, and defines both normal and abnormal ventricular size and configuration. Changes secondary to infections of the brain and demyelinating diseases are evident on CT, while skull films are rarely helpful in such cases (Tsai and Tsuang, 1978). Thus CT can be a useful evaluation technique, if time and resources allow.

DRUG TOXIC STATES

Drug toxic and drug withdrawal states are commonly seen as psychiatric emergencies and often are a source of confusion to evaluating clinicians. Nearly all drugs, if taken in excess or taken by individuals predisposed to idiosyncratic responses because of concurrent illness, psychological makeup, or ingestion of other drugs, can cause alterations of mood, thought, and behavior. Digitalis toxicity is relatively common and is seen in up to 33 percent of patients hospitalized for medical reasons (Shear and Sacks, 1978). Psychiatric symptoms are, in some instances, the first and only symptoms of potentially lethal digitalis toxicity. These symptoms can include incoherent thinking, disturbed orientation, hallucinations, delusional thoughts, irritability, distractability, labile mood, illusions, and disorientation. Fortunately, they are usually accompanied by other symptoms of digitalis toxicity such as anorexia, nausea, blurred vision, and chromatopsia (a phenomenon in which objects appear to have yellow-green edges or tints).

Certain neuropsychiatric symptoms are increasingly seen with use of cimetidine, a competitive histamine H_2-receptor antagonist used to decrease acid secretion in a variety of gastrointestinal disorders, particularly duodenal ulcers and the Zollinger-Ellison syndrome. They include coma, vivid visual hallucinations, lethargy, delirium, paranoia, agitation, depression, slurred speech, and unsteadiness (Barnhart and Bowden, 1979; Adler, Sadja, and Wilets, 1980; Crowder and Pate, 1980). Factors predisposing a patient to these side effects are older age, high-dose medication, preexisting psychiatric illness, cerebral impairment, poor renal function, and simultaneous treatment with psychotropic drugs. Anticonvulsants, including phenytoin, primidone, clonazepam, and carbamazepine, have been implicated in behavior changes resembling functional psychiatric disorders such as schizophrenia. Usual physical signs of toxicity such as dysarthria, nystagmus, ataxia, and lethargy are not always present (Demers-Decrosiers, Nestoros, and Vaillancourt, 1978; Franks and Richter, 1979; Slaby et al., 1981).

Steroids, such as prednisone, are used in the management of collagen disease, Addison's disease, and allergic and neoplastic diseases. If toxicity occurs, mania, depression, nonspecific psychoses, delirium, dementia, and schizophreniform psychoses may be seen (Goldberg and Slaby, 1981).It is not necessary to discontinue the steroid since antipsychotic medication may be prescribed in doses sufficient to control symptoms.

L-dopa (the precursor of dopamine) and amantadine, which are used in the treatment of patients with idiopathic Parkinson's disease, have been associated with psychiatric symptoms. Mania, depression, delirium, and schizophreniform psychoses have been reported with L-dopa toxicity (Braden, 1977; Moskovitz, Moses, and Klawans, 1978). Psychotic delirium with hallucinations, sometimes in conjunction with other disturbances of mental functioning, has been associated with amantadine (Hausner, 1980). In both instances, dosage reduction or substitution of another drug will relieve symptoms. Meperidine is associated with agitation and confusion if decreased renal clearance (as indicated by elevated creatinine levels) is found. Disorientation, visual disturbances, and dysphoria are symptomatic. Management consists of a switch to methadone or another equally potent analgesic with fewer side effects (Slaby et al., 1981).

Reserpine, methyldopa, propranolol, and other antihypertensives may produce depression, in some instances associated with suicidal ideation. Bromism, which like syphilis and tuberculosis has been called a great masquerader, is still seen in patients. The incidence of side effects associated with bromism is greatly underestimated because clinicians often do not think of bromism as a possible cause and hence fail to look for its presence in the blood. Bromism can cause patients to act demented, depressed, delirious, manic, or schizophrenic and can also cause symptoms of a number of other syndromes. The symptoms do not necessarily correlate with serum levels (Brenner and Rheuban, 1978).

Barbiturates and similar-acting hypnotics can cause a variety of psychiatric symptoms when administered at therapeutic levels, at toxic levels, and upon withdrawal. Delirium tremens, for instance, is associated with withdrawal from barbiturates, methaqualone, meprobamate, etchlorvynol, glutethimide, and methyprylon (Epstein, 1980; Heston and Hastings, 1980; Goldberg and Slaby, 1981; Slaby et al., 1981). Another drug associated with psychiatric symptoms is phenylpropanolamine, found as an active ingredient in several newer over-the-counter diet aids. Acute psychotic episodes and paranoia have been reported following use of phenylpropanolamine as a decongestant (Slaby et al., 1981).

Most of the pharmacologic agents used in the management of psychiatric illness, even given at therapeutic levels, have been associated with psychiatric symptoms (Heiser and Wilbert, 1974; Newton, 1975; Rainey, 1977; Biggs, Spiker, Petit, et al., 1977; Rampling,

1978; Brenner and Rheuban, 1978; Krauthammer and Klerman, 1978; Sheehy and Maxmen, 1978; DeBard, 1979; Nelson, Bowers, and Sweeney, 1979; Van Scheyen and Van Kammer, 1979; Chouinard and Jones, 1980; Arnold, Rudd, and Kirshner, 1980; Mitchell and Matthews, 1980). Benztropine mesylate, the tricyclic antidepressants, phenothiazines, and hypnotics such as glutethimide have prominent anticholinergic side effects and can produce an atropine psychosis characterized by agitation, blurred vision, dry mouth, talkativeness, rapid pulse, and hot, flushed skin (Slaby et al., 1981). Untoward aggressiveness has been reported as a side effect of the benzodiazepines and (though rarely) of the tricyclic antidepressant imipramine (Rampling, 1978). Monoamine oxidase inhibitors have been implicated in the production of psychosis, mania, delusions of parasitosis, and delirium (Liebowitz et al., 1978).

Baclofen, structurally related to gamma aminobutyric acid (GABA), has led, when discontinued abruptly, to depersonalization, auditory and visual hallucinations, paranoia, euphoria, and mania (Arnold et al., 1980). It is used in the treatment of a number of spastic disorders and recently suggested as beneficial in the treatment of schizophrenia. Disulfiram may cause side effects of psychosis, catatonia, depression, and loss of libido (Rainey, 1977; Weddington et al., 1980). Premoline, a relatively new medication used to treat hyperactivity, has been shown to cause insomnia, anorexia, mild depression, and ticlike movements resembling Gilles de la Tourette's syndrome (Mitchell and Matthews, 1980).

Vulnerability to prolonged psychotic states after low doses of psychotomimetic drugs is not necessarily due to a patient's psychogenetic factors (Bowers, 1977). The pharmacological data relating amphetamines and potent antipsychotic medication to dopaminergic systems, as well as the literature on amphetamine-exacerbated psychoses implicate dopaminergic hyperactivity or supersensitivity in the pathogenesis of some paranoid psychoses (Gold and Bowers, 1978).

Cocaine and amphetamines, while not addictive, may cause a profound depression during withdrawal that may even require the use of antidepressants or electroconvulsive treatment (Slaby et al., 1981). Phencyclidine, a potent hallucinogen new to the drug scene in the past few years, can cause a bizarre clinical picture that is sometimes confused with schizophrenia (Showalter and Thornton, 1977; Allen and Young, 1978; Rappolt, Gay, and Farris, 1979; Rosen, 1979). Phencyclidine was marketed in 1978 as a veterinary anesthetic with sympathomimetic properties. It is a white crystalline solid that may be ingested, snorted, or injected; ingestion is rare among sophisticated users except as a suicide attempt. Onset of symptoms is rapid; symptoms can be quite incapacitating, and patients may harm themselves or others.

The clinical picture following phencyclidine use seems less dependent on the user's personality than the clinical pictures of other drugs. Phencyclidine intoxication is always considered a serious medical emergency until proven otherwise, and medical consultation should be sought if there is any question of physical complications or a worsening in condition. Patients who have taken large doses of the drug may develop status epilepticus and adrenergic crises. Respiratory failure is a late sequelium (Rappolt et al., 1979).

Nitrous oxide, or laughing gas, causes mild euphoria and lightheadedness. It can be obtained from aerosol cans of whipping cream for a quick high (Block, 1978). Volatile nitrites such as amyl nitrite, used for the relief of angina pectoris, may cause alterations of mood and behavior; they are sold in "head" shops, pornography stores, and novelty shops and through mail-order houses under the trade names of Heart-on, Poppers, Toilet Water, Bullet, Gas, Rush, and Aroma of Men. Volatile nitrites have been used by artists to expand creativity; they have also been used to intensify sexual experiences. As with all drug toxic states, the clinical picture will vary depending on the amount of drug taken and its pharmacology, the user's expectations and personality, the setting, and the effects of any concurrent illnesses (Sigell, Kapp, Fusaro, et al., 1978). Symptoms generally disappear once usage is stopped.

Nutmeg, one of the oldest spices used in cooking, can cause visual hallucinations, changes in time and space perception, and agitation when used to excess. The psychoactive substance in nutmeg is myristicine, found in the seed coat and oil. Death due to fatty degeneration of the liver has been reported in severe cases of myristicine poisoning (Faguet and Rowland, 1978).

The toxic syndromes caused by the use of angel's trumpet, opiates, alcohol, hallucinogens, cannabis, and caffeine will not be discussed here, but are described, along with their management, in the literature (Greden, 1974; Hall, Popkin, and McHenry, 1977; Siegel, 1978;

Schaffer and Pauli, 1980; Goldberg and Slaby, 1981; Slaby et al., 1981).

Sudden death has been reported in patients taking neuroleptic medications. Patients on neuroleptics have been said to die of seizures and asphyxiation, vasodilation and hypotension, hyperpyrexia, laryngeal-pharyngeal dystonia, cardiac toxicity, and other unrelated medical illnesses (Solomon, 1977; Nies, Robinson, Friedman, et al., 1977; Flaherty and Lahmeyer, 1978; Coryell and Sherman, 1980; Smith, Low, and Nasrallah, 1980; Craig, 1980). Given the wide variability in the rate patients metabolize routine doses of tricyclics, we can expect that cardiac toxicity occasionally is caused by changes in conduction and contractibility of the heart rather than by an intentional overdose (Coryell and Sherman, 1980).

Central nervous system effects may also occur. Chlorpromazine acts directly on midbrain autonomic centers, producing sympathetic ganglion blockage and hypotension (Flaherty and Lahmeyer, 1978). In older people, and in others with compromised cerebral or cardiovascular status, chlorpromazine may cause strokes or myocardial infarctions. In addition, patients treated with phenothiazines have a diminished gag reflex that may result in aspiration asphyxia secondary to regurgitation (Slaby et al., 1981). Asphyxia, when it occurs, has been linked to a combination of dopamine blockage and strong anticholinergic effects leading to impairment of swallowing. Drug monitoring minimizes this possibility, and training staff in the Heimlich maneuver may help in resuscitation efforts (Craig, 1980).

Emotional factors alone can cause death in individuals not predisposed by immediate physical factors (Dimsdale, 1977). For example, a man might die of a heart attack when told his wife and children were killed in a car accident. Studies with animals have found that extreme emotional stress increases the risk of ventricular fibrillation (Lawn, Desilva, and Reich, 1980). Voodoo death is a particular subtype of sudden death that has been reported (Golden, 1977). In such instances, the victim must believe in the power of the person who places the curse and must know that he has been hexed.

DRUG WITHDRAWAL STATES

Physiological and psychological changes have been reported following the abrupt withdrawal of antianxiety agents, antidepressants, antipsychotic agents, anticonvulsants, and stimulants (Woody, O'Brien, and Greenstein, 1975; Dysken and Chan, 1977; Demers-Decrosiers et al., 1978; Pevnik, Jasinski, and Haertzen, 1978; Brown, Stancer, Moldofsky, 1978; Gardos, Cole, and Tarsy, 1978; Preskorn and Denner, 1979; Rosenfeld, 1979; Gualtieri and Stave, 1979; Winokur, Rickels, Guenblatt, et al., 1980; Stewart, Salem, and Springer, 1980; Luchins, Freed, and Wyatt, 1980; Gawin and Markoff, 1981; Goldberg and Slaby, 1981; Mirin, Schartzberg, and Creasey, 1981; Slaby et al., 1981). In some instances, these symptoms differ significantly from those seen in alcohol withdrawal. Dysphoria, weight loss, gastrointestinal upset, increase in pulse rate, acute organic brain syndromes, grand mal seizures, and prolonged coma have been reported following sudden withdrawal of large amounts of benzodiazepines (Woody et al., 1975; Dysken and Chan, 1977; DeBard, 1979; Preskorn and Denner, 1979; Winokur et al., 1980). Delirium has been reported as long as eight days after withdrawal from diazepam. These findings are consistent with the fact that symptoms are slower in developing after discontinuation of barbiturates or alcohol. Withdrawal symptoms of the longer-acting benzodiazepines, including chlordiazepoxide and diazepam, tend to occur three to four days after the drug is stopped, with a peak in symptomatology on the fifth. Symptoms of withdrawal from short-acting agents such as oxazepam and lorazepam occur earlier.

Individuals with histories of chronic alcohol or sedative abuse are particularly prone to develop symptoms of benzodiazepine withdrawal. Following withdrawal from antidepressants, a number of psychiatric symptoms have been reported in addition to gastrointestinal dysfunction (Gawin and Markoff, 1981; Mirin et al., 1981). Panic anxiety has been reported during the withdrawal from a number of tricyclic antidepressants, most frequently imipramine (Gawin and Markoff, 1981). Although relapse to depression is more common, both hypomania and mania have been reported in patients who discontinued tricyclics (Mirin et al., 1981).

Changes in the turnover rate of individual neurotransmitters, and the shifts in equilibrium between various transmitters that accompany withdrawal have been implicated in the affective changes. In the first two weeks following cessation of neuroleptics, nausea, vomiting, diaphoresis, restlessness, and insomnia are often reported. Some of these symptoms are seen during the withdrawal of anticholinergic agents among patients with Parkinson's disease, and are attributed to increase in cholinergic activity. It is thought that the neuroleptic withdrawal syndrome may be caused by rebound cholinergic sensitivity (Luchins et al., 1980).

Cessation of neuroleptics can bring on tardive dyskinesia as well as psychotic relapse or deterioration, which also is thought to reflect cholinergic overactivity and changes in dopamine-acetylcholine balance in the basal ganglia. These changes, called "supersensitivity psychosis" (Chouinard and Jones, 1980) or "covert" dyskinesia mimicking symptoms of psychotic exacerbation (Gardos et al., 1978), are also seen when neuroleptic dosage is decreased, as at the end of the injection interval of depot neuroleptics. Concomitant signs of dopamine supersensitivity (that is, tardive dyskinesia) are seen during neuroleptic withdrawal. The central nervous system tolerance for the drug also increases, requiring a gradual increase in dosage to maintain therapeutic effect. As with tardive dyskinesia, the most efficacious way to ameliorate symptoms is treatment with the causative agent, the neuroleptic. Symptoms usually disappear in 6 to 12 weeks. Dyskinesia uncovered at the time of abrupt drug withdrawal may be an early sign of tardive dyskinesia (Slaby et al., 1981).

Abrupt discontinuation of stimulant drugs, such as amphetamines and methylphenidate, may result in profound suicidal depression requiring hospitalization and management with antidepressants or electroconvulsive treatment (Rosenfeld, 1979). Discontinuation of anticonvulsants has been reported to lead to psychotic symptoms characterized by a clear sensorium with markedly increased electroencephalographic abnormalities (Slaby et al., 1981). Individuals withdrawing from alcohol, barbiturates, meprobamate, ethchlorvynol, and related sedative-hypnotics are prone to schizophreniclike psychoses as part of delirium tremens. It is usually thought that those taking 0.4 g per day or less of secobarbital or pentobarbital (or equivalent doses of related drugs) are unlikely to have any symptoms. However, the patient's sex, age, weight, physical condition, and personality must be taken into account since persistent mild hallucinosis and other symptoms suggestive of withdrawal have been reported with lower doses (Epstein, 1980). Duration of symptoms also varies; the schizophreniclike psychosis and organic delirium seen with ethchlorvynol withdrawal may last well beyond the 3 to 12 days usually seen (Heston and Hastings, 1980).

In most cases, symptoms following abrupt withdrawal of psychotropic drugs disappear upon reinstitution of the drug. Subsequent gradual withdrawal is usually successful. Gastrointestinal symptoms alone usually are not sufficiently severe to warrant represcribing the drug (Goldberg and Slaby, 1981; Slaby et al., 1981).

MANAGING THE ACUTELY PSYCHOTIC

The first step in the management of acutely psychotic patients is the taking of a history and a complete physical and psychiatric examination (Andersen and Kuehnle, 1974; Slaby et al., 1981). When patients are unable to provide a history themselves, the clinician should seek out family, friends, lovers, employers, police officers, therapists, or others to obtain as much information on the patient's history and previous treatment as possible. When others are not available and the patient is too psychotic to give an adequate history, diagnosis will depend on physical and psychiatric examination supplemented by laboratory tests.

If the acutely psychotic patient remains a diagnostic problem, hospitalization for further evaluation may be necessary even if a patient's symptoms are controllable by medication. Hospitalization is always indicated if a patient is acutely destructive or dangerous to himself or others, or if the psychosis is uncontrolled by ordinary psychopharmacotherapy (Andersen and Kuehnle, 1974; Slaby et al., 1981). Acute psychosis is painful to the individual; delay in treatment is not a humane alternative (Andersen and Kuehnle, 1974).

When diagnosis is established, specific treatment should be provided whenever possible. The clinician should choose his options carefully to avoid making the patient's condition worse. If an individual has an atropine psychosis or appears psychotic because of the akathisia associated with the use of antipsychotic medication, the administration of antipsychotic drugs, with anticholinergic properties and the potential for extrapyramidal side effects, will worsen the patient's condition.

On the whole, high-potency antipsychotic agents such as trifluoperazine, fluphenazine haloperidol, and perphenazine are preferred in emergency situations. The dosage of haloperidol and perphenazine is 5 to 10 mg when given intramuscularly. This dose may be repeated hourly up to five times if blood pressure and pulse allow and the extrapyramidal side effects are sufficiently controlled (Andersen and Kuehnle, 1974; Slaby et al., 1981). If fluphenazine is given intramuscularly, the hydrochloride form should be used. The decanoate and enanthate forms are long acting (10 to 14 days) and cannot be easily titrated in an emergency (Slaby et al., 1981). Fifty mg of chlorpromazine may also be given intramuscularly, but is more sedating than the higher potency antipsychotics and tends to cause more hypotension. Sedation is usually less important than the antipsychotic effects of the drugs, and may even confuse the patient. Hypotension is seen less frequently with piperazine phenothiazines, haloperidol, and thiothixene.

The choice of antipsychotic agents depends on the patient's age and weight, the severity of the illness, the degree of sedation desired, the patient's past response to drugs (including any allergies), and the risk of extrapyramidal and other side effects (Slaby et al., 1981). Side effects should be monitored. Oral medication is preferred. If it is questionable that the patient can or will swallow the medication, the liquid form should be used. It may be necessary to repeat the dosage hourly in the acute stage until improvement occurs. For example, 5 to 10 mg of haloperidol may be given every hour (up to about a total of 60 mg) until a patient's symptoms decrease or he falls asleep (Andersen and Kuehnle, 1974; Donlon, Hopkin, and Tupin, 1979).

Extrapyramidal effects can be quite frightening to an individual already terrified by the chaos within, and can cause him to discontinue both medication and treatment. It is recommended that appropriate antiparkinsonism agents, such as benztropine mesylate, be administered at a dose of 0.5 to 1 mg t.i.d. or q.i.d. After a few weeks, the antiparkinsonism agent can be withdrawn to see if it is really needed. Antiparkinsonism agents, like antipsychotic medication, have anticholinergic properties and increase constipation, blurred vision, dry mouth, and the risk of postural hypotension and iatrogenic psychosis. Dystonic reactions can be managed with 50 to 100 mg of diphenhydramine or 1 or 2 mg of benztropine mesylate given intramuscularly. Benztropine administered intravenously does not take effect significantly more rapidly.

If there is little or no improvement in major nonspecific psychotic or schizophrenic symptomatology after six hours of pharmacologic treatment, the patient should be hospitalized (Andersen and Kuehnle, 1974).

In the past few years a number of new antipsychotic agents have been introduced that have specific advantages to recommend them. Molindone has a weight-reducing property attributed to a central anorexigenic effect (Gardos and Cole, 1977). Clozapine is said to have strong hypnotic and anxiolytic properties with a low incidence of extrapyramidal side effects; however, it has other side effects that make patients uncomfortable, including hypersalivation, hypotension, and sedation (Shopsin, Klein, Aaronson, et al., 1979). Penfluridol is reported to show a low overall incidence of side effects (Lapierre, 1978).

SELF-DESTRUCTIVE BEHAVIOR

The evaluation and management of suicidal behavior cause considerable anxiety for a psychiatrist. Fortunately, unlike the evaluation of violent behavior toward others, studies have identified a number of epidemiologic and sociodemographic variables that can help guide decisions on whether or not to hospitalize a possibly suicidal patient (Beck, Beck, and Kovacs, 1975; Frederick, 1977; Donlon and Tupin, 1977; Avery and Winokur, 1978; Frederick and Lague, 1978; Croughan, Woodruff, and Reich, 1979).

The United States' suicide rate of about 12 per 100,000 population is about average worldwide (Slaby et al., 1981). Suicide rates generally have increased over the past two decades. Weissman found a nearly twofold increase in suicide attempts in a number of cities in America, Australia, and the United Kingdom between 1960 and 1970 (Weissman, 1974). Other studies indicate that each successive birth cohort starts with a higher suicide rate than the previous, and that at each successive five-year interval it has a higher rate than the preceding cohort at the same age (Hellon and Solomon, 1980; Murphy and Wetzel, 1980; Solomon and Hellon, 1980). Previous attempts are an accurate predictor of future suicide. Since the risk of both depression and suicide increases with age, we may expect the current upward trend to continue, placing considerable stress on emergency psychiatric care systems.

Marital status continues to be a major factor in evaluation of suicide risk. Widowed and divorced people have the highest rates of suicide (four to five times those of married couples); the widowed are at especially great risk during the first year of their bereavement. Singles have twice the suicide rate of the married. The married with children have the lowest rate. An exception to the rule is single teenage girls, who have lower rates than married female adolescents (Winokur, 1972–1973). Women make more suicide attempts, but men succeed more often. This pattern is changing as women, especially professional women, show increasing rates of suicide, alcoholism, and coronary heart disease (Murphy and Wetzel, 1980). A recent study in Boston found that attempted suicide by drug overdose, a method favored in the past by women, was occurring at equal rates for men and women (O'Brien, 1977).

Suicide risk and age have been correlated in the past, but marked changes have been found over the past two decades. Adolescents are now killing themselves more, and older people are killing themselves less. Between 1950 and 1970 there was at least a 250 percent increase in suicides among males aged 15 to 24 (from 6.8 per 100,000 to 17.4 per 100,000 per year), while rates for the elderly decreased; this finding suggests that the attention given in recent years to social supports for the elderly is helping make them less depressed.

Jews and Catholics, particularly if active in a religious organization, have lower suicide rates than Protestants and nonreligious individuals. Rates are high at both ends of the socioeconomic scale, particularly among physicians (Pitts, Schuller, and Rich, 1979), business executives, and other professionals. Half of the suicides by physicians occur during the most productive decades of 35 to 54. After retirement, physicians are 12 times more likely to kill themselves; divorced physicians over 65 are 13 times more likely to kill themselves than are their married colleagues (Slaby et al., 1981). Whites have tended to kill themselves more than blacks, but rates for blacks, especially blacks in urban areas, are beginning to approach those of whites. Some tribes of Native Americans have suicide rates five times the national average (Frederick and Lague, 1978).

Depression increases the risk of suicide; self-inflicted death is 500 times more common among the seriously depressed. Physical illness, hypochondriasis, or recent surgery or childbirth also increases the risk, while suicide is rare during pregnancy. Other factors that increase the risk are severe insomnia, alcohol and drug abuse, schizophrenia

(Tsuang et al., 1980), a predominantly homosexual orientation, a family history of suicide or a personal history of previous attempts (Pederson, Aruad, and Kindler, 1973), and a recent loss of a loved one. A patient who lacks any future plans, who is unemployed or in financial difficulties, who hallucinates commands to kill himself, who disburses his personal property, or who has used an especially lethal method in a past suicide attempt is also at high risk for suicide. Finally, patients whose level of tension was not reduced during initial psychiatric evaluation or who seem to lack an apparent secondary gain from the suicide are at high risk.

If an individual has attempted suicide, the first step in management is evaluating the immediate risk of another attempt. If the risk is significant, the patient should be hospitalized; if not, and there are sufficient social supports, the individual may be treated as an outpatient. The decision of whether or not to hospitalize is based on assessments of the severity of depression, history of past attempts, the availability of social supports, the patient's current living arrangements, and the effect of evaluation and beginning of treatment. A moderately suicidal patient may be managed outside a hospital if supportive friends and family are available, but one without such support may require hospitalization. If the depression and suicidal tendency are secondary to an organic process, such as the effects of antihypertensive medication or of cocaine or amphetamine withdrawal, appropriate medical treatment should begin.

If a suicidal patient is to be managed as an outpatient, social support should be rallied and appropriate psychotherapy, sociotherapy, and psychopharmacotherapy begun. The patient and his family and friends should be given the emergency clinician's telephone number and that of his backup clinician and the name of an emergency room if the clinician is unavailable. Family and friends should be allowed to ventilate their feelings so that they can work better with the patient, and they should be alerted to ominous signs such as increasing withdrawal, preoccupation, and moroseness. A return visit should be scheduled, possibly as soon as the next day.

The central goals of crisis work with self-destructive patients are opening lines of communication, identifying and exploring resources and options, establishing or renewing social supports, and beginning therapeutic interventions (Slaby et al., 1981).

MANAGING VIOLENT BEHAVIOR

The evaluation of a patient's potential for violence toward others remains a problem and is considerably less reliable than the assessment of suicidal potential (Cocozza and Steadman, 1974; Martin, Cloninger, and Guze, 1978; Monahan, 1978; Skodol and Karasu, 1978; Good, 1978; Slaby et al., 1981). Previous psychiatric hospitalizations and diagnoses are not necessarily indicators of violence. Age is related to violence: nearly 80 percent of violent acts are performed by those under age 50. Violent behavior is caused more frequently by individuals who have a number of previous arrests, juvenile police records, or a history of a conviction for a violent crime. The more severe the original offense, the greater the likelihood of future violence.

Those who are violent have a higher incidence of both self-mutilation and violence toward others. While in psychiatric practice wrist-cutters tend to be women, two-thirds of wrist-cutters encountered by the police are men (Bach-y-Rita, 1974; Bach-y-Rita and Veno, 1974). Adults who commit violent acts are often described as being impulsive and stimulus-seeking as children, even to the extent of setting fires. Their home life often is characterized by violence and deprivation. Individuals who live in subcultures characterized by violence tend to act violently at times of stress. Finally, the majority of murders are committed by a relative or close acquaintance of the victim. The majority of aggravated assaults occur within a family, among neighbors, or among acquaintances (Slaby et al., 1981).

All these factors, while providing clues to the potential of patients for future violence, are really less important today, given existing commitment statutes, than is developing a plan for diagnostic workup and management of patients who have already committed a violent act (Skodol and Karasu, 1978). Just as depression, anxiety, and thought disorders may be a symptom of a number of medical and psychological disorders, so too is violence symptomatic of numerous disorders (Slaby et al., 1981). The differential diagnosis of violent behavior includes temporal lobe epilepsy and other temporal lobe pathology, other organic brain syndromes, drug toxic states (especially those associated with phencyclidine and amphetamine use), intermittent explosive disorder, paranoid states, schizophrenia (especially paranoid schizophrenia and catatonic excitement), alcohol intoxication and withdrawal, antisocial personality, homosexual panic, affective illness (Skodol and Karasu, 1978), side effects of benzodiazepine and other drug use (such as barbiturates or antidepressants), dissociative states, decompensating obsessive–compulsive neuroses, hypoglycemia, and uncontrollable violence secondary to interpersonal stress.

Unfortunately, most violent behavior is due not to a potentially treatable medical or psychological illness, but to social maladjustment without manifest psychiatric disorder, and it falls within the domain of the legal system rather than the medical care sector. While a patient is undergoing medical and psychological evaluation of the aggressive behavior, medication should be given in doses adequate to minimize the need for more intrusive restraints. Typical medications and doses used in the emergency setting are haloperidol (5 to 10 mg IM or 5 to 20 mg p.o.), thiothixene (10 to 20 mg IM or 15 to 40 mg p.o.), chlorpromazine (50 mg IM or 100 to 200 mg p.o.), sodium amytal (125 mg to 375 mg IM), diazepam (15 to 45 mg p.o. or 5 to 15 mg IM or IV) and paraldehyde (10 ml IM or 8 to 12 ml p.o.).

If the clinician decides not to hospitalize a patient, he should tell family members or friends what risks exist. Those at whom the violence may be directed, such as a wife abused by an alcoholic husband, should be made aware of what behavior changes will necessitate immediate hospitalization and how to arrange it (say, by calling the police to have the patient arrested and brought to the emergency room for disposition to a psychiatric hospital).

Violent outbursts in the emergency evaluation area should be prevented whenever possible by prompt medication and by structure in the area. Emergency room staff should have written policies and procedures on the management of assaultive behavior. The emergency psychiatric area where violent patients are assessed should be large enough to provide each patient his "private" space, thus minimizing the provocation of violence; the area should be well-lit, should have an alarm system, and should be readily accessible to security officers. The interviewing room should have multiple exits and a minimum of dangerous materials and furnishings that could double as weapons. Self-defense courses have been suggested for clinicians working with violent patients.

When violence does occur, clinicians should document any physical injuries to themselves and to bystanders as well as to equipment and furnishings. Waiting-room attendants and other patients should be told what is happening. The information gathered should then be reviewed by staff to see what steps should be taken to avoid further occurrences.

BURNOUT

Burnout is the occupational hazard of emergency psychiatric clinicians (Freudenberger, 1975; Shubin, 1978; Pines and Maslach, 1978; Slaby et al., 1981). It occurs when excessive demands are placed on clinicians' energy or resources.

Symptoms of burnout include irritability, depression, cynicism, dread of going to work, and overt anger. Burnt-out emergency clinicians appear to others as losing their spirit and to themselves as losing their ability to heal or lead. They are hyperexcitable and they view everything as a crisis. Paranoia comes to the fore, and patient interests become submerged under increasing concern that someone may be impinging on the clinician's territory. They are disillusioned, disquieted, and increasingly ineffective at work. They dread organization and lose their innovation and creativity. Their sleep becomes disturbed, and physical symptoms, such as headache, indigestion, diarrhea, and tearfulness, may appear.

Other objective signs include an increase in the number of sick days taken, the canceling of conferences, declining appearance of self and work area, and devotion of more time to talk with other staff instead of inpatient care. There is a defensiveness about burnt-out clinicians that drives others away; further, they may try, ineffectively, to keep others from seeing how burnt out they really are.

Pines and Maslach (1978) have identified a number of factors that contribute to burnout. A staff–patient ratio that is insufficient to allow good interaction prevents staff members from fully enjoying and feeling fulfilled in their work. The greater the number of staff meetings, the more negative the staff's attitudes toward patients. Longer hours and lack of time to refocus work efforts can lead to more staff stress and to negative feelings toward work. The more time spent in administrative activities and away from direct contact with patients (except for chronic schizophrenic patients) the less job satisfaction and the greater the chance for burnout.

The most effective approach to prevent burnout is diversification of activities, such as outpatient work with individuals in longer term therapy or groups. Emergency psychiatric care should be provided by the team approach: teams composed of individuals from other services such as outpatient clinics, inpatient units, and consultation-liaison services can work on rotation one-half to one day a week on the emergency service.

This approach serves three purposes. First, it allows integration of emergency services with other services in a hospital or mental health center, thus breaking down barriers and facilitating patient flow. Second, it helps to develop and maintain clinicians' skills in crisis handling and diagnostic psychiatry. Even if one's primary interest is long-term outpatient therapy, the evaluative and management skills applied in emergency situations may be needed when a patient's behavior changes suddenly, a chronically depressed person becomes self-destructive, or an individual becomes psychotic. Finally, it lets clinicians deal with a mix of patients. Clinicians become particularly burned out when they see only one kind of patient, especially chronic cases. Maintaining a good patient mix aids in preventing burnout and helps clinicians approach each patient as an individual.

MORE THAN SKILL NEEDED

Nowhere in psychiatry is more skill demanded or more stress placed on a practicing clinician than in an emergency or crisis setting. However, nowhere else does the clinician have such an immediate opportunity to touch so many lives at a moment that may echo months and years later, long after the crisis subsides. To work effectively in an emergency psychiatric situation takes not only great technical skill in assessment, diagnosis, and management but also a special sensitivity to the complexity of what patients' lives are and, indeed, what we all are as human beings struggling in a world in which much is beyond our control. We must be able to confront others' pain as well as our own and, through that confrontation, help others.

REFERENCES

Adler, L. E., Sadja, L., & Wilets, G. (1980), Cimetidine toxicity manifested as paranoia and hallucinations. *Amer. J. Psychiat.*, 137:1112–1113.

Allen, R. M., & Young, S. J. (1978), Phencyclidine-induced psychosis. *Amer. J. Psychiat.*, 135:1081–1084.

Andersen, W. H., & Kuehnle, J. C. (1974), Strategies for treatment of acute psychosis. *J. Amer. Med. Assn.*, 229:1884–1889.

Arnold, E. S., Rudd, S. M., & Kirshner, H. (1980), Manic psychosis following rapid withdrawal from Baclofen. *Amer. J. Psychiat.*, 137:1466–1467.

Avery, D., & Winokur, G. (1978), Suicide, attempted suicide, and relapse rates in depression: Occurrence after ECT and antidepressant therapy. *Arch. Gen. Psychiat.*, 35:749–753.

Bach-y-Rita, G. (1974), Habitual violence and self-mutilation. *Amer. J. Psychiat.*, 131:1018–1020.

——— Veno, A. (1974), Habitual violence: A profile of 62 men. *Amer. J. Psychiat.*, 131:1015–1018.

Barnhart, C. C., & Bowden, C. L. (1979), Toxic psychosis with cimetidine. *Amer. J. Psychiat.*, 136:725–726.

Baxter, S., Chodorkoff, B., & Underhill, R. (1968), Psychiatric emergencies: Dispositional determinants and the validity of the decision to admit. *Amer. J. Psychiat.*, 124:1542–1546.

Beck, A. T., Beck, R., & Kovacs, M. (1975), Classification of suicidal behaviors: I. Quantifying intent and medical lethality. *Amer. J. Psychiat.*, 132:285–287.

Biggs, J. T., Spiker, D. G., Petit, J. M., et al. (1977), Tricyclic antidepressant overdose: Incidence of symptoms. *J. Amer. Med. Assn.*, 238:134–138.

Binder, R. I., & Dickman, W. A. (1980), Psychiatric manifestations of neurosyphilis in middle-aged patients. *Amer. J. Psychiat.*, 137:741–742.

Block, S. H. (1978), The grocery store high. *Amer. J. Psychiat.*, 135:126–127.

Bond, T. C. (1980), Recognition of acute delirious mania. *Arch. Gen. Psychiat.*, 37:553–554.

Bowers, M. B. (1977), Psychoses precipitated by psychotomimetic drugs: A follow-up study. *Arch. Gen. Psychiat.*, 34:832–835.

Braden, W. (1977), Response to lithium in a case of L-dopa-induced psychosis. *Amer. J. Psychiat.*, 134:808–809.

Brenner, I., & Rheuban, W. J. (1978), The catatonic dilemma. *Amer. J. Psychiat.*, 135:1242–1243.

Brown, G. M., Stancer, H. C., Moldofsky, H., (1978), Withdrawal from long-term high-dose desipramine therapy. *Arch. Gen. Psychiat.*, 35:1261–1264.

Chouinard, G., & Jones, B. D. (1980), Neuroleptic-induced super-sensitivity psychosis: Clinical and pharmacologic characters. *Amer. J. Psychiat.*, 137:16–21.

Cocozza, J. J., & Steadman, J. (1974), Some refinements in the measurement and prediction of dangerous behavior. *Amer. J. Psychiat.*, 131:1012–1014.

Coryell, W., & Sherman, A. (1980), Slow tricyclic metabolism, polypharmacy, and cardiac arrest. *Amer. J. Psychiat.*, 137:108–109.

Craig, T. J. (1980), Medication use and deaths attributed to asphyxia among psychiatric patients. *Amer. J. Psychiat.*, 137:1366–1373.

Croughan, J. L., Woodruff, R. A., & Reich, T. (1979), The management of patients with undiagnosed psychiatric illness. *Arch. Gen. Psychiat.*, 36:341–346.

Crowder, M. K., & Pate, J. K. (1980), A case report of cimetidine-induced depressive syndrome. *Amer. J. Psychiat.*, 137:1451.

DeBard, M. L. (1979), Diazepam withdrawal syndrome: A case with psychosis, seizure, and coma. *Amer. J. Psychiat.*, 136:104–105.

Demers-Decrosiers, L. A., Nestoros, J. N., & Vaillancourt, P. (1978), Acute psychosis precipitated by withdrawal of anticonvulsant medication. *Amer. J. Psychiat.*, 135:981–982.

Demuth, G. W., & Rand, B. S. (1980), Atypical major depression in a patient with severe degenerative dementia. *Amer. J. Psychiat.*, 137:1609–1610.

Dimsdale, J. E. (1977), Emotional causes of sudden death. *Amer. J. Psychiat.*, 134:1361–1366.

Donlon, P. T., & Tupin, J. P. (1977), Successful suicides with thioridazine and mesoridazine: A result of probable cardiotoxicity. *Arch. Gen. Psychiat.*, 34:955–957.

——— Hopkin, J., & Tupin, J. P. (1979), Overview: Efficacy and safety of the rapid neuroleptization method with injectable haloperidol. *Amer. J. Psychiat.*, 136:273–278.

Dysken, M. W., & Chan, C. H. (1977), Diazepam withdrawal psychosis: A case report. *Amer. J. Psychiat.*, 134:573.

Epstein, R. S. (1980), Withdrawal symptoms from chronic use of low-dose barbiturates. *Amer. J. Psychiat.*, 137:107–108.

Errera, P., Wyshak, G., & Jarecki, H. (1963), Psychiatric case in a general hospital emergency room. *Arch. Gen. Psychiat.*, 9:105–112.

Faguet, R. A., & Rowland, K. F. (1978), Spice cabinet intoxication. *Amer. J. Psychiat.*, 135:860–861.

Flaherty, J. A., & Lahmeyer, H. W. (1978), Laryngeal-pharyngeal dystonia as a possible cause of asphyxia with haloperidol treatment. *Amer. J. Psychiat.*, 135:1414–1415.

Franks, R. D., & Richter, A. J. (1979), Schizophrenia-like psychosis associated with anticonvulsant toxicity. *Amer. J. Psychiat.*, 136:973–974.

Frederick, C. J. (1977), Current trends in suicidal behavior in the United States. Paper presented at the 13th scientific meeting of the Association for the Advancement of Psychotherapy, Toronto, Canada.

——— Lague, L. (1978), Dealing with the crisis of suicide. New York: Public Affairs Committee, City of New York.

Freudenberger, J. L. (1975), The staff burn-out syndrome in alternative institutions. *Psychother. Theory, Res. & Pract.*, 12:73–82.

Gardos, G., & Cole, J. O. (1977), Weight reduction in schizophrenics by molindone. *Amer. J. Psychiat.*, 134:302–304.

——— ——— Tarsy, D. (1978), Withdrawal syndromes associated with antipsychotic drugs. *Amer. J. Psychiat.*, 135:1321–1324.

Gawin, F. H., & Markoff, R. A. (1981), Panic anxiety after abrupt discontinuation of amitriptyline. *Amer. J. Psychiat.*, 138:117–118.

Gelenberg, A. J. (1976), The catatonic syndrome. *Lancet*, 1:1339–1341.

——— Mandel, M. R. (1977), Catatonic reactions to high-potency neuroleptic drugs. *Arch. Gen. Psychiat.*, 34:947–950.

Gerson, S., & Bassuk, E. (1980), Psychiatric emergencies: An overview. *Amer. J. Psychiat.*, 137:1–11.

Gold, M. S., & Bowers, M. B. (1978), Neurobiological vulnerability to low dose amphetamine psychosis. *Amer. J. Psychiat.*, 135:1546–1548.

Goldberg, R. J., & Slaby, A. E. (1981), Diagnosing disorders of mood, thought, and behavior. New Hyde Park, NY: Medical Examination Publishing Company.

Golden, K. M. (1977), Voodoo in Africa and the United States. *Amer. J. Psychiat.*, 134:1361–1366.

Good, M. I. (1978), Primary affective disorder, aggression, and criminality: A review and clinical study. *Arch. Gen. Psychiat.*, 135:954–960.

Greden, J. F. (1974), Anxiety or caffeinism: A diagnostic dilemma. *Amer. J. Psychiat.*, 131:1089–1092.

Gross, H. S., Herbert, M. R., Knatterud, G. L., et al. (1969), The effect of race and sex on the variation of diagnosis and disposition in a psychiatric emergency room. *J. Nerv. & Ment. Dis.*, 148:638–642.

Gualtieri, C. T., & Stave, J. (1979), Withdrawal symptoms after abrupt cessation of amitriptyline in an eight-year-old boy. *Amer. J. Psychiat.*, 136:457–459.

Hall, R. C. W., Gardner, E. R., Stickney, S. K., et al. (1980), Physical illness manifesting as psychiatric disease: II. Analysis of a state hospital inpatient population. *Arch. Gen. Psychiat.*, 37:989–995.

——— Popkin, M. K., Devaul, R. A., et al. (1978), Physical illness presenting as psychiatric disease. *Arch. Gen. Psychiat.*, 35:1315–1320.

——— ——— McHenry, L. E. (1977), Angel's trumpet psychosis: A central nervous system anticholinergic syndrome. *Amer. J. Psychiat.*, 134:312–314.

Hanson, G. D., & Babigian, H. M. (1974), Reasons for hospitalization from a psychiatric emergency service. *Psychiat. Quart.*, 48:336–351.

Hausner, R. S. (1980), Amantadine-associated recurrence of psychosis. *Amer. J. Psychiat.*, 37:240–242.

Heiser, J. F., & Wilbert, D. E. (1974), Reversal of delirium induced by tricyclic antidepressant drugs with physostigmine. *Amer. J. Psychiat.*, 131:1275–1277.

Heller, S. S., Kornfeld, D. S., Frank, K. A., et al. (1979), Post-cardiotomy delirium and cardiac output. *Amer. J. Psychiat.*, 136:337–339.

Hellon, C. P., & Solomon, M. E. (1980), Suicide and age in Alberta, Canada, 1951 to 1977: The changing profile. *Arch. Gen. Psychiat.*, 37:505–510.

Heston, L. L., & Hastings, D. (1980), Psychosis with withdrawal from ethchlorvynol. *Amer. J. Psychiat.*, 137:249–250.

Jarvik, L. F., Ruth, V., & Matsuyama, S. S. (1980), Organic brain syndrome and aging: A six-year follow up of surviving twins. *Arch. Gen. Psychiat.*, 37:280–286.

Johnson, D. A. W. (1968), Evaluation of routine physical examination in psychiatric cases. *Practitioner*, 200:686–691.

Kantor, J. S., Zitrin, C. M., & Zeldis, S. M. (1980), Mitral valve prolapse syndrome in agoraphobic patients. *Amer. J. Psychiat.*, 37:467–469.

Koranyi, E. K. (1979), Morbidity and rates of undiagnosed physical illness in a psychiatric clinic population. *Arch. Gen. Psychiat.*, 36:414–419.

Krauthammer, C., & Klerman, G. L. (1978), Secondary mania: Manic syndromes associated with antecedent physical illness or drugs. *Arch. Gen. Psychiat.*, 35:1333–1339.

Lapierre, Y. D. (1978), A controlled study of penfluridol in the treatment of chronic schizophrenia. *Amer. J. Psychiat.*, 135:956–959.

Lawn, B., Desilva, A., Reich, P., (1980), Psychophysiologic factors in sudden death. *Amer. J. Psychiat.*, 137:1325–1335.

Liebowitz, M. R., Nuetzel, E. J., Bowser, A. E., et al. (1978), Phenelzine and delusions of parasitosis: A case report. *Amer. J. Psychiat.*, 135:1565–1566.

Luchins, D., Freed, W. J., & Wyatt, R. J. (1980), The role of cholinergic supersensitivity in the medical symptoms associated with withdrawal of antipsychotic drugs. *Amer. J. Psychiat.*, 137:1395–1398.

MacKenzie, T. B., & Popkin, M. K. (1980), Psychological manifestations of nonbacterial thrombotic endocarditis. *Amer. J. Psychiat.*, 137:972–973.

Maguire, G. P., & Granville-Grossman, K. L. (1968), Physical illness in psychiatric patients. *Brit. J. Psychiat.*, 114:1365–1369.

Martin, R. L., Cloninger, R., & Guze, S. B. (1978), Female criminality and the prediction of recidivism: A prospective six year follow-up. *Arch. Gen. Psychiat.*, 35:207–214.

Mirin, S. M., Schartzberg, A. F., & Creasey, D. E. (1981), Hypomania and mania after withdrawal of tricyclic antidepressants. *Amer. J. Psychiat.*, 138:87–89.

Mitchell, E., & Matthews, L. L. (1980), Gilles de la Tourette's disorder associated with pemoline. *Amer. J. Psychiat.*, 137:1618–1619.

Monahan, J. (1978), Prediction research and the emergency commitment of dangerously mentally ill persons: A reconsideration. *Amer. J. Psychiat.*, 135:198–201.

Moskovitz, C., Moses, H., & Klawans, H. L. (1978), Levadopa-induced psychosis: A kindling phenomenon. *Amer. J. Psychiat.*, 135:669–675.

Murphy, G. E., & Wetzel, R. D. (1980), Suicide risk by birth cohort in the United States, 1949–1974. *Arch. Gen. Psychiat.*, 37:519–523.

Nelson, J. C., Bowers, M. B., & Sweeney, D. R. (1979), Exacerbation of psychosis by tricyclic antidepressants in delusional depression. *Amer. J. Psychiat.*, 136:574–576.

Newton, R. W. (1975), Physostigmine salicylate in the treatment of tricyclic antidepressant overdosage. *J. Amer. Med. Assn.*, 231:941–944.

Nies, A., Robinson, M. J., Friedman, M. J., et al. (1977), Relationship between age and tricyclic antidepressant plasma levels. *Amer. J. Psychiat.*, 134:790–793.

O'Brien, J. P. (1977), Increase in suicide attempts by drug ingestion: The Boston experience. *Arch. Gen. Psychiat.*, 34:1165–1169.

Pariser, S. F., Pinta, E. R., & Jones, B. A. (1978), Mitral valve prolapse syndrome and anxiety neurosis panic disorder. *Amer. J. Psychiat.*, 135:246–247.

Pederson, A. M., Aruad, G. A., & Kindler, A. R. (1973), Epidemiological differences between white and nonwhite suicide attempters. *Ment. Health Digest*, 5:27–29.

Pevnik, J. S., Jasinski, D. R., & Haertzen, C. A. (1978), Abrupt withdrawal from therapeutically administered diazepam: Report of a case. *Arch. Gen. Psychiat.*, 35:995–998.

Pines, A., & Maslach, C. (1978), Characteristics of staff burnout in mental health settings. *Hosp. & Commun. Psychiat.*, 29:233–237.

Pitts, F. N., Schuller, A. B., Rich, C. L., (1979), Suicide among U.S. women physicians, *Amer. J. Psychiat.*, 136:694–696.

Preskorn, S. H., & Denner, L. J. (1979), Benzodiazepines and withdrawal psychosis: Report of three cases. *J. Amer. Med. Assn.*, 237:36–38.

Rainey, J. M. (1977), Disulfiram toxicity and carbon disulfide poisoning. *Amer. J. Psychiat.*, 134:371–378.

Rampling, D. (1978), Aggression: A paradoxical response to tricyclic antidepressants. *Amer. J. Psychiat.*, 135:117–118.

Rappolt, R. T., Gay, F. R., & Farris, R. D. (1979), Emergency management of acute phencyclidine intoxication. *J. Col. Emerg. Phys.*, 8:68–76.

Rosen, A. (1979), Case report: Symptomatic mania and phencyclidine abuse. *Amer. J. Psychiat.*, 136:118–119.

Rosenfeld, A. A. (1979), Depression and psychotic regression following prolonged methylphenidate use of withdrawal: Case report. *Amer. J. Psychiat.*, 136:226–228.

Schaffer, C. B., & Pauli, M. W. (1980), Psychotic reaction caused by proprietary oral diet agents. *Amer. J. Psychiat.*, 137:1256–1257.

Schwartz, M. D., & Errera, P. (1963), Psychiatric care in a general hospital emergency room: II. Diagnostic features. *Arch. Gen. Psychiat.*, 9:113–121.

Shader, R. I., Binstock, W. A., Ohly, J. I., et al. (1969), Biasing factors in diagnosis and disposition. *Comp. Psychiat.*, 10:81–89.

Shear, M. K., & Sacks, M. H. (1978), Digitalis delirium: Report of two cases. *Amer. J. Psychiat.*, 135:109–110.

Sheehy, L. M., & Maxmen, J. S. (1978), Phenelzine-induced psychosis. *Amer. J. Psychiat.*, 135:1422–1423.

Shopsin, B., Klein, H., Aaronson, M., et al. (1979), Clozapine, chlorpromazine, and placebo in newly hospitalized, acutely schizophrenic patients: A controlled, double-blind comparison. *Arch. Gen. Psychiat.*, 36:657–664.

Showalter, C. V., & Thornton, W. E. (1977), Clinical pharmacology of phencyclidine toxicity. *Amer. J. Psychiat.*, 134:1234–1238.

Shubin, S. (1978), Burnout: The professional hazard you face in nursing. *Nursing*, 8:23–27.

Siegel, R. K. (1978), Cocaine hallucinations. *Amer. J. Psychiat.*, 135:309–314.

Sigell, L. T., Kapp, F. T., Fusaro, G. A., et al. (1978), Popping and snorting volatile nitrites: A current fad for getting high. *Amer. J. Psychiat.*, 135:1216–1218.

Skodol, A. E., & Karasu, T. B. (1978), Emergency psychiatry and the assaultive patient. *Amer. J. Psychiat.*, 135:202–205.

Slaby, A. E., & Perry, P. L. (1980), Use and abuse of psychiatric emergency services. *Internat. J. Psychiat. & Med.*, 10:1–18.

——— Wyatt, R. J. (1974), Dementia in the presenium. Springfield, IL: Charles C. Thomas.

——— Lieb, J., & Tancredi, L. R. (1981), *Handbook of Psychiatric Emergencies*, 2nd ed. New Hyde Park, NY: Medical Examination Publishing Company.

Smith, R. E., Low, N. N., & Nasrallah, H. A. (1980), Haloperidol and an unrelated sudden death. *Amer. J. Psychiat.*, 137:843–844.

Solomon, K. (1977), Phenothiazine-induced bulbar palsy-like syndrome and sudden death. *Amer. J. Psychiat.*, 134:308–311.

Solomon, M. I., & Hellon, C. P. (1980), Suicide and age in Alberta, Canada, 1951 to 1977: A cohort analysis. *Arch. Gen. Psychiat.*, 37:511–513.

Stewart, R. B., Salem, R. B., & Springer, P. K. (1980), A case report of lorazepam withdrawal. *Amer. J. Psychiat.*, 137:1113–1114.

Summers, W. K., & Reich, T. C. (1979), Delirium after cataract surgery: Review and two cases. *Amer. J. Psychiat.*, 136:386–391.

Tsai, L., & Tsuang, M. T. (1978), Computerized tomography and skull X rays: Relative efficacy in detecting intracranial disease. *Amer. J. Psychiat.*, 135:1556–1557.

Tischler, G. L. (1966), Decision-making process in the emergency room. *Arch. Gen. Psychiat.*, 14:69–78.

Tsuang, M. T., Woolson, R. F., & Fleming, A. (1980), Premature deaths in schizophrenia and affective disorders: An analysis of survival curves and variables affecting the shortened survival. *Arch. Gen. Psychiat.*, 137:979–983.

Van Scheyen, J. D., & van Kammer, D. P. (1979), Clomipramine-induced mania in unipolar depression. *Arch. Gen. Psychiat.*, 36:560–565.

Weddington, W. W., Marks, R. C., & Verghese, P. (1980), Disulfiram encephalopathy as a cause of the catatonia syndrome. *Amer. J. Psychiat.*, 137:1217–1219.

Weissman, M. M. (1974), The epidemiology of suicide attempts: 1960–1971. *Arch. Gen. Psychiat.*, 30:737–746.

Winokur, A. (1972–1973), Females lead suicide attempts. *NAMH Reporter*, Winter:1.

——— Rickels, K., Guenblatt, D. J., et al. (1980), Withdrawal reaction from long term low dosage administration of diazepam: A double-blind, placebo-controlled case study. *Arch. Gen. Psychiat.*, 37:101–105.

Woods, S. W. (1980), Catatonia in a patient with subdural hematomas. *Amer. J. Psychiat.*, 137:983–984.

Woody, G. E., O'Brien, C. P., & Greenstein, R. (1975), Misuse and abuse of diazepam: An increasing common medical problem. *Internat. J. Addict.*, 10:843–845.

Commentary

Meyer Sonis, M.D., and Ben Zimmer, M.D.

It seems incongruous that ones whose principal focus of interest and service is community psychiatry, and especially the mental health of the rural areas, should be asked to comment on the lead, general review article of this anthology. But the problems of this segment of our community in the 1970s and 1980s, unfortunately, has become more obvious and make the connection more clear. Rural America is an often neglected arena where biopsychosocial forces intersect to create some unbelievable stress. Jeffery L. Pasley (1986) effectively, and sometimes dramatically, recently summarized the problem.

> American farmers are reported to be the most efficient and productive in the world. Family farmers keep labor costs very low because the family provides the bulk of the labor. . . . "Child labor laws do not apply to family farms because family farms must have child labor to survive." From a very early age, family farm children participate in every phase of the operation, from work with dangerous heavy equipment to close contact with carcinogenic chemicals and disease-carrying animals. [Like their dads], they may be poisoned by the nitrogen dioxide gas that accumulates in grain silos, or have their lungs permanently damaged from breathing the air in enclosed hog pens. They may be crippled by "farmer's lung disease," caused by moldy grain dust. They may develop leukemia from contact with herbicides used on corn. (Iowa farmers contact leukemia 24% more frequently than the average American.) . . . [Labor] practices that would be outrageous at a textile mill

> suddenly become all warm and cuddly when they appear on the family farm [p. 26].
>
> Family farmers . . . achieve efficiency through a draconian work schedule that no self-respecting union would allow. "The farm family does physically demanding and highly stressful work at least 14 hours a day (18 hours during harvest season), seven days a week, three hundred sixty-five days a year without a scheduled vacation or weekends off. . . . The farmer must endure all of this without the benefit of a health plan, safety regulations, a retirement plan, workmen's compensation or any of the benefits that most U.S. labor unions demand. . . ." Many farmers are permanently tied to their farms. A dairy farmer cannot just take a two-week vacation and not milk his cows. Farmers lost perspective on the other things in life, the farm literally consumes them [p. 27].

Pasley points out further that some may say that all the above can be tolerated because of

> the good-old-fashioned-lemonade values and the supportive friendliness of a rural community. [Unfortunately] many small towns appear to suffer from teenage pregnancy, alcoholism, and other social maladies (including other drugs) at rates that are higher than average. One New England study showed relatively high suicide rates among farmers during a period antedating the [recent] farm crisis. Rural communities have not always stood by their financially troubled members . . . at a "town meeting" in New Marker, Minnesota, with Representative Tim Penny, Democrat from Minnesota, farmers ridiculed the idea of slightly higher property taxes to improve the area's meager school system practically in the same breath that they demanded subsidies for themselves [p. 27].

The drama of the above is confirmed by the data. Pasley also stated that according to the National Safety Council, in 1983 farming had 55 job-related deaths per 100,000 workers, or five times the rate for all major industries combined (Pasley, 1986). While 30 percent of all Americans live in rural areas, they have only 17 percent of all primary care physicians. There are 30 percent fewer nurses per 100,000 population in rural areas than in urban areas. Twenty percent of rural residents must travel more than one-half hour to medical care. Our own state of Pennsylvania, having one of the largest rural populations of any state in the nation, has six counties without a hospital. Ten counties do not have any primary health care facilities and two counties do not have any type of long-term care facility. About 360 of 2,400 community water systems in Pennsylvania have deficiencies in their distribution systems. Up to one-third of Pennsylvania's water facilities are in need of maintenance, expansion, and improvements that would cost a total of $580 million. On a national level infant mortality rates are as much as 10 percent higher in rural areas than in urban areas. In some rural areas, infancy mortality rates are 70 percent above the national average and yet federal funds covering local programs for material and infant care, nutrition, and sewage treatment have been cut by as much as one-third (Wright, 1983).

The above should serve as an alternative viewpoint as one reads Slaby's article. In reviewing the article, Slaby has most adequately overviewed the field of psychiatric emergencies. This article is written in a clear and comprehensive manner though at times is encyclopedic in its scope. He focuses on a biopsychosocial approach to diagnosis as the keystone of emergency psychiatric care. Within the framework he deals with acute psychopathological cases, management issues, and staffing concerns.

While the facts of diagnosis and treatment in this article are most instructive and, it is hoped, can be developed for utilization by the larger number of personnel who see psychiatric emergencies beyond the psychiatrist, we hope the reader pays attention to Slaby's issues of "burnout" and "the more than skill needed."

"In our highly independent society, rural problems quickly become urban problems and vice versa. Neither the urban nor rural portions of our society can flourish for long while the other languishes behind" (Dillman, 1982).

References

Dillman, D. A., & Hobbs, D. J. (1982), Rural Society in the U.S.—Issues for the 1980's. Boulder CO: Westview Press, p. 414.

Pasley, J. L. (1986), The idiocy of rural life. *The New Republic*, Dec. 8, pp. 24–28.

Wright, D. R. (1983), Critical Issues for Rural Pennsylvania. Statement of Policy, House Democratic Caucus, Majority Policy Committee, May 2.

Annotated Bibliography

Gerson, S., & Bassuk, E. (1980), Psychiatric emergencies: An overview. *Amer. J. Psychiat.*, 137:1–11.

A comprehensive overview of the field of psychiatric emergencies written a little earlier than Slaby's chapter. The authors, well known in the area of emergency psychiatry, critically review the literature in this field, focusing on the way services are used, the milieu of the emergency room, and the process of disposition decision making. On the basis of their review they suggest a model for emergency services. They focus less on subtle diagnostic considerations and more on the evaluation of the patient's competence within his community.

Feinsilver, D., & Hall, R. (1982), The new crisis psychiatry: An overview. *Psychiat. Ann.*, 12:757–761.

A brief introductory paper redefining the role of the emergency psychiatrist. The new position, according to the authors, will be fostered by developments in differential diagnostic capabilities, new technology, social restructuring of care-giving institutions, and the development of new financial realities. This new crisis psychiatry is inscribed within the movement to emphasize the identity of psychiatry as a medical specialty.

2

Emergency Psychiatry and Crisis Intervention: Some Legal and Ethical Issues

Laurence R. Tancredi, M.D., J.D.

There are no psychiatric situations more problematic to the clinician than diagnosing and formulating an appropriate treatment plan for patients during emergencies and when crisis intervention is indicated. These cause problems not only because of the precision of clinical judgment necessary to assess a patient's status rapidly, but also because decisions must often be made before a meaningful therapist–patient relationship has been established. Unless the emergency involves a patient already in treatment with the evaluating therapist, the foundation for a therapeutic relationship is often difficult, if not impossible, to create during a short period of contact. As a result, the following two ethical and legal responses have occurred:

1. By virtue of the exigencies involved there appears to be more tolerance for the quality of medical decision making. Greater weight is given to the therapeutic discretion of the clinician in the light of minimal diagnostic data than might be acceptable under more carefully

This chapter was first published in *Psychiatric Annals* (1982), 12:799–806, and it is reprinted by permission.

controlled circumstances such as when a patient is in long-term treatment. The margin of error, therefore, for clinical decision making during emergencies is more flexible and permissive than in the non-emergency situation.

2. The insubstantial nature of the relationship between the emergency clinician and the patient makes it even more important that patients' rights be carefully considered. The clinician has to be especially sensitive to the impact that the emergency has on the accuracy of his assessment and the according of the rights of patients. He must balance competing interests, on the one hand, being responsive to the patient's rights to autonomy and self-determination, but, on the other, asserting his therapeutic "power" where necessary in deciding between commitment or outpatient care. The tension between patients' rights and medical factors associated with emergency care can be intense, particularly when the clinician can acceptably consider alternative treatments, though he feels, on balance, that the patient would do better in the inpatient setting. Where the tradeoffs between the patient's rights and good medical care are not clearly defined, the clinician is faced with a difficult choice. In such cases, particularly where limited information is available, medical judgment would likely thrust the clinician in the direction of the most conservative posture, which may result in any one situation in the patient's admission to a hospital. This may not necessarily be ideal from an ethical or legal perspective, but in the clinician's judgment is the most appropriate for good medical care. However, it is essential that the clinician grapple appropriately with the ethical and legal considerations involving the rights of patients before deciding on measures that restrict those prerogatives.

Legal and ethical considerations apply at various points in the course of evaluating and treating patients during emergencies. Three areas of concern, however, seem particularly troublesome in defining the responsibilities and potential liabilities of clinicians: wrongful commitment and refusing treatment; handling the suicidal patient; and informed consent during emergencies and crisis intervention.

WRONGFUL COMMITMENT AND REFUSING TREATMENT

Psychiatrists involved in emergency care are confronted daily with issues relevant to the commitment of patients who are seriously disturbed. In recent years, with the many changes in the commitment laws, particularly the criteria justifying commitment, there has been a growing awareness of the medical and psychiatric bases for confining patients against their will. The criteria in most states have shifted decidedly away from more subjective tests predicated on a parens patriae (the State as father or guardian) theory, such as "in need of care and treatment," or "for the benefit of the patient," toward "objective" criteria, which include the presence of a mental disease or defect and the determination that the patient is dangerous to himself or others (Horhan and Guerrini, 1981). Cases during the 1970s such as the *Lessard* decision (*Lessard v. Schmidt,* 1974) have addressed the standard of proof that must be present to justify civil commitment of the mentally ill. In that case, the standard of proof was beyond a reasonable doubt (90 percent or better proof) that the patient was likely to be dangerous to himself or others. In 1979, the United States Supreme Court, in the *Addington* case (*Addington v. Texas,* 1979), held that clear and convincing evidence (75 percent or better proof) of mental illness and likelihood of danger to self and others rather than the higher criminal standard, is the appropriate threshold for determining the justification of committing patients against their will to a mental institution. In articulating this standard the United States Supreme Court explicitly referred to the lack of certainty of psychiatric diagnoses, which would preclude the application of a proof as stringent as "beyond a reasonable doubt."

Nonetheless, this move in the direction of relaxing the quantum of proof for the commitment of seriously disturbed, mentally ill patients has done little to relieve the tensions of the psychiatric therapist who is attempting to make such decisions in the emergency room. Evaluating psychiatrists are often concerned that they are going to be held unreasonably accountable for justifying commitment of the mentally ill. The *Addington* case, among other things, alludes to the inappropriateness of requiring infallibility in something as complex as psychiatric diagnosis. This decision seems to support the position that psychiatrists should not be held to rigid standards for commitment and that they should be appropriately seen more as care-givers than deprivers of essential civil rights.

On the more practical level, courts seem to come out in favor of psychiatrists where suits have been brought based on the theory of wrongful commitment (Slaby, Lieb, and Tancredi, 1981). An aggrieved patient may bring a suit arguing defamation or false imprisonment or malicious prosecution, but here, for the most part, patients are unsuccessful unless they can establish that the psychiatrist has deflected egregiously from appropriate standards of care or from the statutory requirements. For example, there have been successful cases against psychiatrists for inadequately examining the patient, or completely avoiding the examination process, but relying instead on reports and the opinion of family members or others in the community. The problem with bringing a wrongful commitment proceeding is that success for negligence actions are predicated for the most part on errors of fact rather than errors of judgment (Horhan and Guerrini, 1981). Where the treating psychiatrist has obtained all the information that he is capable of obtaining in his evaluation and shows a reasonable logic for his decision to admit the patient to the hospital, then the fact that he may have made the "wrong" choice in that decision would probably be seen as an error of judgment rather than of fact. What is of importance is that he clearly documents in his records the underlying basis for his decision to commit the patient.

Occurring at the same time as these developments regarding the application of due process rights to mental patients in the commitment process, there has also been a movement in the direction of the rights of patients once admitted to refuse medication and other treatments (Tancredi, 1980). In a case in New Jersey, *Rennie v. Klein* (1979), the district court held that mental patients involuntarily committed and competent have a limited right of refusal of treatment, but that this can be overridden by an appropriate procedure such as review by a psychiatrist as long as that psychiatrist is not a member of the treatment team involved with the patient's care. In this case the court was apparently concerned with the quality of psychiatric care being provided in the institution, so that requiring a second psychiatrist to make the treatment decision essentially provides a system of consultation for the benefit of the patient (Stone, 1981). This case relied heavily on the theory that the administration of neuroleptic drugs against a patient's will essentially invades that patient's constitutionally protected privacy rights. This right of privacy, as well as the first amendment guarantee of freedom of speech (interpreted to include thought) and the eighth amendment right against cruel and unusual punishment have served in many cases as the theoretical bases for affirming the patient's rights against psychotropic medication. The U.S. Court of Appeals (Third Circuit) on reviewing this decision upheld the constitutional right to refuse treatment, but rejected the requirement for an adversarial hearing before an independent psychiatrist. It returned to previous proceedings that rely on a final decision being made by the medical director of the hospital.

A second case, *Rogers v. Okin* (1981), recently before the United States Supreme Court (*Mills v. Rogers*)[1] takes a stronger position on the patient's rights to refuse psychotropic medication. This case as affirmed by the Court of Appeals for the First Circuit (*Rogers v. Okin*, 1980) relies heavily on the right of privacy theory also articulated in the New Jersey case, and focuses predominantly on neuroleptic medications particularly because of the danger of the patient developing tardive dyskinesias. The involuntarily committed, competent patients' rights against neuroleptic medications can be trumped, however, if an emergency ensues. The lower court defined an emergency as "a substantial likelihood of physical harm to that patient, other patients or to the staff." The higher court ruled that this definition of emergency was far too restrictive, and that a more flexible definition was appropriate that would give greater discretion to the treating psychiatrist.

Both of these cases seem to recognize the importance of flexibility in decision making for the treating physician in the emergency situation when the rights of the involuntarily committed patient may be trumped in favor of appropriate treatment. The definition of when an emergency occurs needs to be clarified in the *Rogers v. Okin* case. In *Rennie v. Klein* at the district court level four factors were considered important for establishing when the patient's rights to refuse psychotropic medication can be overruled in a nonemergency:

1. The physical threat of the patient to other patients and staff of the institution;
2. The patient's capacity to decide on a particular treatment;
3. The availability (and existence) of less restrictive alternatives; and
4. The nature and extent of risk of permanent side effects for the treatment being proposed.

[1]On June 18, 1982 the Supreme Court ruled to remand the case to the lower court so that the court could decide if Massachusetts state law resolves the issues.

These factors are decidedly patient rights oriented. The Court of Appeals rejected these and returned to previous criteria to be considered by the medical director that seem to be based more on the therapeutic advantages of medication, and thus provide greater discretion to the treating clinicians. The Supreme Court has yet to decide whether to grant *certiorari* in this case.

In both the commitment process as well as the medicating of patients, the psychiatrist is obligated to consider the rights of patients. The justifications for commitment or infracting the rights of patients when administering psychotropic medication must be relatively clear, and the factual basis as complete as possible given the context of the emergency evaluation. This obligation requires the clinician to resort to the more intrusive treatments such as confinement and neuroleptic medication only after other less intrusive alternatives have been truly exhausted. In the case of psychotropic medications, the patient's right to refuse treatment, pending the state laws, may prevail. Even though the higher courts appear to be coming out in favor of flexibility for psychiatric decisions, it will still be ethically imperative that treating clinicians be aware of those countervailing factors that would justify the patient's position regarding refusal of treatment.

THE SUICIDAL PATIENT

The evaluation and treatment of the suicidal patient is one of the most difficult emergency problems. When a patient enters an emergency room or a crisis intervention center, it is incumbent upon the evaluating psychiatrist to explore, as thoroughly as possible, the suicidal potential or risk of that patient. In most cases, this would require that the psychiatrist or other mental health professional probe into the suicidal tendencies of the patient through specific, well-directed questions both with the family and the patient himself. Certain characteristics should alert the psychiatrist to the high suicidal potential of the patient (Waltzer, 1980). He should be aware that successful suicides occur most frequently in older persons (in recent years, however, they are occurring with greater frequency in individuals below the age of 35, and most surprisingly, in adolescents and older children) or those with a history of previous suicide attempts, obsessive thoughts of suicide, recent death or loss of a critical figure in the patient's life, or family history of suicide and alcohol or drug abuse. In cases where a patient fits into a high-risk category, psychiatrists are under a special obligation to establish the suicidal potential of that patient and arrange for an appropriate treatment disposition in the light of that evaluation.

In the past, most of the lawsuits have been brought not against the psychiatrist for a patient's suicide, but against the hospital for failing to observe and properly protect the patient who has been admitted. Where a patient is being treated on an outpatient basis, psychiatrists are rarely held responsible for the death of that patient (Slovenko, 1981). This may be due, in large part, to the fact that the psychiatrist's control over the patient and the patient's environment is significantly more limited than in a hospital context. On the other hand, with deinstitutionalization, short-term hospitalization and the shift toward increasing use of outpatient services, the potential for suits against the treating psychiatrist with regard to malpractice in the evaluation and treatment of the suicidal patient is very real. Also, where the patient is seen frequently by the therapist in an outpatient setting, and there is sufficient evidence to suggest that the patient has a high likelihood of committing suicide, the psychiatrist may be liable for not intervening and placing the patient under greater control in a hospital setting.

In a legal action against a psychiatrist for suicide, the psychiatrist is unlikely to be found liable for the consequences of his diagnosis and treatment if he exercised a required degree of skill and care (Twardy, 1978). This test appears to be similar to the standard of care doctrine applied in negligence or traditional malpractice cases that addresses the extent to which the psychiatrist exercised the degree of skill and care in the treatment and diagnosis of the patient that would be employed by a reasonable practitioner of that specialty under similar circumstances. In establishing whether this occurred, a court would be concerned with determining that the psychiatrist was not negligent in his diagnosis of the patient, which would include the eliciting of proper information regarding the patient's suicidal risk, or the establishment of an appropriate treatment regimen, given that risk. Notions that are particularly important for a court would include the "foreseeability" of the suicide of the patient, that is to say, whether at the time of the evaluation and treatment it was "foreseeable" that this patient would likely commit suicide (Waltzer, 1980).

Another issue that the court would concern itself with is the preventability of that injury, especially in terms of whether the therapist exhibited an appropriate degree of care and skill in his handling of the patient. In the absence of negligence, a failure of medical judgment would likely not result in a successful suit against the psychiatrist. Hence, if after evaluating all of the information that has been gleaned from the patient and the family, the psychiatrist or medical staff involved reasonably concludes that the patient is not a high suicidal risk at the time of admission and consequently places the patient on an open ward, then the fact that the patient commits suicide implies at most an error in judgment, not an act of negligence, and would probably not result in a successful suit.

Two other issues that are of particular importance with respect to the responsibility of the psychiatrist in the emergency context are those of vicarious liability and iatrogenic (treatment-induced) suicide. With respect to the former, which is particularly applicable to the psychiatrist practicing in a clinic or hospital setting, the potential exists for vicarious liability based on the negligent supervision or lack of direct involvement in the management of the patient where other mental health professionals are involved. When a psychiatrist is in charge of residents in training or other mental health professionals, he may be held liable for their negligent behavior (Slaby et al., 1981). There was a case in New York State (*Cohen v. New York State,* 1976) where the court addressed the issue of the institution's responsibility for assuring appropriate supervision of mental health professionals by a qualified psychiatrist. This case involved a 23-year-old, third-year medical student who voluntarily admitted himself to a medical center and was diagnosed as having paranoid schizophrenia. The admitting notes contained a statement indicating that the patient had suicidal potential, but he was nonetheless placed in an open ward as part of a therapeutic community. Four months after admission, the treating physician, a first-year resident in psychiatry, determined that the patient no longer needed to be restricted to the ward. The day that these restrictions were lifted the patient committed suicide. The patient's wife brought a suit against the institution, and the court concluded that the resident at this stage in his training lacked the requisite skill, in the absence of supervision, to provide reasonable psychiatric treatment and care for this patient. This case highlights the extent to which a psychiatrist who has delegated responsibilities of the care of patients to those in training or to paraprofessionals has a continuing duty to be directly involved in their care through proper supervision. When this does not occur and an injury results, he may be held liable for the negligence of those under his supervision.

An area of growing concern is the extent to which suicide might be induced by the therapist–patient encounter (Slovenko, 1981). One can speculate on various situations where the intervention triggers such intense conflict and depression in the patient that he commits suicide. For example, a young male ambivalent over his sexuality enters crisis intervention in a condition of increasing anxiety. During the course of a few sessions, the therapist focuses almost totally on the issue of homosexuality, which creates even more conflicts for the patient. In the absence of appropriate support, which may require a more careful delineation of the sexual issues concurrent with the establishment of a meaningful therapist–patient relationship, the patient becomes depressed, is unable to deal with his own conflicts, and commits suicide. In this scenario, the therapist would probably argue that the confrontation was part of the therapeutic process. On the other hand, a proper assessment of the fragility of the patient would likely balance strongly in the direction of a more cautious approach to very highly charged personal issues.

In the case where the therapist abandons a patient, humiliates him in the context of the family or others, or even inadvertently encourages self-destructive behavior, the therapist's negligence is more clear-cut than in the previous example, and might very well lead to a successful malpractice action. One of the difficulties of establishing a successful malpractice suit involving patients undergoing psychotherapy is the complexity of establishing the closeness of connection between the therapeutic process and the injury. This connection may be more obvious in an emergency evaluation involving a one-time encounter, especially if the suicidal act is closely related in time to the interchange between the psychiatrist and patient.

INFORMED CONSENT

When informed consent emerged as an ethical and legal requirement in the physician–patient relationship, it was viewed by scholars and practitioners alike to be an important advance in the protection of the patients' rights in the medical care system (Tancredi, 1981). Many legal developments have occurred since the first cases appeared in the 1950s to provide, through informed consent, even greater power for the patient in medical decision making. Most particularly, the *Canterbury v. Spence* (1972) case modified the standard of disclosure of information from the physician disclosure standard, still the prevailing test in the United States, to a more patient-centered standard for information disclosure. The physician disclosure standard obligates the physician to disclose that information that similarly situated physicians would disclose to patients in like circumstances. In contrast, the test resulting from the *Canterbury* case, requires a disclosure of information that would "materially affect" a patient's decision based on what a reasonable person would want to know under similar circumstances.

Even with developments to improve the effectiveness of informed consent, serious conceptual problems remain (Katz, 1980), most particularly, those involving the "competency" of patients to understand the medical and psychiatric information presented to them. Studies conducted on the general nonpsychiatric population have demonstrated repeatedly the problems that patients have in understanding information regarding the benefits, risks, and alternatives of diagnostic and treatment procedures. In a study involving 200 cancer patients who were given information on chemotherapy, radiation therapy, and surgery as alternative treatments for their conditions, questionnaires filled out the following day indicated that only 55 percent were able to identify even one major complication from these treatments, and less than one-half actually read the forms carefully (Cassileth, Zupkis, and Sutton-Smith, 1980). Other studies corroborate these observations (Muss, 1979; Priluck et al., 1979).

Mental patients share these difficulties in comprehending psychiatric information. There have been only a few studies involving the efficacy of informed consent in psychiatric treatment, and the results have been equally unimpressive (Palmer and Wohl, 1972; Olin and Olin, 1975; Roth, 1981). In the emergency situation involving psychiatric patients, there can be little surprise that comprehension would be even further compromised. The tendency of patients when confronted with a crisis is to regress to a predominantly passive and help-seeking stance, relying heavily on the discretion of the treating clinician. Hence, information regarding alternative medication, hospitalization or outpatient care, or the application of various diagnostic or treatment procedures may be essentially ignored, as the patient strongly desires that others take control of his condition.

The awareness of the tendency toward regression and inattentiveness during informed consent proceedings places an added burden on the therapist or psychiatrist to make every effort conceivable to convey the pros and cons of various treatment options. The overall benefits to be gained from allowing patients to participate directly in medical decisions are so important that even if relatively few are actually capable under compromised conditions of engaging actively in informed consent, the mere fact that it is done ensures that everyone in the mental health care system will have their rights protected. Furthermore, it forces the clinician to reflect, once again, on his diagnostic and treatment recommendations. It may be important in some circumstances to repeat the information at more than one sitting if time permits. Of course, in an emergency where the patient is in no condition to exercise judgment for himself, full disclosure is impossible, in which case it would be necessary, if possible, to involve the next of kin or other family members in the decision-making process (Shea, 1979).

CONCLUSION

This discussion has addressed a few of the many ethical and legal issues affecting emergency evaluation and crisis intervention. The emphasis has been on the responsibility of the treating psychiatrist to administer quality care in an atmosphere that demonstrates sensitivity to the needs and rights of patients. Throughout the diagnostic and treatment process, therapists must be constantly aware of the patient's rights to self-determination and autonomy. This is most effectively assured when high standards of psychiatric care are employed in determining commitment, assessing suicidal potential, and in actively bolstering the effectiveness of informed consent under these difficult circumstances. When conflicts occur between what the therapist considers to be quality psychiatric care and the rights of patients, the therapist should defer, as much as possible, to the patients' desires, except in those circumstances where commitment is warranted, or where the patient has been considered incompetent, in which case, the next of kin or court-appointed guardian would need to be consulted.

REFERENCES

Addington v. Texas (1979), 99 *Supreme Court Reporter:* 1804.

Canterbury v. Spence (1972), 464 F2d.

Cassileth, B. R., Zupkis, R. V., & Sutton-Smith, K. (1980), Informed consent—Why are its goals imperfectly realized? *N. Engl. J. Med.*, 302:896–899.

Cohen v. New York State (1976), 382 *New York Supplement* 2d 128.

Horhan, D. J., & Guerrini, M. E. (1981), Developing legal trends in psychiatric malpractice. *J. Psychiat. & Law*, 9:65–89.

Katz, J. (1980), Disclosure and consent in psychiatric practice. Mission impossible. In: *Law and Ethics in the Practice of Psychiatry*, ed., E. K. Hofling. New York: Brunner/Mazel, pp. 91–117.

Lessard v. Schmidt (1974), 379 F Supp 1078, vacated 94 Supreme Court 713.

Muss, H. B. (1979), Written informed consent in patients with breast cancer. *Cancer*, 43:1549–1556.

Olin, G. B., & Olin, H. N. (1975), Informed consent in voluntary mental hospital admissions. *Amer. J. Psychiat.*, 132:938–941.

Palmer, A. B., & Wohl, J. (1972), Voluntary admission forms: Does the patient know what he is signing? *Hosp. & Commun. Psychiat.*, 12:250–252.

Priluck, I. A. (1979), What patients recall of the preoperative discussion after retinal detachment surgery. *Amer. J. Ophthalmol.*, 87:620–623.

Rennie v. Klein (1979), 476 F Supp 1294.

Rogers v. Okin (1st cir 1980), 634 F2d 650.

——— (1981), 478 F Supp 1342 (Ed Mass 1979), cert. granted and case argued sub nom Mills v. Rogers, 101 Supreme Court 1972.

Roth, I. (1981), Competency to consent: Implications of some empirical data. Paper presented at the International Symposium of Law and Psychiatry, University of Virginia School of Law, June 11–13.

Shea, I. I. (1979), Legal standard of care for psychiatrists and psychologists. *Western State Univ. Law Rev.*, 6:71–99.

Slaby, A. E., Lieb, J., & Tancredi, I. R. (1981), *Handbook of Psychiatric Emergencies*, 2d ed. New Hyde Park, NY: Medical Examination Publishing Company.

Slovenko, R. (1981), Malpractice in psychiatry and related fields. *J. Psychiat. & Law*, 9:18–19.

Stone, A. A. (1981), The right to refuse treatment. *Arch. Gen. Psychiat.*, 38:358–362.

Tancredi, L. R. (1980), The right to refuse psychiatric treatment: Some legal and ethical considerations. *J. Health Polit. Policy Law*, 5:514–522.

——— (1981), Informed consent: The dilemma. In: *Biomedical Innovations*, eds. E. B. Roberts et al. Cambridge, MA: MIT Press.

Twardy, S. (1978), The issue of malpractice in psychiatry. *Med. Trial Tech. Quart.*, 25:161–176.

Waltzer, H. (1980), Malpractice liability in patient's suicide. *Amer. J. Psychother.*, 34:89–98.

Commentary

George A. Huber, J.D.

In chapter 2, Tancredi raises important issues for consideration by those working in the setting of emergency psychiatry and crisis intervention. Certain of his points are worthy of further elaboration.

Care must be taken in how one interprets the statement that the margin of error for clinical decision making during emergencies is more flexible and permissive than in the nonemergency situation. The degree of confidence that such a statement may provide should be balanced against the significant number of serious incidents and amount of litigation that originate in the psychiatric emergency room alone. Review of these cases shows that "bad results" are not without clinical vulnerabilities. Most common are lack of experience (i.e., junior resident staffing), poor supervision, failure to obtain critical information and help, and timidity in treatment. The psychiatric emergency room is extremely complex not only from the clinical standpoint, but also from the administrative standpoint since it involves the intersection of multiple systems.

It is true that in most states two elements of involuntary commitment are the presence of a mental disease or defect and the determination that the patient is dangerous to himself or others. Not mentioned is a third element, which relates to the first two, that is, when, *as a result of a mental illness,* a person's capacity to exercise self-control, judgment, and discretion in the conduct of his affairs and social relations, or to care for his own personal needs is so lessened that he poses a clear and present danger of harm to others or to himself. In other words, the dangerousness is a *result* of mental illness. For many patients who present themselves, or are presented to the psychiatric emergency room, this can be a most difficult clinical determination, especially for those patients with character disorders. Is dangerousness the result of mental illness? If not, what are the duties of clinicians to protect society, on the one hand, and patient confidentiality, on the other? Should such patients be restrained in the hospital as a commitment, or should they be referred to the criminal justice system? What statutory protections do clinicians have in these cases? These are tough questions to answer now, but even tougher on the line of fire. They require mature and experienced consideration.

In illustrating the difference between an error in judgment and an act of negligence, the author provides the example where after evaluating all of the information that has been gleaned from the patient and the family, the psychiatrist involved reasonably concludes that the patient is not a "high" suicidal risk at the time of admission and consequently places the patient on an open ward. According to the author, the fact that the patient commits suicide implies at most an error in judgment, not an act of negligence, and would probably not result in a successful litigation by the spouses of the deceased. Each case turned on the failure of the emergency room physician (in both cases a first-year resident) to order constant observation initially, at least for a limited period of time, on the open ward for the patient assessed to be a possible, but not "high," suicidal risk. The lesson to be learned is that even though the patient may not be evaluated as "highly" suicidal, other precautions, especially for the newly admitted patient to the open ward, may be appropriate. It should be remembered that bad results are viewed retrospectively by the jury, not prospectively.

To illustrate the importance of appropriate supervision, the chapter provides an example of the first-year resident who lifts patient restrictions with resulting suicide. This is truly a vulnerable area for bad results. Another related area is where professionals perform acts beyond what their license permits (i.e., nurses prescribing medications). In a recent malpractice case involving a suicide, the hospital's and psychiatrist's defenses were weakened by the plaintiff's expert testimony that the medical record reflected that diagnosis in the emergency room appeared to be conducted by nurses, not physicians, who are the only ones licensed to do so.

In concluding, it is suggested that throughout the diagnostic and treatment process, therapists must be constantly aware of the patient's rights of self-determination and autonomy. "When conflicts occur between what the therapist considers to be quality psychiatric care and the rights of patients, the therapist should defer, as much as possible, to the patients' desires. . . ." Good advice! However, this advice should be balanced with other practical considerations. First, mental health procedure acts have placed the psychiatrist in a judgmental position with broad immunities with respect to civil commitment. Second, as to civil commitment and aside from the immunities, I would rather be in the position of arguing before a jury on a charge of false imprisonment or violation of patient rights for the committed patient, than suicide or murder for the prematurely released patient. To restate the point: when in doubt, commit.

Annotated Bibliography

Mills, M., & O'Keefe, A. M. (1983), Legal issues in outpatient treatment. *J. Clin. Psychiat.*, 44:33–40.

An overview of the major aspects of the interface between psychiatry and the law. While the article does not focus specifically on emergency psychiatric issues, its relevance to this area is apparent. Legal issues in clinical management which are touched upon include the areas of civil commitment, the least restrictive setting principle, and informed consent. A discussion of patient confidentiality, including the Tarosoff decision, is presented, as well as caveats for clinicians concerned with legal issues.

Roth, L. (1977), Involuntary civil commitment: The right to treatment and the right to refuse treatment. *Psychiat. Ann.*, 7:244–257.

This classic forensic article written by the Director of the Law and Psychiatry Program at the University of Pittsburgh has much relevance to the area of emergency psychiatry. Roth reviews the area of involuntary civil commitment and ponders on the consequences of psychiatrists' actions. These issues, raised approximately 10 years ago, are still timely.

Julavits, W. (1983), Legal issues in emergency psychiatry. *Psychiat. Clin. N. Amer.*, 6:335–345.

A general review of topics relevant to a psychiatric emergency room including informed consent, the right to treatment, the right to refuse treatment, confidentiality, and commitment. It also offers a broad discussion of standards of care for practitioners in emergency psychiatry.

3

Training Tomorrow's Psychiatrist

Herman Oliver, M.D., and Charles J. Rabiner, M.D.

Emergency room and walk-in clinic psychiatry will come to play an increasingly large part in the working life of tomorrow's psychiatrist. Utilization of these services, where available, has risen steadily and significantly and shows no sign of leveling out. The psychiatric emergency ward is now a chief entry point into the network of mental health services for people in need of help for their problems in living (Gerson and Bassuk, 1980). The ever-increasing number of community clinics, combined with the projected decreased availability of psychiatrists will inevitably emphasize the role of the psychiatrist as organizer, teacher, and consultant. This will require skills that can best be learned in the walk-in clinic and emergency room.

Inevitably, more training time will be spent in these areas with an emphasis on working quickly and productively with families, community agencies, other community resources, and support systems. This mediating, integrating role combined with the application of brief

This chapter was first published in *Psychiatric Quarterly* (1982), 54:33–37, and it is reprinted by permission.

contact, face-to-face work with the nominated patient is the essential model of much of the community psychiatry of the future.

The community mental health movement, largely conceived by psychiatrists to improve standards of mental health care nationally, appears to be going through an evolutionary phase in which there is decreasing utilization of psychiatrists and increasing utilization of other mental health professionals (Winslow, 1979). This deprofessionalization of the community mental health center has many roots, among which is the lack of psychiatrists trained, oriented, and interested in this important aspect of the mental health delivery system. We agree with Fink and Weinstein who indicate that the delivery of services to people with problems, be they mental, family, or schizophrenia related, should at least be monitored, if not delivered, by professionals (Fink and Weinstein, 1979).

Studies show that between 1970 and 1975, the number of full-time equivalent psychiatrists in community mental centers dropped from 6.8 to 4.3 per center even though the total staff of these same centers almost tripled during the same period. While this was happening the number of patients per community mental center increased more than 50 percent, including, of course, a large percentage of patients with major mental disorders. This last group, the chronic severely ill patient, is one of the real challenges to American psychiatry today.

These patients, who have been released from our hospitals, are frequently unable to work, unable to socialize, and live on the fringe of society. They often do not come in contact with mental health agencies unless they run into trouble with the law. When they do seek help, they are often excluded by the bureaucracy of the system, or shuttled off to rehabilitation programs, socialization programs, or similar programs where the medical input is minimal. They rarely see a psychiatrist unless the insurance form requires a physician's signature. These patients are considered to be "unmotivated," "uninteresting," and sometimes even "unpleasant." They are also often "untreated."

How did this all come about? Some see a conspiracy of the other mental health professions who have joined in an attempt to challenge the role of psychiatry and psychiatrists, and seek equality in the treatment of these patients. We suggest that, essentially, we have brought this about ourselves, and we should look within. The majority of our residency training programs have stressed the treatment of the verbal, intelligent, cooperative patient, and have usually assigned the most senior and knowledgeable supervisors to the supervision of these cases. Long-term individual psychotherapy, and the number of hours of supervision are emphasized in training brochures. Residents are often "exposed" to chronically ill patients, but this is done as little as possible because the treatment of these patients is considered a "service need," whereas individual psychotherapy comes under the heading of an "educational experience." The one area where residents frequently encounter chronic patients with acute episodes is in the emergency room, usually at night and on weekends. Here the idea is to dispose of problems as expeditiously as possible. Rarely is this seen as a unique opportunity to provide an educational experience. This is despite the fact that the progression of deinstitutionalization has and will continue to result in the release of many hospitalized patients into the community, and that currently responsibility for these patients has shifted partially to community centers and general hospitals (Lowry, Wintrob, and Borwick, 1961; Greenblatt and Glazier, 1975; Talbott, 1978; Bassuk, 1980).

The thrust of the majority of our training programs then is to indoctrinate our residents with the concept that there are good patients who require psychotherapy and bad patients who can usually be handled by a nonmedical therapist with an occasional consultation with a psychiatrist for case management. However, when these residents go out into the real world, they find there are many more bad patients than good ones, and are often ill-equipped to handle them.

The Hillside Division of the Long Island Jewish-Hillside Medical Center is not very different from most other residency training programs. Historically, individual psychotherapy was emphasized, and when the walk-in clinic was opened, residents vehemently objected to rotations through that service. It was considered to be a repetition of emergency room experience and, therefore, not desirable. Residents felt they were being used to meet a service need and received nothing in return.

The Director of the Outpatient Department examined the rotation and essentially agreed with the residents. Merely to examine patients and refer them elsewhere was not in itself a true learning experience, although one could possibly argue that any clinical experience has some value. Nevertheless, the service was reorganized in an attempt to provide the residents with the same quality of supervision they were receiving on other services.

Rather than assign residents piecemeal, psychiatric interns are assigned for one month. They spend their time doing triage both in the walk-in clinic and the emergency room. They also see patients in crisis intervention. All of this is done under the supervision of full-time psychiatric staff assigned to the clinic. Didactic lectures on emergency psychiatry are given, and there is a weekly case presentation where cases in brief contact therapy and crisis intervention are presented and discussed. These conferences are attended not only by the walk-in clinic staff, but also by the Director and Assistant Director of Adult Outpatient Services.

During 1981–1982, the psychiatric interns assigned to the service considered it to be a very positive experience. Although members of the group tended to differ somewhat in describing the positive and negative aspects of the clinic, interviews with them revealed the following areas of agreement. First, and foremost, all interns emphasized the importance of being able to see a broad range of psychopathology. Most of the first year is spent on the inpatient service, where the interns see acutely disturbed patients, or acute exacerbations of chronic illness. Even an assignment to the emergency room, as an adjunct to a more senior resident, does not appreciably change the patient mix, as the same group of patients utilize an emergency room. However, the walk-in clinic affords the beginning resident an opportunity to see a wide variety of neurotic patients who are not generally admitted to a psychiatric hospital, and are not ordinarily present at night at a psychiatric emergency room. This comes at a time when the interns are beginning to wonder if all psychiatric practice is confined to the treatment of the very sick, and the opportunity to be exposed to an entirely different range of psychopathology is most welcome. The intern, confronted mainly with the psychoses in the hospital, now has the opportunity to differentiate psychotic patients from neurotics, and those with character disorders.

A second area of agreement concerned the ability of the intern to follow the patient through an acute crisis as an outpatient. The intern does the initial triage, and then may follow the patient during the month-long rotation. Here there was some disagreement among the group as to the value of increasing the time in the clinic. Several interns would have preferred a longer rotation so that they could do more follow up and more brief therapy. However, this exposure to crisis intervention helped all interns in terms of making decisions quickly.

Many articles written about supervision in our field deal with the complicated supervisor–supervisee relationship. This relationship includes the transference, the countertransference, and the identification of the supervisee with the patient and/or the supervisor. Indeed these are multifaceted relationships that must be addressed.

The emergency room and the walk-in clinic can provide a more unique teaching mechanism through role-modeling, a means of instruction prominent in other medical specialties but often missing in the psychiatric training program. On-the-spot teaching with immediate discussion of what has been done is more effective, in many instances, than delayed supervision. It is also significantly more popular among many medical students taking clerkships in psychiatry. Medical students can profit educationally from working in these areas (Werkman, Landau, and Wakefield, 1973), and they wish to work in these areas. Recent surveys have indicated that medical students were generally dissatisfied with the psychiatric training they received. Further, among the most frequent complaints listed was limited clinical involvement and inadequate supervision (Kasuboski and Marshall, 1973). There have been some who have reservations related to the quality of service delivered by students. "Patient care is not compromised as long as careful supervision is provided . . . the clinic is the ideal place to learn about psycho-social problems because they are so central to ambulatory patient care" (Gorall, Stoeckle, and Lazare, 1974, pp. 957–962).

This conclusion by Gorall et al. was echoed in similar experiences at Dartmouth by Goodstein and Napoliello (1978), who also found that primary patient-care responsibility in an ambulatory setting was the most frequently articulated positive comment by the student. With the shrinking number of medical students opting for psychiatry today, it is imperative that we listen to the students' complaints. At our medical center this approach has been rather successful as judged by the medical students and residents who have experienced it. Some medical students have requested additional time in their senior year following clerkships spent there. "In general, I believe it to be a growth producing experience. . . ." is how one of our residents described it (Eichler, 1980).

In discussing the methodological maze in teaching methods the American Psychiatric Association (APA) publication, *Psychiatric Education: Prologue to the '80s,* lists six methodological strategies, one of which is "Actual practice under close supervision: to permit skill and knowledge development with close corrective feedback and guidance'' (Rosenfeld, 1976). I can think of no better arena for the implementation of the above than in the emergency room and walk-in clinic. Further, these areas can also provide the opportunity to teach diagnosis and phenomenology. Finally, the student can begin to learn about empathy, a trait that a good psychiatrist must develop. The patient population of the emergency areas and their families frequently present with dispositions that are less than hopeful or even pleasant. The observations of a senior staff member spending time in one of these unpopular or uncomfortable situations is more valuable than any seminar or lecture on the topic.

The teachers working in these areas must be interested in working there and not simply people who are assigned or rotated:

> The best teachers will be eternal learners and as such they will help their students to identify with their activity and their own process of constant growth, rather than with static opinions that become frozen dogmas of limited usefulness. Teaching and learning are then the mutually interdependent two sides of the coin, if it carries the permanent value of professional identity [Ekstein and Wallerstein, 1958].

This prescription by Ekstein and Wallerstein needs no improvement.

In conclusion, the emergency room and the walk-in clinic are areas which should become an integral focus for teaching the psychiatrist of the 1980s. They can fulfill two major training needs. The methods employed are unique to the field and should thus not be overlooked. Second, with the increasing use of these areas and mental health centers as an entree toward getting help, an ongoing program can provide the very manpower it is designed to train.

REFERENCES

Bassuk, E. L. (1980), The impact of deinstitutionalization on the general hospital psychiatric emergency ward. *Hosp. Commun. Psych.*, 31:623–627.

Eichler, S. (1980), Experiences in a psychiatric emergency room. *Bull. Area II District Branches, APA*, 22/8.

Ekstein, R., & Wallerstein, R. S.(1958), *The Teaching and Learning of Psychotherapy*. New York: Basic Books.

Fink, P. J., & Weinstein, S. P. (1979), Whatever happened to psychiatry? The deprofessionalization of community mental health centers. *Amer. J. Psychiat.*, 136:406–409.

Gerson, S., & Bassuk, E. (1980), Psychiatric emergencies: An overview. *Amer. J. Psychiat.*, 137:1–11.

Goodstein, R. K., & Napoliello, M. J. (1978), Clinical psychiatry clerkships and the emergency walk-in service. *Comprehen. Psychiat.*, 19:267–274.

Gorall, A. H., Stoeckle, S. D., & Lazare, A. (1974), Teaching the clinical interview: An experiment with first year students. *J. Med. Ed.*, 49:957–962.

Greenblatt, M., & Glazier, E. (1975), The phasing out of mental hospitals in the United States. *Amer. J. Psychiat.*, 132:453–456.

Kasuboski, D., & Marshall, J. (1973), Responsibility and relevance in a psychiatric clerkship, *J. Med. Ed.*, 48:752–757.

Lowry, F. H., Wintrob, R. M., & Borwick, B. (1961), A follow-up study of emergency psychiatric patients and their families. *Comprehen. Psychiat.*, 12:36–47.

Rosenfeld, A. (1976), *Psychiatric Education: Prologue to the 1980's*. Amer. Psychiatric Assn., Washington, DC/Baltimore, MD: Garomond Pridemark Press.

Talbott, J. A. (1978), *The Chronic Mental Patient*. Washington, DC: American Psychiatric Press.

Werkman, S. L., Landau, S., & Wakefield, H. (1973), Medical students view clinical psychiatry. *Amer. J. Psych.*, 130:562–565.

Winslow, W. (1979), The changing role of psychiatrists in community health centers. *Amer. J. Psychiat.*, 136:24–27.

Commentary

Peter B. Henderson, M.D.

The Oliver and Rabiner chapter is a pungent statement for psychiatric educators in the 1980s. I am in particular agreement that "actual practice under close supervision: to permit skill and knowledge development with close corrective feedback and guidance" is the way to go. Or, it is an important way! In the first (or second, at the latest) year of psychiatric residency, a training and educational experience in an emergency/walk-in clinic is the best approach to teach these observational skills.

The inpatient wards offer much for the training of a beginning psychiatrist, particularly regarding work as a diagnostician and a psychiatric physician in an interdisciplinary team. However, residents there do not have an opportunity to be more autonomous in making critical decisions, and they have supervision, ideally, only once or twice a week, and that is mainly by reporting on care already rendered. Attempts should be made to observe residents as they interview, interact with patients, and explore areas in which they have limited knowledge. These issues are not brought to the attention of the faculty often enough, and the psychiatric resident frequently becomes the scapegoat for other professionals on the unit in his efforts to master these developmental steps.

That is why I think the emergency/walk-in clinic is a splendid psychiatric education sight for dealing with these early learning tasks. Here, regularly, the resident should have an opportunity to interview, in the presence of a member of the psychiatric faculty, with a nursing staff that is appropriately trained in dealing with this unpopular, ''unattractive,'' but very important and prevalent type of patients. Psychiatric residents should have a minimum of one month (and preferably two or three) of this activity as early in their training as possible.

As psychiatry has changed its attitude toward the care of the chronic patient, it is my belief that the orientation of psychiatric residencies should change, indeed, must change. There is still a place for long-term psychotherapy training, but the psychiatric consultant role should extend in particular from the medical and pediatric services to the walk-in clinics. I look forward to the next several years in psychiatric education, for I feel certain that the role of the psychiatric specialist, particularly in the primary care aspects of psychiatry, will be in our emergency rooms and walk-in clinics. Oliver and Rabiner's chapter describes the future of our field.

Annotated Bibliography

Shwed, H. (1980), Teaching emergency room psychiatry. *Hosp. & Comm. Psychiat.*, 31:558–562.

A short and practical article concerning basic didactic principles to be taught in emergency room psychiatry, based on a supervisor's personal experience. In the area of interviewing, the authors differentiate skills necessary for the emergency room from those for other clinical settings. The importance of seeking information from a wide range of informants is stressed along with the importance of a formal mental status examination. Knowledge of community resources is also emphasized as well as the value of looking for general medical and neurologic factors in any psychiatric abnormality.

Fauman, B. (1983), Psychiatric residency training in the management of emergencies. *Psychiat. Clin. N. Amer.*, 6:325–334.

An experienced teacher in psychiatric emergency settings describes various models for health care providers (psychiatrists and nonpsychiatrists). The emergency room can be used to furnish innovative coping techniques to largely normal persons experiencing acute psychiatric stress as well as complementary care for the deinstitutionalized chronically mentally ill. Also, psychiatrists can serve in general hospital emergency rooms as consultants for psychiatric and psychosocial problems.

Melchiode, G., Puryear, D., & Babick, M. (1983), The emergency room as a clerkship site. *Amer. J. Psychiat.*, 140:894–897.

A brief article based on the authors' personal experience as medical student education coordinators, about the successful use of the emergency room as a clerkship (home base) site for training medical students in psychiatry. Sharing the core didactic work of other students placed at more traditional sites, the emergency room students averaged more patient contact, more direct observation, and more supervisory experience. Furthermore, these students had additional seminars in crisis intervention and better orientation to social agencies.

4

The Brief Evaluation Form: Semistructured Assessment of Current Psychiatric Illness

Juan E. Mezzich, M.D., Ph.D.

Efficiency in psychiatric assessment is a prominent concern in busy clinical settings where disposition and management decisions are to be made under considerable time constraints. This concern explains the wide clinical use of the Brief Psychiatric Rating Scale (Overall and Gorham, 1962) and the Mini-Mental State Examination (Folstein, Folstein, and McHugh, 1975) for screening symptomatology and cognitive functioning, respectively.

Of course, efficiency is not the only requirement for adequate clinical evaluation. Of key importance is the use of all sources of information available; that is, the patient, accompanying persons, and archival and current documentation. This requirement is intrinsically connected to the face validity of a diagnostic evaluation, which, as argued by Spitzer (1983), must include consideration of all pertinent data.

Procedures for conducting and recording psychiatric evaluations range from free-format approaches to fully structured arrangements. Using the terminology of Richardson, Dohrenwend, and Klein (1965), procedures are classified first into standardized or not standardized, depending on whether or not they include a clear specification of areas and items to be covered. Standardized procedures are divided into scheduled or not scheduled, depending on whether or not the wording and order of the questions for the subject's interview are fixed. The appropriate degree of structure of an evaluation procedure would depend on its purpose. For example, the exploration of an unknown area as in an anthropological inquiry, would be best performed through a free-format interview conducted by an expert in the field, while the systematic assessment of a well-formulated problem in a research laboratory may be most effectively addressed through a rigidly scheduled procedure.

For most patient evaluation purposes, both in clinical care and in clinical research, the use of semistructured approaches appear to be preferable (Sartorius, 1983). These approaches typically refer to largely standardized procedures with only minimally or flexibly scheduled interviews.

The above considerations are relevant to the design of the Brief Evaluation Form (BEF), a semistructured procedure addressed to the efficient evaluation of the current episode of illness.

A SEMISTRUCTURED APPROACH TO PSYCHIATRIC EVALUATION

Basic Features

The key characteristics of the semi-structured psychiatric evaluation approach originally presented by Mezzich, Dow, and Coffman (1981) include the following.

1. Use of standardized procedures and flexibly scheduled interviewing. The first aspect here involves specification of areas to be covered, definitions for all items included, and guidelines for severity and temporal assessment. The second refers to the provision of broad guidelines for conducting the interview in such a way that patients' feelings and the need to probe unclear reports are considered and articulated by a trained clinician.

2. Use of a recording format containing narrative and structured

components complementing each other. The rationale for including a narrative reflects the consideration that no matter how extensive a checklist mapping of psychopathology may be it would not be able to cover all significant particularities of the patient's condition, especially when clinical care decisions are to be based on the evaluation. Furthermore, the need for narratives even in highly systematic research evaluations has been pointedly noted by Brockington and Meltzer (1982). The side-by-side layout of narrative and structured components is in line with the finding by Laska (1974) that systems involving completely separate narrative and structured forms require a significant amount of duplicate clinical reporting and may, paradoxically, lead to incomplete documentation. One of the advantages of the structured component, in addition to helping the organization of the evaluation process, is its allowing the efficient computerization of key information leading to the development of cumulative data bases of great potential for clinical research and administrative planning.

3. Use of all sources of information. This involves interviewing not only the patient, but also relatives, associates, and social agency staff accompanying the patient and even other individuals who may be available through the telephone. Furthermore, it also includes the use of any charts documenting previous care of the patient as well as current referral notes sent by health and social agencies. The need for multiple information sources has been emphasized by Brockington and Meltzer (1982) and, as mentioned before, is a component of the validity parameters recently proposed by Spitzer (1983) for diagnostic evaluations.

4. Yielding a multiaxial diagnostic formulation along the lines of *The Diagnostic and Statistical Manual of Mental Disorders* (DSM-III) (American Psychiatric Press, 1980), and compatible with ICD-9-CM coding (U.S. National Center for Health Statistics, 1978). Given the flexibility of the semistructured evaluation approach used, it has been possible to cover all diagnostic categories and all axes in DSM-III, plus a sixth axis on current functioning.

The Initial Evaluation Form

The first component of the clinical information system developed according to the semistructured approach outlined above was the Initial

Evaluation Form (IEF) (Mezzich, Dow, Rich, Costello, and Himmelhoch, 1981). A second version was developed in 1982 (Mezzich, Slayton, Dow, Costello, and Himmelhoch, 1983). The IEF is aimed at providing a reasonably comprehensive description of the history and current condition of a new psychiatric patient.

Its major sections include (1) demographic and financial information; (2) history of present and past psychiatric disorders, mental status observations, and an inventory of symptoms which appeared in the past, the current episode, and during the interview; (3) a cognitive functioning inventory; (4) family, personal, and social histories; (5) physical health history and examination; (6) narrative assessment summary, problem list, and recommendations, a DSM-III multiaxial diagnostic formulation; and (7) clinical disposition and legal status.

A study of the interrater reliability of the IEF conducted on a quasi-random sample of 42 general psychiatric patients showed quite substantial reliability figures (kappa coefficients for typological variables and intraclass correlations for dimensional variables); for example, 0.61 for current symptoms, 0.60 for DSM-III Axis I, 0.61 for Axis II, 0.66 for Axis III, 0.55 for specific psychosocial stressors, 0.32 for overall stressor severity (Axis IV), and 0.72 for Axis V.

The factorial structure of the 64 general symptoms contained in the current version of the IEF has been shown to include a set of fifteen clearly interpretable factors, as follows: (1) delusional psychosis, (2) anxiety spectrum symptoms, (3) violence, (4) depression, (5) cognitive impairment, (6) elation/hyperactivity, (7) decreased vegetative functions, (8) increased vegetative functions, (9) hyperactivity, (10) dramatic, dependent, and erratic behaviors, (11) hallucinations, (12) substance abuse, (13) disturbed sexuality, (14) bizarre behavior, and (15) hysterical neurosis.

The IEF is being used with all new patients presenting for care at the Western Psychiatric Institute and Clinic of the University of Pittsburgh since August 1980. This amounts to over 20,000 new patients seen through December 1988. This growing data base is being utilized in a number of studies on diagnostic processes and clinical decisions (Mezzich, Evanczuk, Mathias, and Coffman, 1984a,b; Fabrega, Mezzich, and Mezzich, 1987). The IEF has been translated into Spanish and adapted for standard use at the Peruvian National Institute of Mental Health in Lima (Wharton, Sogi, Mezzich, Lopez-Merino, and Castro, 1988).

The Discharge Summary Form

Another evaluation procedure inscribed within the semistructured approach presented above is the Discharge Summary Form (DSF), the purpose of which is to provide a synopsis of the patient's clinical history, to document assessments and interventions during the treatment period, to summarize the patient's condition at discharge time, and to indicate his disposition.

The DSF is longitudinally coordinated with the IEF, not only by representing an update of the patient's condition originally evaluated with the IEF at the point of admission, but also by having a symptom inventory and a DSM-III diagnostic format identical to those of the IEF (Mezzich, Dow, Ganguli, Munetz, and Zettler-Segal, 1986).

The major sections of the DSF include the following: (1) summaries of psychiatric, family, developmental, social, and physical health histories, concisely incorporating any new information obtained during the course of treatment; (2) assessments (tests, examinations, consultations) conducted during the treatment period, their overall results and need for further evaluation; (3) a description of the treatment course, including a checklist of therapeutic modalities used and their perceived effectiveness, and a rating of the patient's overall cooperation; (4) a symptomatological evaluation comparing admission ratings with those made at discharge; (5) a final diagnostic formulation covering all five axes of DSM-III plus an axis on adaptive functioning at discharge, placed side-by-side, for comparative purposes, with the initial diagnostic formulation; and (6) a dispositional statement including reasons for discharge, referrals for further care, prescriptions and recommendations.

PURPOSE AND DESCRIPTION OF THE BRIEF EVALUATION FORM

The Brief Evaluation Form (BEF) is a semistructured psychiatric assessment procedure focused on the current episode of illness. It was developed to provide an updated evaluative statement on patients entering a new period of care and who had been assessed in the past few years with the more comprehensive and historically extensive IEF. Additionally, the BEF may be useful for screening and time-limited evaluations in straight emergency settings.

The structure of the BEF, like that of the IEF and DSF, involves complementary narrative and standardized components organizing its various content sections. Table 4.1 outlines this structure.

Figures 4.1 through 4.4 exhibit the corresponding pages of the BEF. Some highlighting comments are presented below.

The first page of the BEF (Figure 4.1) begins with a general identification of the patient and the evaluation, chief presenting complaint, and sources of information. Then, it contains a summarized description of the history of present psychiatric illness, with focus on recent problems and events. Complementing this, structured questions on length of psychiatric hospitalization and modalities of mental health treatment in the past 12 months are posed, along with another on recent change or discontinuation of psychotropic medication.

Page 2 (Figure 4.2) presents an inventory of current symptomatology. The first 64 symptoms listed are intended for the evaluation of patients of all ages and cover the following areas: vegetative, substance abuse, and characterological items; general appearance and behavior; speech and thought rate and pattern; mood and affect; thought content and perception; and sensorium, orientation, intellectual functions, and insight. This list is supplemented with 22 items to be used additionally with children and adolescents, covering conduct and emotional disturbances, problems with physical manifestations, and developmental problems. Each symptom is assessed regarding its presence and severity in the current episode and its presence during the

Table 4.1
Structural Components of the Brief Evaluation Form

Narrative	Structured
Identifying Information	Patient's Name and Number, Evaluation Date, and Setting
Summary of Present Illness	Psychiatric History Markers
Mental Status Remarks	Symptom Inventory
Brief Medical History and Examination	Vital Signs
Narrative Assessment Summary; Problems and Recommendations	Diagnostic Summary
Disposition Remarks	Admission and Referrals; Acceptance of Recommendations; Legal status
Evaluators' Signatures	Evaluators' Codes and Signature Dates

interview. Severity is measured on a 4-point scale (absent, mild, moderate, and severe) according to the frequency and intensity of the symptom during the current episode. Symptoms that cannot be assessed adequately are rated as "unknown."

Page 3 (Figure 4.3) starts with space for mental status remarks to complement the standardized symptom ratings. Then, a brief description of current physical disorders, medications, and allergies and a preliminary physical examination are presented, followed by standard vital signs measurements. The page ends with a narrative assessment summary and a short listing of major problems and recommendations.

Finally, page 4 (Figure 4.4) of the BEF contains a diagnostic summary and dispositional information. The diagnostic summary covers all five axes of DSM-III plus a sixth axis on current functioning. For each of the first three axes, psychiatric syndromes, personality, and specific developmental disorders, and physical disorders, a main formulation listing of several diagnoses is available as well as a listing of additional or alternative diagnoses to be ruled out. Instructions and a list of categories and codes for Axes I and II are printed on the back of BEF pages 2 and 3. The latter also contains instructions for Axis III ratings, the codes for which appear in the nonpsychiatric chapters of the current *International Classification of Diseases* (ICD-9-CM).

The psychosocial stressors section of the diagnostic summary includes first slots for a listing of specific stressors, and then a linear scale for circling the overall severity of the stressors (DSM-III Axis IV). For rating adaptive functioning, both regarding highest level in the past year (DSM-III Axis V) and current functioning (occupationally, with family and with other individuals and groups), linear scales are also available in the diagnostic format. Instructions for the assessment of Axes IV, V, and VI are presented on the back of page 4 of the BEF. They broadly follow, but are more specific than, the guidelines offered in DSM-III.

The disposition portion of page 4 covers admission and referral information, acceptance of recommendations by patient and family, and the patient's legal status upon completion of the evaluation.

COMMENT

The validation studies of the IEF outlined earlier in this chapter are relevant to the BEF as the components of this form (e.g., current

Figure 4.1 First page of the Brief Evaluation Form (BEF). (For a larger version of this page, see appendix pages 420 and 421.)

UNIVERSITY OF PITTSBURGH
WESTERN PSYCHIATRIC INSTITUTE AND CLINIC
BRIEF EVALUATION FORM
(5/14/82)

Name: ______________________
WPIC Number ☐☐☐☐☐
Date: ______ M ______ D ______ Y
Evaluation Setting: ______________

☐ Previous (latest) IEF completed at WPIC. Evaluation setting: Date: / /

IDENTIFYING INFORMATION, CHIEF COMPLAINT, AND SOURCES OF INFORMATION:

SUMMARY OF PRESENT ILLNESS *(Describe the history of present psychiatric illness, with focus on the most recent problems and events, and on changes in the patient's course of illness since the last Initial Evaluation Form was completed.)*

1. Number of weeks of psychiatric hospitalization during the past 12 months: ____________ ☐ Unknown
2. Modalities of mental health treatment received during the past 12 months (check all applicable):

☐ None	☐ Family psychotherapy	☐ Minor tranquilizers	☐ Stimulants	☐ Other/Unspecified medication
☐ Individual psychotherapy	☐ Specific behavioral techniques	☐ Antidepressants	☐ Anti-Parkinsonian medication	☐ ECT
☐ Group Therapy	☐ Neuroleptics	☐ Lithium	☐ Anticonvulsants	☐ Other/Unspecified modalities

3. ☐ Recent significant psychotropic medication change or discontinuation.

Figure 4.2 Inventory of current symptomatology on the BEF. (For a larger version of this page, see appendix pages 422–425.)

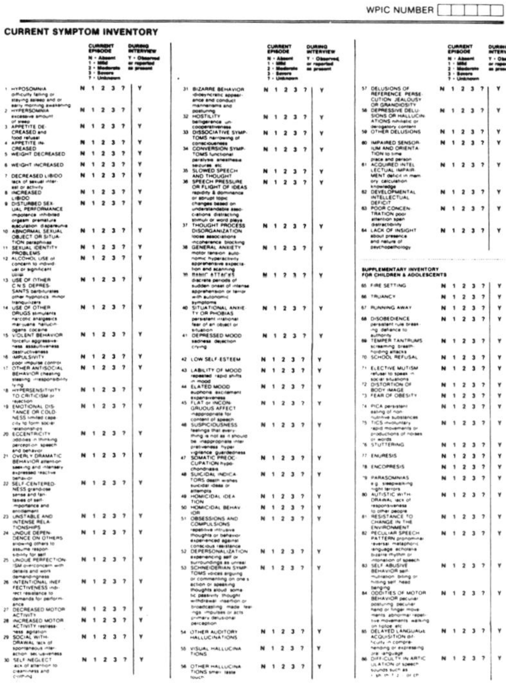
WPIC NUMBER

CURRENT SYMPTOM INVENTORY

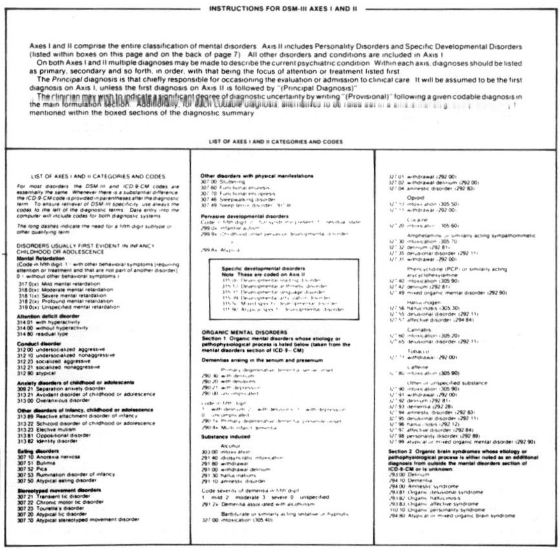
INSTRUCTIONS FOR DSM-III AXES I AND II

Axes I and II comprise the entire classification of mental disorders. Axis II includes Personality Disorders and Specific Developmental Disorders (listed within boxes on this page and on the back of page 7). All other disorders and conditions are included in Axis I.
On both Axes I and II multiple diagnoses may be made to describe the current psychiatric condition. Within each axis, diagnoses should be listed as primary, secondary and so forth, in order, with that being the focus of attention or treatment listed first.
The *Principal* diagnosis is that chiefly responsible for occasioning the evaluation or admission to clinical care. It will be assumed to be the first diagnosis on Axis I, unless the first diagnosis on Axis II is followed by "(Principal Diagnosis)".

LIST OF AXES I AND II CATEGORIES AND CODES

Figure 4.3 Mental status, medical history, and summary on the BEF. (For a larger version of this page, see appendix pages 426–429.)

WPIC NUMBER ☐☐☐☐☐

MENTAL STATUS REMARKS *(Comment on general appearance and behavior, speech and thought rate and pattern, mood and affect, thought content, perception, sensorium, orientation, intellectual functions and insight.)*

BRIEF MEDICAL HISTORY AND EXAMINATION *(Include current physical disorders, medications, allergies and a preliminary physical examination.)*

VITAL SIGNS: Pulse ________ B.P.: _____/_____ Temp.: ________ Resp.: ________

NARRATIVE ASSESSMENT SUMMARY

PROBLEMS *(Psychopathological, physical and social)* **RECOMMENDATIONS** *(Diagnostic studies, treatment modalities, instructions to patient/family)*

LIST OF AXES I AND II CATEGORIES AND CODES (CONTINUATION)

SUBSTANCE USE DISORDERS

Code in fifth digit 1 = continuous, 2 = episodic, 3 = in remission, 0 = unspecified

305 0x Alcohol abuse
303 9x Alcohol dependence (Alcoholism)
305 4x Barbiturate or similarly acting sedative or hypnotic abuse
304 1x Barbiturate or similarly acting sedative or hypnotic dependence
305 5x Opioid abuse,
304 0x Opioid dependence
305 6x Cocaine abuse,
305 7x Amphetamine or similarly acting sympathomimetic abuse
304 4x Amphetamine or similarly acting sympathomimetic dependence,
305 9x Phencyclidine (PCP) or similarly acting arylcyclohexylamine abuse, (3/8 4x
305 3x Hallucinogen abuse,
305 2x Cannabis abuse,
304 3x Cannabis dependence,
305 1x Tobacco dependence,
305 9x Other, mixed or unspecified substance abuse,
304 6x Other specified substance dependence,
304 9x Unspecified substance dependence,
304 7x Dependence on combination of opioid and other non alcoholic substance,
304 8x Dependence on combination of substances, excluding opioids and alcohol,

SCHIZOPHRENIC DISORDERS

Code in fifth digit 1 = subchronic, 2 = chronic, 3 = subchronic with acute exacerbation, 4 = chronic with acute exacerbation, 5 = in remission, 0 = unspecified

Schizophrenia,
295 1x disorganized,
295 2x catatonic,
295 3x paranoid,
295 9x undifferentiated,
295 6x residual,

PARANOID DISORDERS

297 10 Paranoia
297 30 Shared paranoid disorder
298 30 Acute paranoid disorder
297 90 Atypical paranoid disorder

PSYCHOTIC DISORDERS NOT ELSEWHERE CLASSIFIED

295 40 Schizophreniform disorder
298 80 Brief reactive psychosis
295 70 Schizoaffective disorder
298 90 Atypical psychosis

AFFECTIVE DISORDERS

Major affective disorders

Code major depressive episode in fifth digit 6 = in remission, 4 = with psychotic features (the unofficial non ICD 9 CM fifth digit 7 may be used instead to indicate that the psychotic features are mood incongruent), 3 = with melancholia, 2 = without melancholia, 0 = unspecified

Code manic episode in fifth digit 6 = in remission, 4 = with psychotic features (the unofficial non ICD 9 CM fifth digit 7 may be used instead to indicate that the psychotic features are mood incongruent), 2 = without psychotic features, 0 = unspecified

Bipolar disorder,
296 6x mixed,
296 4x manic,
296 5x depressed,

Major depression,
296 2x single episode,
296 3x recurrent,

Other specific affective disorders
301 13 Cyclothymic disorder
300 40 Dysthymic disorder (or Depressive neurosis)

Atypical affective disorders
296 70 Atypical bipolar disorder
296 82 Atypical depression

ANXIETY DISORDERS

Phobic disorders (or Phobic neuroses)
300 21 Agoraphobia with panic attacks
300 22 Agoraphobia without panic attacks
300 23 Social phobia
300 29 Simple phobia

Anxiety states (or Anxiety neuroses)
300 01 Panic disorder
300 02 Generalized anxiety disorder
300 30 Obsessive compulsive disorder (or Obsessive compulsive neurosis)

Post traumatic stress disorder
308 30 acute
309 81 chronic or delayed
300 00 Atypical anxiety disorder

SOMATOFORM DISORDERS

300 81 Somatization disorder
300 11 Conversion disorder (or Hysterical neurosis, conversion type)
307 80 Psychogenic pain disorder
300 70 Hypochondriasis (or Hypochondriacal neurosis)
300 71 Atypical somatoform disorder (300 70)

DISSOCIATIVE DISORDERS (OR HYSTERICAL NEUROSES, DISSOCIATIVE TYPE)

300 12 Psychogenic Amnesia
300 13 Psychogenic fugue
300 14 Multiple personality
300 60 Depersonalization disorder (or depersonalization neurosis)
300 15 Atypical dissociative disorder

PSYCHOSEXUAL DISORDERS

Gender identity disorders

Indicate sexual history in the fifth digit of Transsexualism code

1 = asexual, 2 = homosexual, 3 = heterosexual, 0 = unspecified

302 5x Transsexualism
302 60 Gender identity disorder of childhood
302 85 Atypical gender identity disorder

Paraphilias
302 81 Fetishism
302 30 Transvestism
302 10 Zoophilia
302 20 Pedophilia
302 40 Exhibitionism
302 82 Voyeurism
302 83 Sexual masochism
302 84 Sexual sadism
302 90 Atypical paraphilia

Psychosexual dysfunctions
302 71 Inhibited sexual desire
302 72 Inhibited sexual excitement
302 73 Inhibited female orgasm
302 74 Inhibited male orgasm
302 75 Premature ejaculation
302 76 Functional dyspareunia
306 51 Functional vaginismus
302 70 Atypical psychosexual dysfunction

Other psychosexual disorders
302 00 Ego-dystonic homosexuality
302 89 Psychosexual disorder not elsewhere classified

FACTITIOUS DISORDERS

300 16 Factitious disorder with psychological symptoms
301 51 Chronic factitious disorder with physical symptoms
300 19 Atypical factitious disorder with physical symptoms

DISORDERS OF IMPULSE CONTROL NOT ELSEWHERE CLASSIFIED

312 31 Pathological gambling
312 32 Kleptomania
312 33 Pyromania
312 34 Intermittent explosive disorder
312 35 Isolated explosive disorder
312 39 Atypical impulse control disorder

ADJUSTMENT DISORDER

309 00 with depressed mood
309 24 with anxious mood
309 28 with mixed emotional features
309 30 with disturbance of conduct
309 40 with mixed disturbance of emotions and conduct
309 23 with work (or academic) inhibition
309 83 with withdrawal
309 90 with atypical features

PSYCHOLOGICAL FACTORS AFFECTING PHYSICAL CONDITION

Specify physical condition on Axis III
316 00 Psychological factors affecting physical condition

PERSONALITY DISORDERS

Note: These are coded on Axis II

301 00 Paranoid
301 20 Schizoid
301 22 Schizotypal
301 50 Histrionic
301 81 Narcissistic
301 70 Antisocial
301 83 Borderline
301 82 Avoidant
301 60 Dependent
301 40 Compulsive
301 84 Passive Aggressive
301 89 Atypical, mixed or other personality disorder

V CODES FOR CONDITIONS NOT ATTRIBUTABLE TO A MENTAL DISORDER THAT ARE A FOCUS OF ATTENTION OR TREATMENT

V65 20 Malingering
V62 89 Borderline intellectual functioning (V62 88)
V71 01 Adult antisocial behavior
V71 02 Childhood or adolescent antisocial behavior
V62 30 Academic problem
V62 20 Occupational problem
V62 82 Uncomplicated bereavement
V15 81 Noncompliance with medical treatment
V62 89 Phase of life problem or other life circumstance problem
V61 10 Marital problem
V61 20 Parent child problem
V61 80 Other specified family circumstances
V62 81 Other interpersonal problem

ADDITIONAL CODES

300 90 Unspecified mental disorder (nonpsychotic)
V71 09 No diagnosis or condition on Axis I
799 90 Diagnosis or condition deferred on Axis I

V71 09 No diagnosis on Axis II
799 90 Diagnosis deferred on Axis II

INSTRUCTIONS FOR DSM-III AXIS III: PHYSICAL DISORDERS

Axis III includes any current physical disorders or conditions relevant to the understanding or management of the individual. Such conditions are catalogued in the non-mental disorder sections of the International Classification of Diseases (ICD-9-CM). Physical conditions identified for an individual should be described in standard terms and will be coded later. Past disorders that are not currently active should be described in the Medical History but not listed in the diagnostic formulation.

Figure 4.4 Diagnostic summary and dispositional information on the BEF. (For a larger version of this page, see appendix pages 430–433.)

UNIVERSITY OF PITTSBURGH
WESTERN PSYCHIATRIC INSTITUTE AND CLINIC

BRIEF EVALUATION FORM

Name ______
WPIC NUMBER [| | |]
Date m d y
Evaluation Setting ______

DIAGNOSTIC SUMMARY

I. Clinical psychiatric syndromes *(Instructions and codes on back of pages 2 and 3)*

Main Formulation:	Codes	Alternatives to be ruled out	Codes
1.			
2.			
3.			
4.			

II Personality and specific developmental disorders *(Instructions and codes on back of pages 2 and 3)*

Main Formulation:	Codes	Alternatives to be ruled out:	Codes
1.			
2.			

III. Physical Disorders *(Instructions on back of page 3)*

Main Formulation:	Codes	Alternatives to be ruled out	Codes
1.			
2.			
3.			
4.			

IV. Psychosocial stressors *(Instructions on back of this page)*

A. Ranked list: 1 ______ 2 ______ 3 ______ 4 ______ Codes

B. Overall stressor severity:

1	2	3	4	5	6	7	0
None	Minimal	Mild	Moderate	Severe	Extreme	Catastrophic	Unspecified

V. Highest level of adaptive functioning during the past year *(Instructions on back of this page)*

1	2	3	4	5	6	7	0
Superior	Very Good	Good	Fair	Poor	Very Poor	Grossly Impaired	Unspecified

VI. Current functioning: *(Instructions on back of this page)*

	Superior	Adequate	Slightly Impaired	Moderately Impaired	Markedly Impaired	Unspecified
A. Occupational	1	2	3	4	5	0
B. With family	1	2	3	4	5	0
C. With other indiv. & groups	1	2	3	4	5	0

DISPOSITION

A. Admission or Referrals

Name of program or facility	Date of admission or appointment (month/day/year)	Release of information signed (✓)

Remarks: ______

B. Were referrals and recommendations accepted by patient/family? □ Yes □ No If no, explain ______

C. Legal status after evaluation:
□ Voluntary (regular) □ Voluntary-302 Commitment discontinued □ 302 Commitment in force □ 303 Commitment □ 304 Commitment □ Other involuntary

EVALUATORS *(Who interviewed the patient)*

1. ______ Signature of first clinician ______ Code ______ Date
2. ______ Signature of second clinician ______ Code ______ Date
3. ______ Signature of third clinician ______ Code ______ Date

INSTRUCTIONS FOR DSM-III AXIS IV: PSYCHOSOCIAL STRESSORS

Axis IV assesses psychological stressors (both discrete events and ongoing strains) [illegible] of the present disorder.

First identify relevant stressors during the past 12 months as specifically as possible and list them (up to 4) in order of importance. To accomplish this, ask for a summary of events and strains from the patient, and then probe specifically to clarify the patient's initial report and to inquire about areas of the patient's life which may not have been mentioned spontaneously. Situations which mainly reflect the patient's symptomology or dysfunctions should be excluded.

Please consider the following categories of stressors:

1. **Health:** e.g. acute or chronic physical illness or injury either to the patient or to someone close to the patient; mental illness in significant others. A physical disorder, which is listed as such on Axis III, can also be a psychosocial stressor if it creates a considerable strain on the patient's life.
2. **Bereavement:** e.g. death of parent, extended family member, or significant other
3. **Love and marriage:** e.g. separation, divorce, persistent marital discord
4. **Parental:** e.g. pregnancy, birth of a child, loss of custody of child, behavior problems in children
5. **Family stressors for children and adolescents:** e.g. cold or hostile relationship between parents, cold or hostile parental behavior towards child, stressful family situation
6. **Other familial relationships:** e.g. acute or chronic serious family arguments other than with immediate relative, change in the frequency of family interaction
7. **Other relationships outside the family:** e.g. terminating a close friendship, terminating organizational activities, serious disruptions in social relationships
8. **Work:** e.g. demotion or promotion at work, significant changes in work conditions, having a difficult supervisor, becoming retired, lack of employment opportunities
9. **School:** e.g. began or changed a school or training program, failed an important academic milestone, completing or failing a school or training program
10. **Financial:** e.g. significant decrease in income, took a large loan or mortgage, foreclosure on a loan
11. **Legal:** e.g. court appearances, major lawsuits, arrests, sentenced to (or served) a jail term
12. **Housing/environmental:** e.g. change in residence, significant deterioration in living conditions, eviction or threat of eviction
13. **Miscellanea:** e.g. being victim of a crime or assault, facing a new culture

Next rate the severity (from 1 to 7) of the summed effect of all the psychosocial stressors listed. This rating should be based on your assessment of the "objective" stress represented by the events or strains, not on the patient's subjective vulnerability to the stressors. The level of stress rated should be that likely to be experienced by an "average" person of similar socio-cultural circumstances as the patient [illegible]. The following examples may be used as a guide in making your ratings.

Code	Term	Adult examples	[illegible] examples
1	None	No apparent psychosocial stressors	No apparent psychosocial stressors
2	Minimal	Minor violation of the law, small bank loan	Vacation with family
3	Mild	Argument with neighbor, change in work hours	Change in schoolteacher, new school year
4	Moderate	New career, death of close friend, pregnancy	Chronic parental fighting, change to new school, illness of close relative, birth of sibling
5	Severe	Serious illness in self or family, major financial loss, marital separation, birth of child	Death of peer, divorce of parents, arrest, hospitalization, persistent and harsh parental discipline
6	Extreme	Death of close relative, divorce	Death of parent or sibling, repeated physical or sexual abuse
7	Catastrophic	Concentration camp experience, devastating natural disaster	Multiple family deaths
0	Unspecified	No information or not applicable	No information or not applicable

In summing the effect of all stressors, it may be necessary to take into account [illegible] and the severity of stressors. For example, one moderate stressor would receive a rating of 4, while a combination of 3 moderate stressors might receive a rating of 5 [illegible] same rating which a single more severe stressor would receive.

INSTRUCTIONS FOR DSM-III AXIS V: HIGHEST LEVEL OF ADAPTIVE FUNCTIONING IN PAST YEAR

Axis V assesses an individual's highest level of adaptive occupational and social functioning for at least a few months during the past year.

Recommended rating steps:

1. Identify the best couple of months of adaptive functioning during the past 12 months and focus attention on that period for making the following assessments.
2. Separately judge the individual's performance and degree of impairment in the following two regards:
   a) Occupational Functioning. This encompasses consistency and effectiveness of performance of expected role as worker, student, and/or homemaker. If an individual is unemployed not primarily because of inability to hold a job but because of unavailability of employment, his occupational assessment should focus on alternative roles, e.g. homemaker.
   b) Social Relations. This encompasses frequency and quality of social interaction [illegible] meeting, communicating and sharing common activities with family members and with other individuals and groups.
3. Combine the occupational functioning and social relations ratings [illegible] for obtaining the overall highest level of adaptive functioning in the past year. As noted, use of leisure time is considered only for the highest levels of functioning and essential self care only for the poorest.

Code	Term	Description
1	Superior	Unusually effective functioning in occupational functioning, social relations and use of leisure time
2	Very Good	Better than average functioning in occupational functioning, social relations and use of leisure time
3	Good	No more than slight impairment in either occupational or social functioning
4	Fair	Moderate impairment in either occupational functioning or social relations, or some impairment in both
5	Poor	Marked impairment in either occupational functioning or social relations, or moderate impairment in both
6	Very Poor	Marked impairment in both occupational functioning and social relations
7	Grossly Impaired	Gross impairment in virtually all areas of functioning including essential self care
0	Unspecified	

INSTRUCTIONS FOR AXIS VI: CURRENT FUNCTIONING

Axis VI assesses current levels of functioning at work, school or homemaking, and relations with family, and with other individuals or groups.

Separately judge the individual's performance **during the past month** in the following three regards:

a) Occupational Functioning. This encompasses consistency and effectiveness of performance of expected role as worker, student, and/or homemaker. If an individual is unemployed not primarily because of inability to hold a job but because of unavailability of employment, his occupational assessment should focus on alternative roles, e.g. homemaker.

b) Functioning with Family. This encompasses frequency and quality of interaction with family members (i.e. meeting, communicating, and sharing common activities with them).

c) Functioning with Other Individuals and Groups. This encompasses frequency and quality of interaction with non family individuals and groups (i.e. meeting, communicating, and sharing common activities with them).

Determine the individual's current functioning level in each of these regards by using the scale given below.

Code	Functioning Level	Occupational Functioning	Functioning with Family and with Other Individuals and Groups
1	Superior	Highly regular and competent work	Very frequent and close personal contacts
2	Adequate	Acceptable work regularity and competence	Acceptable frequency and closeness of personal contacts
3	Slightly Impaired	Occasionally misses work and/or has some difficulty with competence	Rather restricted or irregular frequency and closeness of personal contacts
4	Moderately Impaired	Misses work frequently and/or shows moderate incompetence	Infrequent and superficial or troubled personal contacts
5	Markedly Impaired	Works rarely or not at all, and/or is grossly incompetent	Almost non existent or grossly disturbed personal contacts
0	Unspecified		

symptom inventory, multiaxial diagnostic formulation) constitute a subset of the IEF.

The BEF has been used at the Western Psychiatric Institute and Clinic (WPIC) of the University of Pittsburgh since November 1982 for the evaluation of all patients starting a new episode of care who had an IEF completed in the past three years. The multiaxial diagnostic formulation it yields has been found to be helpful for the preparation of comprehensive treatment plans, an experience that is being used extensively in treatment planning workshops organized by WPIC throughout the Western Pennsylvania region.

From an educational viewpoint, the semistructured organization of the BEF has been useful to guide trainees in conducting patient evaluations at WPIC. Furthermore, the BEF has facilitated, by using the checklists, the supervision of trainees by the faculty and of line staff by program leaders.

Furthermore, the applicability of the BEF (as well as that of the IEF and DSF) to regular patient care and the resulting growth of large clinical data bases has furnished the opportunity of enhancing administrative planning and the investigation of diagnostic processes and treatment decisions in a naturalistic clinical environment.

REFERENCES

American Psychiatric Association (1980), *Diagnostic and Statistical Manual of Mental Disorders,* 3rd ed. (DSM-III). Washington, DC: American Psychiatric Press.

Brockington, I. F., & Meltzer, H. Y. (1982), Documenting an episode of psychiatric illnesses: Need for multiple information sources, multiple raters and narrative. *Schiz. Bull.,* 8:485–492.

Fabrega, H., Jr., Mezzich, J. E., & Mezzich, A. C. (1987), Adjustment disorder as a marginal or transitional category of illness in DSM-III. *Arch. Gen. Psychiat.,* 50:31–49.

Folstein, M. F., Folstein, S. E., & McHugh, P. R. (1975), Mini-mental state: A practical method for grading the cognitive state of patients for the clinician. *J. Psychiat. Res.,* 12:189–198.

Laska, M. L. (1974), The multi-state information system. In: *Progress in Mental Health Information System,* eds. J. L. Crawford, D. W. Morgan, & D. T. Gianturco. Cambridge, MA: Ballinger.

Mezzich, J. E., Dow, J. T., & Coffman, G. A. (1981), Developing an efficient clinical information system for a comprehensive psychiatric institute. I. Principles, design and organization. *Behav. Res. Meth. & Instrument.,* 13:459–463.

——— ——— Ganguli, R., Munetz, M. R., & Zettler-Segal, M. (1986), Computerized initial and discharge evaluations. In: *Clinical Care and Information Systems in Psychiatry,* ed. J. E. Mezzich. Washington, DC: American Psychiatric Press.

——— ——— Rich, C. L., Costello, A. J., & Himmelhoch, J. M. (1981), Developing an efficient clinical information system for a comprehensive psychiatric institute. II. The Initial Evaluation Form. *Behav. Res. Meth. & Instrument.,* 13:464–478.

——— Evanczuk, K. J., Mathias, R. J., & Coffman, G. A. (1984a), Symptoms and hospitalization decisions. *Amer. J. Psychiat.,* 141:764–769.

——— ——— ——— ——— (1984b), Admission decisions and multiaxial diagnosis. *Arch. Gen. Psychiat.,* 41:1001–1004.

——— Slayton, R. I., Dow, J. T., Costello, A. J., & Himmelhoch, J. M. (1983), A semi-structured psychiatric evaluation procedure. Paper presented at the Symposium on New Developments in Systematic Clinical Evaluation, 136th Annual Meeting of the American Psychiatric Association, New York.

Overall, J. E., & Gorham, D. R. (1962), The brief psychiatric rating scale. *Psychol. Rep.,* 10:799–812.

Richardson, S. A., Dohrenwend, B. S., & Klein, D. (1965), *Interviewing: Its Form and Functions.* New York: Basic Books.

Sartorius, N. (1983), The experience of the World Health Organization with psychiatric scales. Paper presented at the Symposium on Comprehensive Psychopathological Scales, VII World Congress of Psychiatry, Vienna, Austria.

Spitzer, R. L. (1983), Psychiatric diagnosis: Are clinicians still necessary? *Comprehen. Psychiat.,* 24:399–411.

U.S. National Center for Health Statistics (1978), *International Classification of Diseases,* 9th rev., Clinical Modification (ICD-9-CM). Ann Arbor, MI: Commission on Professional and Hospital Activities.

Wharton, D., Sogi, C., Mezzich, J. E., Lopez-Merino, I., & Castro, J. (1988), Experience with the semi-structured Initial Evaluation Form in Peru and the United States. In: *International Classification in Psychiatry,* eds. J. E. Mezzich & M. von Cranach. Cambridge, U.K.: Cambridge University Press.

Commentary

Shawn C. Shea, M.D.

In this well-written and concise paper Mezzich attempts to review some of the basic principles that define the characteristics of the clinical interview. Following his description of standardized and nonstandardized interview formats, he discusses the development of a flexible style of interview, while also illustrating the document utilized to record the information yielded by this technique. One of the most striking attributes in the creation of this interviewing format is the fact that it was developed entirely within an actual clinical setting. In short, it is practical.

In this regard, Mezzich has stood as a pioneer in advocating the importance of a well-rounded data base in the approach to treatment planning. The Initial Evaluation Form (IEF) reflects this position. Areas for recording information range from the standard history of the present illness to an extensive evaluation of social history and interpersonal functioning. These latter categories provide ready avenues into the exploration of personality dysfunction. Other critical areas such as the medical review of systems and the physical exam are afforded adequate space for exploration. The expected data, suggested by the structure of the recording document, leads the clinician to understand the patient in a true biopsychosocial context.

Along the lines of the IEF, Mezzich subsequently developed the

Brief Evaluation Form (BEF), which is the focus of chapter 4. The BEF arose from the need to interview efficiently and subsequently document the information gained from patients in a busy emergency room and admission center setting. The BEF clarifies for the clinician the critical areas needed during a rapid assessment including identifying information, the history of the present illness, the mental status and lethality assessment, medical exam, medical review of systems, the psychiatric review of symptoms, and the diagnostic assessment summary.

The use of collaborative sources of information including family members, friends, therapists, and past records is emphasized. Indeed, in an emergency room setting such collaborative sources are critical, for it becomes crucial to gain valid information concerning issues such as lethality or the presence of a psychotic process. The patients themselves may not provide reliable or valid information with regard to such concerns.

In the emergency room, the clinician must learn to focus on obtaining pertinent triage information, while avoiding extended exploration of data that ultimately may be of interest but is not needed for triage. When pressed for time, clinicians frequently become inefficient because of a compulsive need to finish "the clinical picture," but the emergency room is not a finishing room.

The handling of the family history represents a prime area where valuable time may be lost. It is not uncommon to observe trainees, in an emergency room, methodically exploring a detailed family history, perhaps checking for major depression in all family members even after it has already been established that the patient is acutely suicidal and warrants immediate admission. Instead, the emergency room clinician should be guided by the following principle, "Is the question I am about to ask going to affect my decision on triage or immediate treatment?" If the answer is negative, then the proposed question is probably not appropriate, unless being asked for specific engagement purposes.

By way of example, suppose a patient presents with soft signs suggesting an underlying psychosis. The patient may display a hint of delusional material and some signs of increased agitation such as pacing and difficulty falling asleep. The emergency room clinician is faced with deciding between aggressive outpatient therapy or hospitalization. In this type of circumstance it is of value to explore for a history of schizophrenia in other family members, for the presence of schizophrenia in family members may sway the clinician toward hospitalization, especially if these family members demonstrated rapid deterioration with their first breaks.

On the other hand, suppose a patient presents with an adjustment disorder demonstrating no psychotic symptoms. The patient requests outpatient therapy and seems relatively stable and motivated. In the hectic emergency room setting, there is no reason to explore a family history of psychosis with this patient, for this information will have probably no impact on triage or immediate treatment planning. In later interviews, the patient's treating clinician will actively explore this area.

Another important point to remember while reading this paper is that the order of the items in the IEF and the BEF does not necessarily suggest the order in which the information should be gathered. The clinician is expected to approach each patient creatively, gathering the data in the fashion best suited for such a patient. For example, the symptom inventory is not expected to be covered in a checklist fashion. Instead, these symptoms are largely explored following leads presented by the patient. In a similar light, trained clinicians do not typically refer to the IEF or BEF during the interview itself. Notes may be written on tablet paper as needed. The forms do not represent a schedule of when to ask what questions. This substantial flexibility provides for a more valid data base, while allowing the clinician to develop a strong rapport with the patient.

At present, collaborative work is well under way at Western Psychiatric Institute and Clinic in developing refined flexible ways of handling interviews, based on many of the principles emphasized by the IEF and the BEF. In this regard, no matter what the clinical situation, three factors remain of paramount importance in determining the style of the interview: (1) the tasks specific to the clinical situation, (2) the need to gather information efficiently while engaging the patient, and (3) the importance of attending to the validity of the data base. All three factors are very important whether the interview is a research interview or an emergency room interview. Moreover, all of these factors inextricably depend on the clinician's ability to establish a sound and rapid rapport with the patient. Flexibility remains the key word. Without it, serious doubts must be cast on the validity of so-called "research interviews," which adhere to rigidly scheduled formats. The IEF and the BEF stand as important first steps toward the realization of an interviewing style that will serve as an equally powerful tool in both research and clinical settings. Such a tool is long overdue.

Annotated Bibliography

Summers, W., Munoz, R., & Read, M. (1981), The psychiatric physical examination—Part I: Methodology. *J. Clin. Psych.*, 42:95–98.

This paper presents a practical physical examination of the patient experiencing behavior abnormalities. It was written in response to the need for reasonably thorough medical assessment in psychiatric clinics. Significantly, its authors are internists and psychiatrists.

II

SPECIFIC BEHAVIORAL EMERGENCIES

This part reviews various forms of behavioral emergency, some of which involve widely recognized psychopathological disorders as they present in emergency settings, while others involve highly sensitive suicidal and violent behaviors. The presentation of behavioral emergencies in early and late developmental stages are reviewed. Finally treated are special situations such as repeated visitors to and death and dying in the emergency unit.

Issues addressed in Part II include the following: how to identify organically based behavioral disturbances; how to conduct a differential diagnosis of organic brain syndromes in a way that would enhance management; how to assess and help substance abusers in the emergency department, both regarding cognitive impairment induced by drugs and the patterns of their abuse; what the most frequent forms of acute psychosis are and how they can be elucidated in an immediate care setting; how dramatic clinical syndromes such as hysteria and borderline personality disorder present in the emergency department and what complications they create there; what epidemiological patterns can be noted for dangerous behaviors, and how their prediction can be advanced within the framework of short-term clinical care; what are the psychological features and contextual factors of behavioral emergencies presented by children and adolescents and by geriatric patients.

All in all, an attempt will be made to facilitate understanding of the problematic behaviors of patients presenting for emergency care.

5

The Differential Diagnosis of Organic Based Psychiatric Disturbance in the Emergency Department

Michael A. Fauman, M.D., Ph.D., and Beverly J. Fauman, M.D.

INTRODUCTION

The emergency physician frequently encounters patients with behavioral abnormalities including severe agitation, withdrawal, confusion, extreme fear or anxiety, disruptive, combative, psychotic, bizarre, or inappropriate behavior. The physician must first establish control over the patient's behavior by reassurance, talking, and, if necessary, physical restraint. He must then determine whether the patient's abnormal behavior is a result of a psychological ("functional") process, an acute or chronic organic based disorder, or both. Many potentially life-threatening organic disorders may have a behavioral disturbance as their most obvious and striking symptom. Therefore, the physician must be

This chapter was first published in the *Journal of the American College of Emergency Physicians* (1977), 6:315–323, and it is reprinted by permission.

aware of the possibility of an underlying organic disorder in a patient with abnormal behavior and not dismiss the patient as merely "crazy," a "turkey," or a "crock."

DEFINITIONS

Several terms have been used to describe alterations in mental status secondary to an organic process and their use has been confusing and contradictory.

According to the American Psychiatric Association (1968), an "organic brain syndrome" is "a basic mental condition characteristically resulting from diffuse impairment of brain tissue function from whatever cause" (DSM-II). It must include symptoms of impairment of orientation, memory, all intellectual functions, judgment, and lability and shallowness of affect. Behaviorial disorders having an organic basis but not these five characteristics are not organic brain syndromes. They will be referred to as organic based behavioral disturbances, organic brain disturbance, organic based behavioral disorder, organic based behavioral abnormality, organic brain disease, or organic brain disorder. These latter terms include the more specific *organic brain syndrome* within them which may be subdivided into acute organic and chronic organic brain syndromes. A diagnosis of an acute organic brain syndrome implies the rapid onset of a temporary, reversible, diffuse disturbance of brain function which may present as delirium, stupor, or coma and which always ends with some resolution of the organic symptoms. Chronic brain syndrome comes on slowly, may include a dementia, delirium, stupor, or coma, and is due to an irreversible diffuse disturbance of brain tissue resulting in some permanent alteration in brain function and often terminating in death.

Delirium is a syndrome produced by a transient diffuse disturbance in brain tissue function characterized by a disturbance of consciousness, and a global impairment of cognition, memory, and perception (Lipowski, 1967; Sandok, 1975). In their early studies Engel and Romano (1959) referred to delirium as a syndrome of "cerebral insufficiency" and defined its properties as a reduction of the level of cognition and a characteristic slowing of the electroencephalogram. The symptoms of delirium are similar to those of the organic brain syndrome and if the delirium state reverses completely with no neurological residual, the patient can be considered to have had an acute organic brain syndrome. If the delirium state does not reverse and there is a neurological residual, the patient has a chronic brain syndrome.

As opposed to delirium, dementia usually implies a slow, progressive, global impairment of the patient's cognitive processes with particular emphasis on memory and intellectual functions. Changes in awareness or state of consciousness usually occur in a dementia at the end of a long period of progressive deterioration. If a dementia is shown to be irreversible, it can be a chronic brain syndrome. However, a number of dementias exist, such as that associated with pernicious anemia, which may go on for many years, but still be reversible. Finally, it is not unusual to find a delirium state superimposed upon a chronic brain syndrome or a dementia. This is usually seen when an abrupt change occurs in the patient's consciousness or awareness with further anxiety accompanied by further deterioration of the cognitive processes.

After the patient's behavior is under control, the most important step is to obtain a complete medical and psychiatric history and to give the patient a physical examination emphasizing the neurological examination. During the examination to diagnose an organic based behavioral abnormality, the physician should pay particular attention to evaluating 12 areas (Table 5.1).

MEDICAL AND PSYCHIATRIC HISTORY

First, any preexisting illnesses that might produce behavioral abnormalities must be elucidated, including head trauma, cardiovascular and pulmonary disorder, metabolic and endocrine disorders, infections, neoplasm, seizure disorders, and other less frequent disorders such as connective tissue diseases. Typical signs of organic brain syndromes such as disturbances in judgment, orientation, memory, cognitive functioning, and lability or shallowness of affect are not unusual accompaniments of cerebral hypoxia secondary to myocardial infarction, severe congestive heart failure, arthrosclerotic vascular disease, lupus erythematosus cerebrovascular inflammation, and severe chronic obstructive lung disease (American Psychiatric Association, 1968; Peterson and Martin, 1973; Steinhilber, Peterson, and Martin, 1966; Sandok, 1975). Seizure disorders and neoplasms of the central nervous

Table 5.1
Guidelines for Diagnosis
Organic Brain Disorder (OBD)

Medical and Psychiatric History

1. Preexisting medical illness with potential associated OBD
2. Previous psychiatric illness
3. Medication with potential OBD side effect
4. History of alcohol or other drug abuse

Physical Signs and Symptoms and Laboratory Tests

5. Abnormal vital signs
6. Onset of incontinence of urine or stool
7. Lateralizing neurological signs, ataxia, tremor, seizures
8. Abnormal metabolic values

Mental Status Signs and Symptoms

9. Fluctuating level of awareness or consciousness
10. Impairment of orientation, memory judgment or cognition
11. Lability of affect and other organic behaviors
12. Ego-dystonic hallucinations, olfactory or tactile hallucinations

system, especially the temporal lobe region, may produce many psychiatric symptoms including changes in perception, self-awareness, thought processes, mood and affect, and complex hallucinatory experiences (Ervin, 1975). Metabolic and endocrine disorders such as hypoglycemia, secondary to an excess of insulin (case 4) and hypocalcemia secondary to hypoparathyroidism (case 3) are not uncommon causes of altered mental functioning (Dale, 1975).

Also, the physician must be aware that a new disease diagnosed through his history and physical may also have behavioral concomitants. The patient's behavioral disorder may be a psychological reaction to his or her illness with or without an organic brain disorder.

A previous history of psychiatric disorder or psychiatric hospitalization allows the physician to determine whether the patient's present behavioral disorder is long-standing or recent. If this particular episode of behavioral disturbance is similar to past episodes, especially those that have been successfully treated with psychotherapy or psychoactive medication, the physician has more evidence of a psychological rather than organic diagnosis. Nevertheless, even in patients with a previous psychiatric disturbance (case 3) the reappearance of similar symptoms may indicate an organic disorder. Therefore, it is essential that the physician does not immediately assume that the patient's behavioral disorder is purely psychological because of evidence of previous psychiatric disorder in the history.

There are three separate groups of medications the physician should ask about specifically: those prescribed by other physicians for internal or external organic medical problems, those prescribed for psychiatric or behavioral problems, and over-the-counter preparations (Table 5.2). It is important to ask about over-the-counter medication because many patients do not consider these preparations as medication. Bromide preparations such as Nervine and compounds containing atropinelike agents such as Sominex, Sleep-Eze, or Compoz have the potential to produce organic brain disorders. Several medically prescribed agents also have psychiatric side effects. With prolonged use stimulants like amphetamine and its derivatives can produce a paranoid schizophreniclike syndrome and they may be associated with a severe depression and suicidal ideation on withdrawal. Anticonvulsive agents like diphenylhydantoin (Dilantin) cause an organic brain disorder in high doses while ethosuximide (Zarontin) has side effects that include paranoid psychoses, and depressive syndromes. Belladonna alkaloids may produce an "atropine psychosis," and L-dopa, commonly used in the treatment of Parkinson's disease, can produce a delirium, depression, or psychosis. Cardiovascular agents such as digitalis may cause a delirium state including hallucinations with toxic doses. Reserpine, methyldopa, procainamide, and propranolol produce severe depression. The two latter drugs have also been reported to produce psychotic behavior. Hormones such as adrenocorticotropic hormone (ACTH), cortisol, and prednisone may produce a "steroid psychosis." Overdoses of insulin may produce hypoglycemia with accompanying organic brain disorder as seen in case 4 (Table 5.2, A–F) (Goodman and Gilman, 1970; Angrist and Gershon, 1972; Goodwin, 1972; Goodwin, Ebert, and Bunney, 1972; Greenblatt and Shader, 1972; Shader, 1972; Shader and Greenblatt, 1972; Wallach and Gershon, 1972; Peterson, 1975).

Table 5.2
Psychiatric Side Effects

A. Cardiovascular Drugs[a]

Symptoms / Drugs	Digitalis	Reserpine	(Pronestyl) Procainamide	(Inderal) Propranolol	(Aldomet) Methyldopa	(Apresoline) Hydralazine
OBS delirium	●					●
Confusion	●		●			●
Disorientation	●					●
Depression	●	●	●	●	●	●
Psychosis			●	●		
Hallucination	●		●	●		
Euphoria						
Mania-Hypomania						
Withdrawal seizures						
Toxic seizures	●					
Withdrawal syndrome	NO	NO	NO	NO	NO	NO

B. Antiinfection Drugs

Symptoms / Drugs	Isoniazid	Cycloserine	Iproniazid	Sulfonamides	IV Penicillin
OBS delirium	●	●	●		
Confusion	●	●		●	
Disorientation	●	●			
Depression		●		●	
Psychosis	●	●		●	●
Hallucination	●	●			●
Euphoria	●		●		
Mania-Hypomania			●		
Withdrawal seizures					
Toxic seizures	●	●			●
Withdrawal syndrome	NO	NO	NO	NO	NO

Table 5.2 cont.

C. Neuropharmacological Drugs

Symptoms / Drugs	(Dilantin) Diphenyl-hydantoin	(Zarontin) Ethosuxi-mide	L-Dopa	Belladonna Alkaloids Anticholinergics 1-hyoscine (Scopolamine) *d*, 1-hyposcyamine (Atropine) Trihexyphenidyl (Artane) Benztropine (Cogentin)	(Benadryl) Diphenhydramine
OBS delirium	●		●	●	
Confusion	●		●	●	
Disorientation	●		●	●	●
Depression	●	●	●		
Psychosis		●	●	●	●
Hallucination	●		●	●	●
Euphoria		●			●
Mania-Hypomania			●	●	
Withdrawal seizures					
Toxic seizures	●			●	●
Withdrawal syndrome	NO	NO	NO	NO	NO

D. Psychiatric and Abused Drugs

Symptoms / Drugs	**Amphet-amine**	**Barbiturates**	**(Librium) Chlordiazepoxide (Valium) Diazepam**	**Pheno-thiazines**	**(Elavil) Amitriptyline (Tofranil) Imipramine**	**Lithium**
OBS delirium	●	●[c]	●	●	●	●
Confusion	●	●[c]	●	●	●	●
Disorientation	●	●[c]	●	●	●	
Depression	●[b]			●		
Psychosis	●	●[c]				
Hallucination	●	●[c]	●		●	
Euphoria	●	●				
Mania-Hypomania					●	
Withdrawal Seizures		●[c]	●			
Toxic Seizures	●			●	●	●
Withdrawal Syndrome	YES	YES	YES	NO	NO	NO

Table 5.2 cont.

E. Sedative-Hypnotic Abused Drugs

Symptoms / Drugs	(Quaalude) Methaqualone	(Doriden) Glutethimide	Bromides
OBS delirium	●[d]		●
Confusion			●
Disorientation			●
Depression			●
Psychosis			●
Hallucination			●
Euphoria			
Mania-Hypomania			●
Withdrawal Seizures	●	●	
Toxic Seizures	●	●	
Withdrawal Syndrome	YES	YES	NO

F. Miscellaneous Drugs

Symptoms / Drugs	Steroids	Salicylates	(Indocin) Indomethacin	Insulin	Disulfiram	Aminophylline
OBS delirium		●	●	●	●	●
Confusion	●	●	●	●	●	●
Disorientation					●	
Depression	●		●		●	
Psychosis	●	●	●	●	●	
Hallucination		●	●			
Euphoria	●					
Mania-Hypomania						
Withdrawal Seizures						
Toxic Seizures		●	●	●		●
Withdrawal Syndrome	NO	NO	NO	NO	NO	NO

[a] Peterson, 1975; Goodman and Gilman, 1970; Greenblatt and Shader, 1972.
[b] Symptom of withdrawal mainly.
[c] Symptom of toxicity and withdrawal.
[d] Symptom of withdrawal only.

Psychiatric medications also have potent behavioral side effects. Barbiturates, minor tranquilizers, and major tranquilizers such as chlorpromazine (Thorazine), thioridazine (Mellaril), trifluoperazine (Stelazine), and antidepressants such as imipramine (Tofranil) and amitriptyline (Elavil) can produce delirium states in high doses. Lithium carbonate has a small therapeutic index with toxic symptoms when lithium levels rise above 2 mEq/liter. These side effects include agitation, delirium, and neurological signs with higher serum concentrations (Goodman and Gilman, 1970; Peterson, 1975).

It is important to inquire about the patient's potential alcohol or drug abuse history including hallucinogens such as lysergic acid diethylamide (LSD), mescaline, dimethoxymethylamphetamine (STP) or phencyclidine (PCP, Sernyl) (Fauman, Aldinger, and Fauman, 1976). Patients in a state of alcohol withdrawal may present with paranoid ideation and hallucinations that look like paranoid psychosis or paranoid schizophrenia (case 2). Phencyclidine (PCP) abuse may lead to an organic brain syndrome and, with high doses, to death (Fauman et al., 1976). Other abused drugs such as barbiturates, chlordiazepoxide (Librium), and diazepam (Valium) may produce toxic confusional states and disorientation in high doses. All three drugs may produce severe withdrawal symptoms including confusion, anxiety, seizures, and acute delirium states (Peterson, 1975).

CASE REPORTS

Case 1

A 44-year-old white woman entered a hospital for evaluation and treatment of systemic lupus erythematosus and unexplained hypertension. She had psychiatric consultation because she appeared agitated, complained of periodic inability to move, and vigorously denied her illness. The psychiatric consult service felt that these symptoms were consistent with a primitive hysterical personality structure but cautioned that they might be secondary to lupus cerebritis. The patient was discharged to outpatient follow-up on Aldomet, propranolol, hydralazine, Diuril, and 20 mg of prednisone per day.

Nine days later she returned to the emergency department with severe headache, right neck pain, and sudden left-sided weakness. Her blood pressure was 164/100, pulse rate 56/minute, respirations 12/minute, temperature 36.2 C (97.2 F). A neurological examination showed cranial nerves II through XII intact, normal bilateral reflexes, no abnormal reflexes, and a negative Babinski sign. She complained of decreased sensation to pinprick and light touch over the left side. No other focal or lateralizing neurological signs were found. The patient was admitted to rule out the possibility of a left-sided hemiplegia secondary to a cerebrovascular accident, although the resident physician felt that the vagueness of the patient's complaints of weakness and sensory loss made the diagnosis of hemiplegia unlikely. He felt that the most likely diagnosis was a hysterical conversion reaction.

Nevertheless, a neurological workup included a computerized tomography (CAT) scan during the next two days. While she waited for tests, the patient continued to complain of a headache. During the evening of the second day she became progressively more obtunded. An emergency CAT scan was ordered on the third day after admission and revealed a deep intracerebral bleed on the left side at the parietal, frontal junction. The patient was started on mannitol and Decadron and transferred to the neurosurgery service where an emergency craniotomy was performed with evacuation of a right frontoparietal hematoma. Following surgery, the patient continued to have a mildly elated affect with continued denial of her illness. Her left-sided hemiparesis gradually began to resolve.

In this case, the patient's apparent hysteric behavior and childlike denial of her illness confused and may have delayed the diagnosis of a cerebrovascular accident. Yet, this anxious childlike behavior and massive, almost delusional, denial of illness, is a relatively common behavioral component of organic brain disease (Weinstein and Kahn, 1959). It is important to remember this when the patient has a preexisting medical illness that may affect the central nervous system.

Case 2

A 32-year-old black man wandered alone into the emergency department and complained to the physician that the police were out to get him. He appeared anxious, diaphoretic, tremulous, "very paranoid," and admitted to having visual hallucinations. He had been hospitalized in the past for "nerves" and had quit taking the medication prescribed. He did not remember the name of his "nerve" medication but indicated that he was on NPH insulin, U-40 insulin, and Aldomet. His blood pressure was 183/124, pulse rate 124/minute, respirations 20/minute and his temperature was 37.3 C (98.7 F). Glucose, red blood cell count, hemoglobin, hematocrit reading, electrolyte, blood urea nitrogen, creatinine, calcium, magnesium, and amylase were all within normal limits. His blood test was negative for alcohol and salicylates. Blood gases were within normal limits.

The emergency physician made a provisional diagnosis of paranoid psychosis. A psychiatric consultation was called. When the psychiatrist arrived he found an extremely anxious, diaphoretic, and hyperalert young black man. The psychiatrist and the emergency physician interviewed the patient in an adjoining room.

When the psychiatrist began to question the patient, he suddenly started screaming "God save the King," looked around anxiously and got up and left the room. Upon further questioning, the physicians learned that he had had a history of heavy alcohol abuse. The patient insisted that he had not had a drink in many weeks. He also denied any previous history of delirium tremens.

Both physicians had the initial impression that the patient was suffering from a paranoid psychosis. The emergency physician felt that his elevated vital signs could be attributed to anxiety. The patient's old chart indicated he had been treated for alcohol withdrawal on three separate occasions in the past year. He was restrained on a litter and treated with 100 mg thiamin intramuscularly, 5 percent dextrose 0.5 *N* saline with multivitamins, and intravenous Librium. The following morning his agitation and paranoia were substantially decreased. He stated that it was time for him to leave, refused admission for further treatment, and was discharged on oral Librium with a follow-up appointment.

Patients suffering from alcohol withdrawal or delirium tremens commonly present with hallucinations, delirium and paranoid delusions. Since untreated delirium tremens has a high mortality rate, misdiagnosing this disorder as a paranoid psychosis can be a lethal mistake. If a patient with abnormal behavior has a reported history of alcohol abuse, alcohol withdrawal is a distinct possibility even if the patient consistently denies that he has recently been drinking.

When a patient with a behavioral disorder has abnormal vital signs, the physician should investigate the possible medical basis for the abnormalities and not attribute them to anxiety. Case 2 is a good example of a patient whose abnormal vital signs were a clue to the correct diagnosis of alcohol withdrawal. Hypertension in a patient suffering from an amphetamine psychosis may be a similar clue to the organic nature of the patient's behavioral disturbance. Recent onset of incontinence of urine or stool is another important physical symptom. Although it is not uncommon to see chronic schizophrenic patients who are incontinent, they have usually had a long, progressively deteriorating psychiatric history with long-term psychiatric hospitalization.

Even with such patients, organic disorder is a possibility if incontinence is of recent onset. In general, the onset of incontinence of urine or stool accompanied by mental status changes is a serious indicator of potential organic brain disease. Lateralizing neurological signs, including ataxia, seizures, tremors, and visual defects, when associated with behavioral disturbances, should also alert the physician to a potential organic basis for the patient's psychological disorder. Ataxia is such an indicator in case 3.

Finally, abnormal metabolic values should increase suspicion of an organic disorder. Delirium states associated with hyponatremia, hypoglycemia, hyperglycemia, and uremia are well known (Dale, 1975). Other metabolic abnormalities such as hypocalcemia may commonly produce hallucinations (case 5).

Case 3

A 74-year-old black woman was brought to the emergency department by her daughter who complained that the patient was "going downhill," since her discharge from the same hospital three weeks previously. During that admission she had intention tremors of the right arm and leg and fell to the right while standing. A diagnosis of cerebellar infarction was made and corroborated by CAT scan. After a week in the hospital, her neurological signs resolved.

She had been hospitalized for depression nine years previously at the death of her husband. During her entire recent hospital admission her physician felt that she was also profoundly depressed. He reported that she rarely spoke and that when she did she complained that "God is punishing my lack of faith." She was usually seen with her head lying in her food tray. She was discharged to the care of her daughter when her neurological signs resolved.

During the three-week period between her discharge and her presentation to the emergency department, the patient became more retarded and experienced the onset of incontinence of stool and urine. There was no evidence of further paralysis or tremor. The physician who saw her in the emergency department was one who had cared for her while she had been in the hospital. He felt that her new symptoms indicated that her depression had intensified.

On examination, her blood pressure was 150/90, pulse rate 68/minute, respirations 16/minute, and temperature 36.6 C (97.9 F). Her neurological examination indicated a right-sided hypereflelxia, a positive snout reflex, and a positive suck reflex. She appeared very retarded with her head on her chest and responded to questions with snarls or screams.

The consulting psychiatrist felt that the recent onset of incontinence in conjunction with the patient's history of stroke and previous ataxia indicated the intensification of an organic brain syndrome with a possible component of depression. The patient was readmitted to the medical service where a repeat CAT scan showed a definite posterior fossa tumor that had caused a significant obstructive hydrocephalus. She was immediately transferred to the neurosurgery service for an operation to place a ventricular shunt to reduce the intracerebral pressure. The operation resulted in a moderate improvement in the patient's mental status.

Although withdrawal accompanies depression, it is also a common finding in patients with an organic brain syndrome (Weinstein and Kahn, 1959). In these cases, it is difficult to separate out which part of the behavior is due to depression and which is organically based. Symptoms such as incontinence and lateralizing neurological signs offer some clue to the diagnosis of the organic component of these behavioral disorders.

Case 4

A 38-year-old black woman was brought to the emergency department by a friend who told the physician that he thought the patient had taken some "pills" because "she acted strange like this when she took my codeine pain pills a year ago." The patient was a known diabetic and was receiving insulin therapy and in the past had been reported to "malinger."

Her blood pressure was 134/70, her pulse rate 60/minute and respirations 12/minute. Positive findings included small, slightly reactive pupils and an altered mental status. The patient was alert, oriented times three, uncooperative, struggling, and yelled and screamed while being questioned and examined.

She was given four ampules of Narcan by intravenous (IV) push over a period of one hour with no response. She continued to scream, struggle, and be uncooperative. A dextrostix indicated a blood glucose level between 0 and 25. Blood was drawn for a complete blood count, glucose, electrolytes, and a salicylate level. The patient was restrained, and given 2 ampules of 50 cc of 50 percent glucose (IV) push. While the glucose was being administered, she continued to struggle and managed to pull out her intravenous line. The emergency physician called a psychiatric consult on the basis of the patient's reported overdose attempt, agitation, and lack of cooperation and the minimal effect of the glucose or Narcan on her mental status.

During the psychiatric interview the patient repeatedly denied that she had taken an overdose. The emergency physician felt that the patient was malingering because she was arousable when he stimulated her and then would scream and curse at him. Initial laboratory tests indicated that the patient had blood glucose of 25 mg/100 ml. A new IV was started and the patient was given 2 more ampules of 50 cc each of 50 percent glucose. Over the next two to three hours the patient became more alert, less agitated, stopped screaming, and became more cooperative. She was discharged with a follow-up medical appointment to reevaluate her diabetes.

This case again illustrates the importance of knowledge of the patient's preexisting illness and present medication and the need for routine clinical chemistry tests when the physician suspects that the altered mental status is secondary to an organic process. These tests should include electrolytes, calcium, CBC, glucose, BUN, and creatinine.

This case also illustrates the problems of communication between the patient or his relatives and the physician with regard to the nature of the patient's "overdose." Regardless of the patient's history, the medical staff believed that the patient had taken a conscious overdose of medication presumably in a suicide attempt and did not consider other causes of an altered mental status. Patients who are in a mild delirium state are easily arousable, belligerent, and abusive. The physician thought that the patient was malingering because she was able to respond to stimuli. If the patient is assumed to have taken a deliberate overdose and is at the same time abusive and hostile, the stage is set to regard the patient as a behavioral problem with little important organic disorder.

MENTAL STATUS SIGNS AND SYMPTOMS

Changes in mental status are often the most sensitive and yet at times the most subtle indicators of an organic brain disorder. A fluctuating level of awareness, consciousness, and cognitive function—a sign of a delirium state—may easily be missed or attributed to a conscious psychological ("functional") cause. In mild forms of this state the patient appears to drift off, fall asleep, and, while easily aroused, may be angry or abusive when stimulated to full awareness. This is often interpreted as an indication of the patient's lack of cooperation with the medical staff and may lead to a description of the patient as a "malingerer" (case 4). If the patient needs constant stimulation to remain alert and responsive to the physician, it indicates a potential organic brain disorder and not a personality disturbance, particularly when it is necessary to slap or pinch the patient to gain his attention.

To evaluate a patient with a suspected organic brain syndrome, the patient's orientation to person, place, and time, concentration and cognitive function—such as serial subtraction of sevens, simple calculation, and a series of names of objects to remember—have been routinely used. Other psychological tests, such as parts of the Wechsler Adult Intelligence Scale (WAIS) or the Reitan-Halsted battery, may take from an hour to one or two days to administer (Benton, 1975). These tests are far too extensive for the emergency physician who needs a brief, reliable series of mental status questions that can be administered quickly at the bedside. Kahn, Pollack and Goldfarb (1961; Kahn, 1971) have designed a ten question mental status questionnaire (MSQ), which will quickly evaluate the patient's orientation, memory, cognitive functioning, and knowledge of general information (Lipowski, 1967).

The questions are:

1. What is the name of this place (or where are you now)?
2. Where is this place located (address)?
3. What is today's date?
4. What is the month now?
5. What year is it?
6. How old are you?
7. When were you born (month)?
8. When were you born (year)?
9. Who is the President of the United States?
10. Who was the President before him?

Kahn feels that the first five questions are evaluations of disorientation while the last five measure cognitive impairments. This test was devised to evaluate organic brain disorders in the elderly but it can be applied equally well to any patient with a potential organic brain syndrome.

Kahn scores the MSQ as follows, "Clinically, an aged person who makes 0 to 2 errors can be regarded as having no or mild brain syndrome, 3 to 8 errors as moderate brain syndrome, and 9 or 10 errors as severe brain syndrome" (Kahn, 1971).

Another useful brief test of an organic brain disorder is the Face-Hand test devised by Bender (1973). This test depends on the patient's perception of simultaneous tactile stimuli. The Face-Hand test takes approximately five minutes to administer and is a fairly sensitive indicator of organic brain disease (Kahn, 1971; Bender, 1973).

Patients with organic brain disease may show lability or change of affect as well as other "organic" behaviors. These may include euphoria, paranoia, irritability, anger, and abusive behavior. The patient's sensorium or cognitive functions may also be completely clear for short intervals between periods of disorientation and intellectual impairment.

The patient's degree of depression must be assessed by asking him about his mood, his appetite, weight loss, sleep disturbances, decreased energy, constipation, interest in sexual activity. Elderly patients who are depressed may appear to have an organic brain disorder. If no major organic impairment exists, treatment with antidepressant medication may be appropriate. Patients with organic brain disease also have an element of depression.

Weinstein and Kahn (1959) have described a series of organic behaviors related to the patient's denial of his organic brain impairment. Explicit denial is often seen in stroke patients with a hemiparesis who deny any weakness on the affected side. Confabulation, where the patient makes up a story to deny a medical illness, physical, or mental impairment, is seen in Korsakoff's syndrome as well as other organic brain disorders. Paraphasia is a mode of behavior where the patient misidentifies objects in his environment. This often occurs with a medically related object as when a patient calls a stethoscope a "telescope." Inappropriate sexual behavior and propositioning is a common behavior related to organic brain syndrome. Families and friends may report that the patient, who had always been relatively "proper," has recently begun to make overt sexual remarks or lewd comments. Finally, patients may attempt to deny their illness by withdrawal. This is commonly mistaken for depression but, although depression may be present, withdrawal can also be seen with organic brain syndromes where the patient is attempting to deny a catastrophic change in his physical or mental process (Weinstein and Kahn, 1959; Kahn, 1971).

Hallucinations may be another important indicator of organic brain disease. Some patients, such as the one in case 5, may experience hallucinations that are ego-dystonic, meaning that they are alien to their personality. When they report them to another person they express surprise about the nature of the hallucination rather than recognizing it as consistent with their personality. Hallucinations that are predominantly olfactory or tactile are usually of organic cause. Olfactory hallucinations in particular are indicative of a temporal lobe focal seizure or lesion.

Case 5

A 60-year-old black woman was transferred to the emergency department from another hospital at the request of her family. Four months prior to her presentation she began having hallucinations of ghosts, huge dogs, and other objects. Periods of hallucinations alternated with normal periods. Three weeks prior to presentation she developed a severe cold and substernal chest pains and was admitted to another hospital where lung scans indicated multiple pulmonary emboli. She was treated with heparin but instead of improving, became progressively weaker and suffered further mental deterioration. The only other significant past medical history was a thyroidectomy 40 years previously.

Upon presentation to the emergency department, the patient's blood pressure was 180/110, her pulse rate 90/minute, respirations 15/minute, and temperature 37 C (98.6 F). She was described as "euphoric" and was oriented to person, place, but not to the year. Cranial nerves were intact and she had normal muscle strength and tone bilaterally. The result of sensory examination and reflexes were normal with the exception of a 4+ Chovstek bilaterally. Multiple clinical chemistry tests were normal with the exception of an elevated lactic dehydrogenase, creatine phosphokinase, and amylase. In addition, her serum phosphorus concentration was 9.2 mg/100 ml and calcium 4.2 mg/100 ml. The patient was diagnosed as having hypoparathyroidism, pulmonary embolism, and cataracts. She was started on calcium lactate, 3.9 gm three times a day, 100,000 units of vitamin D per day, and Basaljel to lower her blood phosphorus. Over a period of several days her calcium rose to 8.1 mg/100 ml and her phosphorus concentration decreased.

While on the medical ward the psychiatric consultant interviewed the patient who described her hallucinations: "Doctor, it was amazing, wasn't it? One day my daughter and I were washing clothes in the basement, she would hang some clothes up and I was sorting some out and all of a sudden I heard this sound like a box dragging on the floor and I jumped around to see what it was. I couldn't say anything, I just stood there looking and there was this laminated great dog. He was bigger than a dog but I will say a dog. He was as big as a calf. Then all of a sudden, he said, 'I want a drink of water.' He didn't have any head and all of a sudden he disappeared."

The striking characteristic is the patient's surprise at the content of the hallucinations and the fact that she is having them. They make no sense to her, emotionally or cognitively. These are ego-dystonic hallucinations because the majority of the patient's personality regards the hallucination as unusual and not really belonging to her. Hallucination in patients with purely psychological behavioral disorders usually have meaning to the patient within the context of his personality.

DISCUSSION

Organic based behavioral disorders can be divided into two groups on the basis of etiology and symptomatology. The first, the organic brain syndrome, is produced by diffuse organic impairment in brain tissue function and must have the five behavioral criteria. The second includes behavioral disturbances such as hallucinations, thought disorders, depression, or other disturbances of affect that do not meet the five criteria. This second group is produced by nondiffuse brain diseases, such as focal seizures or lesions, toxic agents, or organic diseases of the body, exclusive of the central nervous system, which have been associated with them. Specific behavioral disturbances of thought, mood, or perception are associated with the group and are alleviated by treating the noncentral nervous system organic disease.

The behavior associated with an organic brain syndrome stems from a combination of the patient's preexisting personality and his present organic disease. The patient's paranoia or excess irritability may be an organic amplification of his previous suspiciousness and irritability. In addition, the patient's paranoia or anger may be a denial of or reaction to his awareness of his intellectual deficits. Many of the behavioral symptoms of organic brain disease may also be produced by severe psychological stress (Weinstein and Kahn, 1959). Patients with mild organic brain disease may adapt relatively well to their environment and show no behavioral abnormalities or intellectual deficits until an added psychological stress, such as hospitalization, is superimposed over a nonsymptomatic organic brain disease.

Delirium and organic brain syndromes are two of the most commonly misdiagnosed disorders on medical services particularly in patients who are anxious, disruptive, or combative. For two reasons, many physicians view these patients as uncooperative or psychologically disturbed. First, the physician appears to be angered by the patient's inability to cooperate in the treatment protocol. This anger then stands in the way of the physician's objective analysis of the basis of the patient's behavior and leads the physician to describe the patient as "uncooperative" or "crazy." Second, and perhaps most important, the physician finds it difficult to think of psychological abnormalities as stemming from an organic cause. Physicians are more accustomed to seeing organic brain diseases reflected in physical neurological signs and symptoms. Since this bias is widespread, the physician must include an organic based behavioral disorder in the differential diagnosis of behavioral disturbances that appear in the emergency department.

REFERENCES

American Psychiatric Association (1968), *Diagnostic and Statistical Manual of Mental Disorders,* 2nd ed. Washington, DC: American Psychiatric Press.

Angrist, B. M., & Gershon, S. (1972), Psychiatric sequelae of amphetamine use. In: *Psychiatric Complications of Medical Drugs,* ed. R. I. Shader. New York: Raven Press, pp. 173–199.

Bender, M. R. (1973), The incidence and type of perceptual deficiencies in the aged. In: *Neurological and Sensory Disorders in the Elderly,* ed. W. S. Fields. New York: Stratton Intercontinental.

Benton, A. L. (1975), Psychological tests for brain damage. In: *Comprehensive Textbook of Psychiatry,* 2nd ed., eds. A. M. Freedman, H. I. Kaplan, & B. J. Sadock. Baltimore, MD: Williams and Wilkins, pp. 757–767.

Dale, A. J. D. (1975), Organic brain syndromes associated with disturbances in metabolism, growth and nutrition. In: *Comprehensive Textbook of Psychiatry,* 2nd ed., eds. A. M. Freedman, H. I. Kaplan, & B. J. Sadock. Baltimore, MD: Williams & Wilkins, pp. 1078–1085.

Engel, G. L., & Romano, J. (1959), Delirium, a syndrome of cerebral insufficiency. *J. Chronic Dis.,* 9:160–277.

Ervin, F. R. (1975), Organic brain syndromes associated with epilepsy. In: *Comprehensive Textbook of Psychiatry,* 2nd. ed., eds. A. M. Freedman, H. I. Kaplan, & B. J. Sadock, Baltimore, MD: Williams & Wilkins, pp. 1138–1157.

Fauman, B. J., Aldinger, G., & Fauman, M. A., (1976), Psychiatric sequelae of phencyclidine abuse. *Clin. Toxicol.,* 9:529–538.

Goodman, L. S., & Gilman, A. (1970), *The Pharmacological Basis of Therapeutics,* 4th ed. New York: Macmillan.

Goodwin, F. K. (1972), Behavioral effects of L-dopa in man. In: *Psychiatric Complications of Medical Drugs,* ed. R. I. Shader. New York: Raven Press, pp. 150–174.

——— Ebert, M. H., & Bunney, W. E. (1972), Mental effects of reserpine in man: a review. In: *Psychiatric Complications of Medical Drugs,* ed. R. I. Shader. New York: Raven Press, pp. 73–101.

Greenblatt, D. J., & Shader, R. I. (1972), Digitalis toxicity. In: *Psychiatric Complications of Medical Drugs,* ed. R. I. Shader. New York: Raven Press, pp. 25–47.

Kahn, R. L. (1971), Psychological aspects of aging. In: *Clin. Geriatrics,* ed. I. Rossman. Philadelphia: J. B. Lippincott, pp. 107–113.

——— Pollack, M., & Goldfarb, A. I. (1961), Factors related to individual differences in mental status of institutionalized aged. In: *Psychopathology of Aging*, eds. P. Hock & J. Zubin. New York: Grune & Stratton.

Lipowski, M. B. (1967), Delirium, clouding of consciousness and confusion. *Nerv. Men. Dis.*, 145:227–255.

Peterson, G. C. (1975), Organic brain syndromes associated with drug or poison intoxication. In: *Comprehensive Textbook of Psychiatry*, 2nd. ed., eds. A. M. Freedman, H. I. Kaplan, & B. J. Sadock. Baltimore, MD: Williams & Wilkins, pp. 1108–1120.

Peterson, H. W., & Martin, M. J. (1973), Organic disease presenting as a psychiatric syndrome. *Postgrad. Med.*, 54:78–82.

Sandok, B. A. (1975), Organic brain syndromes: Introduction. In: *Comprehensive Textbook of Psychiatry*, eds. A. M. Freedman, H. I. Kaplan, & B. J. Sadock. Baltimore, MD: Williams & Wilkins, pp. 1060–1064.

——— (1975), Organic brain syndromes associated with circulatory disturbances. In: *Comprehensive Textbook of Psychiatry*, 2nd. ed., eds. A. M. Freedman, H. I. Kaplan, & B. J. Sadock. Baltimore, MD: Williams & Wilkins, pp. 1065–1077.

Shader, R. I., ed. (1972), *Psychiatric Complications of Medical Drugs*. New York: Raven Press.

——— Greenblatt, D. J. (1972), Belladonna alkaloids and synthetic anticholinergies: Uses and toxicity. In: *Psychiatric Complications of Medical Drugs*, ed. R. J. Shader. New York: Raven Press, pp. 103–147.

Steinhilber, R. M., Peterson, H. W., & Martin, M. J. (1966), Emotional states caused by organic diseases. *Postgrad. Med.*, 39:621–630.

Wallach, M. G., & Gershon, S. (1972), Psychiatric sequelae to tuberculosis chemotherapy. In: *Psychiatric Complications of Medical Drugs*, ed. R. I. Shader. New York: Raven Press, pp. 201–212.

Weinstein, E. A., & Kahn, R. L. (1959), Symbolic reorganization in brain injuries. In: *American Handbook of Psychiatry*, ed. S. Arieti. New York: Basic Books, pp. 964–981.

Commentary

Charles F. Reynolds III, M.D.

The proposed guidelines for the differential diagnosis of organically based psychiatric disturbance remain as useful in the mid-1980s as when they were formulated in the mid-1970s.

In the light of DSM-III, several points merit greater emphasis in the diagnosis of delirium. I refer particularly to the presence of psychomotor disturbance (not only agitation, but also retardation), fever, and recent severe disruption of the sleep schedule. Physicians also need to be alert to the heightened risk of suicide in delirious patients, who may run into traffic or jump through a hospital window in response to panic, hallucinations, or agitation. The possibility of drug–drug reactions, particularly in multiply medicated elderly patients, should not be overlooked in the differential diagnosis of delirium.

Fauman and Fauman may have understood the potential value of serial EEGs in monitoring the progress and reversibility of acute organic mental status changes. The EEG is a sensitive indicator of encephalopathy as well as of ictal and postictal states.

Certainly, however, the authors are correct in their insistence that time is of the essence when the physician is confronted with organically based psychiatric disturbance. The patient's safety, as well as the reversibility of organic mental status changes, often depend on adequate (i.e., specific) treatment. The latter, in turn, rests upon swift judgment of the more likely causes of organic mental status changes. As psychiatrists, we can and do make important contributions to this area of patient care and research. In-depth treatment of this area is available in monographs by Lishman (1978) and Flor-Henry (1983).

References

Flor-Henry, P. (1983), *Cerebral Basis of Psychopathology*. Bristol, U.K.: John Wright, PSG.

Lishman, W. A. (1978), *Organic Psychiatry*. Oxford: Blackwell Scientific Publications.

Annotated Bibliography

Seltzer, B., & Sherwin, I. (1978), Organic brain syndromes: An empirical study and critical review. *Amer. J. Psych.*, 135:13–21.

The authors note that 20 percent of cases admitted to mental hospitals and more than 50 percent of the geriatric population may be diagnosed as having an organic brain syndrome. They studied a random sample of 80 patients who had been given the diagnosis of organic brain syndrome, in an attempt to formulate a more specific diagnosis. This proved feasible in the large majority of the cases, using only conventional diagnostic techniques. The authors emphasize the utility of differential diagnosis in this area for both clinical management and research.

Gross, D. A. (1981), Medical origins of psychiatric emergencies: The systems approach. *Internat. J. Psychiat. in Med.*, 11:1–24.

This is a comprehensive and readable review of general medical causes of psychiatric emergencies. While the emphasis is on physiological etiologies, the author also provides a short and substantial discussion of the relationship between psychic and somatic distresses.

Purdie, F. R., Honogman, B., & Rosen, P. (1981), Acute organic brain syndrome: A review of 100 cases. *Ann. Emerg. Med.*, 10:455–461.

This paper looks retrospectively at 100 patients admitted with the diagnosis of organic brain syndrome. Again, the need for precise diagnosis is pointed out and the value of drug screens in the emergency room is discussed. The authors use the cases studied to offer a brief discussion of specific etiologies of organic brain syndrome.

Dubin, W. R., Weiss, K. J., & Zeccardi, J. A. (1983), Organic brain syndrome, the psychiatric imposter. *JAMA*, 249:60–62.

This paper reports on 1,140 patients who presented after general medical clearance to a psychiatric emergency room. The authors were able to detect 38 cases of organic brain syndrome by using four screening criteria: disorientation, abnormal vital signs, clouded consciousness, and age; that is, older than 40 without previous psychiatric history.

Fauman, M. A. (1983), The emergency psychiatric evaluation of organic mental disorders. *Psych. Clin. N. Amer.*, 6:233–255.

Using DSM-III concepts, this paper rather comprehensively reviews the area of organic brain syndromes in the context of an emergency setting. Fauman discusses the efficacy of a structured organic screening procedure for all emergency psychiatric patients which may help the physician detect a large proportion of organic mental disorders that, on the surface, appear to be caused solely by psychological processes.

6

Aiding the Drug Abuser

Sidney H. Schnoll, M.D., Ph.D.

In recent years, drug abuse has become an increasingly significant medical problem. No longer are we dealing with a problem primarily confined to those in their teens and early twenties or in minority groups. Today drug abusers include people of all ages, sexes, and ethnic and socioeconomic groups. Not all of these abusers are purchasing their drugs through illicit sources. Many abusers are skillful at manipulating physicians to obtain their drugs. In addition, people in several health care professions have easy access to drugs.

Because of the large number of drug-abusing patients who present themselves for medical care, physicians must be familiar with the signs and symptoms of abuse, modes of therapy for acute intoxication with drugs, and syndromes produced by their withdrawal. This article describes methods of recognition and treatment of acute and chronic drug problems (including opiates, barbiturates and other sedative-hypnotics, stimulants, and hallucinogens) that may serve as guidelines for the care of such patients.

RECOGNIZING THE DRUG ABUSER

It is always easiest to recognize the problem of drug abuse when a patient presents with the request to get off drugs. However, because

This chapter was first published in *Hospital Medicine* (1983), 19:116–155, and it is reprinted by permission.

of the stigma associated with drug abuse, few patients feel comfortable presenting in this way. When this does occur, the physician should be prepared to seize this opportunity and initiate treatment or refer the patient to an appropriate treatment program. The names, locations, and telephone numbers of programs can be obtained by calling the state drug abuse authority or local mental health center.

It is advisable to call or visit any drug abuse treatment program before making referrals there. Sending a 50-year-old suburban woman dependent on benzodiazepines to a center treating inner city opiate addicts will almost insure a treatment failure.

All of your patients are potential drug abusers, and you will only make the diagnosis if you think of it, especially in the ones who request increased doses of prescribed abusable drugs or request refills more frequently than anticipated. Tolerance develops to almost all drugs of abuse. Therefore, patients abusing drugs desire increasing amounts. Every patient can lose a prescription once, but the patient who repeatedly presents excuses for running out of medication should be suspected of being drug dependent.

A method of verifying your suspicion is to call the pharmacy where the patient's prescriptions are filled and check whether prescriptions are being filled for the same drugs from other physicians. Or call other physicians treating the patient to find out what they are prescribing and how frequently. Many pharmacists will call physicians to alert them to the problem of multiple prescriptions. Don't assume that because Mr. Jones has been a patient for 20 years and is president of the local chamber of commerce that he can't be addicted.

Another clue is a sudden change in your patient's behavior. A patient who is normally docile and now becomes aggressive, or vice versa, should be evaluated for drug abuse, among other things. The same may be true of a patient who is normally fastidious in his or her appearance but who now appears more slovenly. Sudden loss of a job or frequent job changes for no apparent reason should arouse suspicion. Unexplained financial or family problems can also be a result of drug abuse.

Certainly the patient who presents in your office exhibiting toxic behavior yet adamantly denies drug use should be considered a potential abuser. (Patients may also present because of trauma from accidents due to intoxication.)

Almost all drugs of abuse alter sexual function as well as other behaviors. Although many patients believe that drugs will enhance their sexual performance, in reality they usually decrease it and may even cause impotence or other dysfunction. Any patient presenting with complaints of sexual dysfunction should be evaluated for possible drug abuse as a contributing cause.

Chronic drug abusers will often develop medical sequelae. If your patient is an intravenous drug abuser, infections are common, such as endocarditis or hepatitis. Needle marks may be present on the skin from recent injections, or "tracks" may be present over veins from repeated injections. If your suspicion is aroused, don't confine your investigation for needle marks to the obvious sites. Many affluent users, in an attempt to hide their drug problem, will inject in the axilla, under the tongue, under the breast, in the legs, and even into the dorsal vein of the penis.

Those who smoke their drugs (e.g., marijuana, hashish, or free-base cocaine) may present with chronic bronchitis or throat irritations. Drugs taken by insufflation (snorting) often cause irritation and lesions of the nasal mucosa. Unexplained nasal stuffiness or postnasal drip can also occur from insufflation of drugs.

Although many of these signs and symptoms can be caused by other diseases, once your suspicion is aroused, steps should be taken to verify whether or not the patient is a drug abuser. One method is to express to your patient in a nonaccusatory tone that you suspect drug abuse and that help is available. Give concrete examples of why you are suspicious. Many patients will be relieved that they no longer have to hide their problem and that help is available. Others will adamantly deny having a problem even in the face of overwhelming evidence. In all cases, a urine sample should be collected for a drug screen to confirm or contradict your suspicion.

Once the diagnosis of drug abuse is made, both acute and long-term treatment are necessary; simple admonitions to stop are insufficient. Therapy for drug abuse most often begins with withdrawal, or detoxification, but this is merely the first step in overall treatment.

It is the job of the physician to motivate the patient to seek treatment. Compliance is a problem with all chronic disease therapies, and this is also true in addiction. Threatening the patient is not the answer, but being firm and utilizing the assistance of family and employers can be helpful. Waiting until the patient is "ready" for treatment or has "hit bottom" may be too late (Schnoll, 1980a).

ACUTE OPIATE POISONING

Clinical Findings

The most common findings in a patient who has taken an overdose of opiates include miosis, hypotension, depressed respiration and level of consciousness, bradycardia, and hypothermia (Figure 6.1). Pulmonary edema is also frequently present. While the miotic pupil is the sign most commonly sought to indicate opiate overdose, the pupil may be dilated rather than constricted if the patient has experienced prolonged anoxia. The patient who has overdosed with meperidine may present with a dilated rather than miotic pupil.

Therapy

Intravenous naloxone is presently the drug of choice in the treatment of narcotic overdose because it is a relatively pure narcotic antagonist; it has also been shown to be effective in treating overdoses with propoxyphene (Kersh, 1973) and the mixed agonist–antagonist narcotics, for example, pentazocine, nalbuphine, and butorphanol (Martin, 1976).

If an opiate overdose is suspected, 0.4 mg (1.0 ml) of naloxone should be administered intravenously. If there is no response (to the initial dose of naloxone) within one or two minutes, a second or third dose may be administered. If there is no improvement in the patient's condition after three intravenous doses of naloxone, it can be assumed that the patient has not taken an opiate overdose, since the majority of patients who have taken opiates respond after one or two doses of naloxone.

In treating narcotic poisoning with naloxone, it is important to remember that the duration of action of this antagonist when given intravenously is *one to two hours*—whereas heroin's duration of action is *four to six hours,* and that of methadone is *24 to 36 hours*. Because of this, the patient who has responded to naloxone may relapse into coma unless he or she is carefully watched.

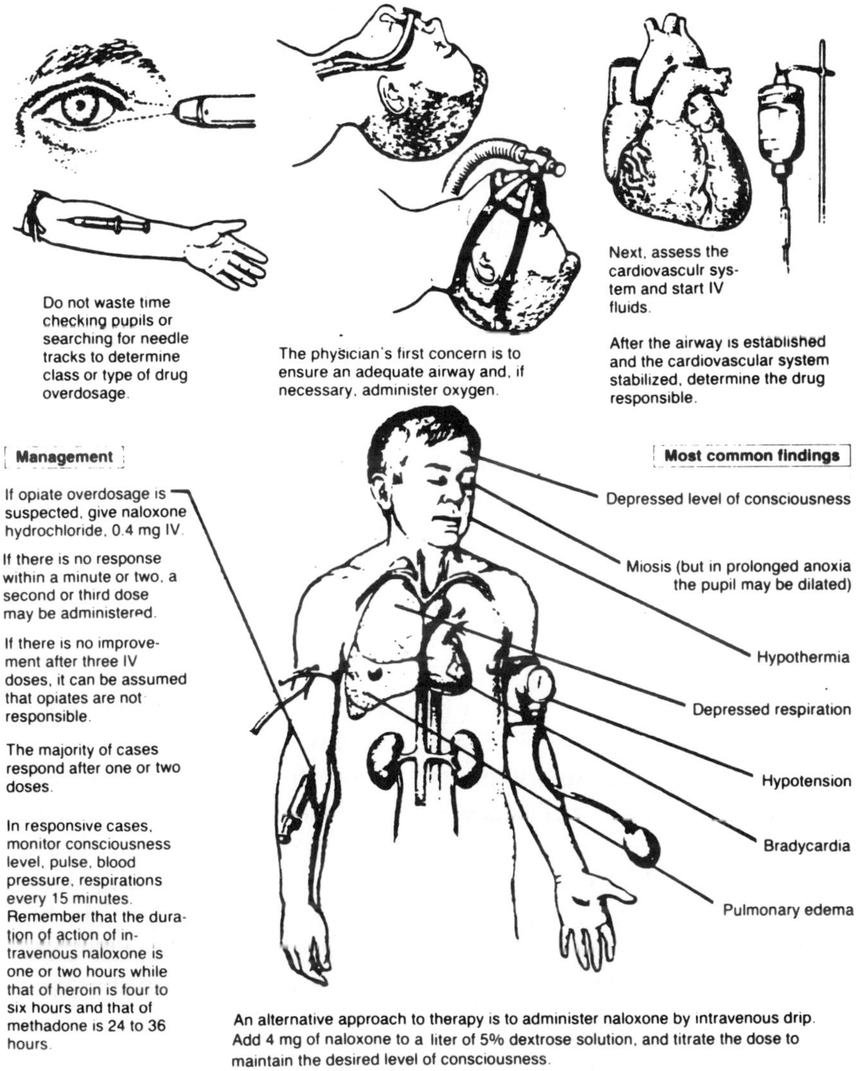

Figure 6.1 Acute opiate poisoning: Important considerations. Reproduced from *Hospital Medicine,* August 1983, with permission of Hospital Publications, Inc.

The patient who has responded favorably should be monitored for level of consciousness, respirations, pulse, and blood pressure at least every 15 minutes. If the patient appears to be relapsing into coma, additional naloxone should be administered. An alternative form of therapy is to administer naloxone by intravenous drip. Add 4 mg of naloxone to a liter of 5 percent dextrose solution, and titrate the dose to deliver the amount of naloxone per hour necessary to maintain the desired level of consciousness (Fraser, 1972).

The patient with acute opiate poisoning should be observed for at least 24 hours before being released from the hospital. Plans for long-term management of the drug problem should be made as well; psychiatric consultation is frequently indicated.

CHRONIC OPIATE ADDICTION

Although "cold turkey" withdrawal from heroin usually produces physical effects no worse than a bad case of influenza, this form of therapy is not justifiable because of the extreme anxiety produced in opiate users by sudden cessation of the drug. The most commonly used treatment for opiate withdrawal is substitution of methadone for the opiate, followed by gradual withdrawal of methadone.

Methadone is used for the following reasons: (1) Its long duration of action requires that it be administered only once or twice per day; (2) it can be given orally; and (3) its withdrawal symptoms are less intense than those produced by heroin or other shorter-acting narcotics, although they persist for a longer period of time.

A problem in substituting methadone for heroin is how to determine what dose of methadone is approximately equivalent to the dose of opiate being used by the patient. Although there is no clear-cut evidence at this time that the severity of withdrawal symptoms is related to the amount of opiate being used, the following method has been used extensively to titrate methadone with opiate withdrawal, without producing oversedation or severe discomfort to the patient during withdrawal.

Method for Determining the Dose of Methadone Required for Opiate Withdrawal

It is important to base the evaluation on as many objective signs of withdrawal as possible. The dose of methadone required to suppress withdrawal should be determined by rating the following signs and symptoms: pupillary dilation, rhinorrhea, lacrimation, piloerection, nausea and vomiting, diarrhea, yawning, cramps and restlessness, and subjective evaluation. Each of these should be rated zero if not present, 1 point if present in mild form, and 2 points if present in severe form. The score for the particular evaluation period should be added up, and for each 5 points the patient should receive 5 mg of methadone. The maximum dose of methadone that can be administered during any evaluation period is 20 mg.

The patient should be evaluated in a similar manner every 6 hours for a 24-hour period. Each evaluation period should be independent of the previous period, so the dose of methadone administered in one period is not necessarily repeated in subsequent evaluation periods. If no signs of withdrawal are present or the score is less than 5, the patient should receive no additional medication; if the score totals 5, the patient would receive 5 mg of methadone, and so on.

After 24 hours, the total dose of methadone that has been administered to the patient is computed. This dose of methadone is approximately proportional to the dose of opiate the individual was taking. In our experience with this method of evaluation, users of ''street'' heroin have rarely received more than 20 mg of methadone per day. After being stabilized on the appropriate dose of methadone, the patient can be withdrawn by reducing the dose of methadone 5 mg a day.

The patient who is known to have been receiving methadone in a methadone program should be withdrawn from that daily dose in increments of 5 mg per day. The dose of methadone should be verified by calling the program. Do not rely on the patient's knowledge of the dose.

In an outpatient setting, it is much more difficult to determine the dose of methadone a patient should receive because the patient cannot be observed for 24 hours. In outpatient cases, we use a challenge of naloxone 0.2 mg intravenously, evaluate the patient 5 minutes later (with the scoring system outlined above), and double the score achieved to determine the dose of methadone to be administered. This method has proven safe, and since the acute withdrawal effects precipitated by naloxone wear off within 20 to 30 minutes, the patient is not uncomfortable for a prolonged period of time. Methadone can be administered as soon as the dose is determined. This reduces the withdrawal symptoms.

If the patient is on a *known dose* of another narcotic and is to be withdrawn, he or she can be switched to an equivalent dose of methadone to make the withdrawal easier, or the dose of the original narcotic can be reduced gradually. If the latter method is chosen, it is best to reduce the total daily intake by approximately 10 percent per day, maintaining the *dosing frequency* as long as possible. By reducing the frequency (increasing the interval between doses) at which the drug is given, especially with short-acting narcotics like meperidine and hydromorphone, the patient goes into withdrawal repeatedly, making the process uncomfortable and difficult.

Methadone can be given as a single daily dose, or the dose can be divided in half and given morning and evening. (Giving the evening dose before the patient goes to bed facilitates sleep and thus obviates the use of sedative-hypnotic sleep preparations.)

Once a withdrawal schedule is determined, it should not be altered unless the patient shows objective signs of worsening. During the withdrawal period, we never tell the patient what dose of methadone he or she is receiving. If the patient is aware of receiving a low dose prior to drug discontinuance, anxiety frequently causes symptoms of withdrawal. Therefore, it is sometimes worthwhile to administer a placebo even after withdrawal is complete.

Use of Analgesics Concurrently with Methadone

Frequently patients receiving methadone require analgesic medication for coexisting medical problems. In most cases, attempts should be made to control the pain through the use of nonnarcotic analgesics. If this is not possible, the dose of methadone that the patient is receiving should be used as a baseline, and additional narcotic analgesics should be added in standard therapeutic doses to control the pain. The use of hydroxyzine or amitriptyline potentiates the narcotic analgesic action, thus alleviating the need for large doses of additional narcotics.

It is important to remember that neither pentazocine, nalbuphine, nor butorphanol should be administered to any patient taking pure agonists such as methadone because these drugs have antagonistic properties and can precipitate an immediate withdrawal.

ACUTE SEDATIVE-HYPNOTIC INTOXICATION

Clinical Findings

Findings that indicate barbiturate or other sedative-hypnotic intoxication include respiratory depression, depressed level of consciousness, nystagmus, hypotension, ataxia, dysarthria, depressed deep tendon reflexes, confusion, coma, and shock (Figure 6.2).

Management

The patient who has taken an overdose of sedative-hypnotics should be treated initially like any other patient with drug intoxication: Provide an adequate airway and ventilation, and maintain the cardiovascular system. Once these initial measures have been carried out, perform gastric lavage.

If barbiturates are the cause of the overdose, administer a sufficient amount of intravenous sodium bicarbonate to alkalinize the patient's urine. The dose of bicarbonate will vary depending on the patient's metabolic state. This alkalinization increases the rate of excretion of barbiturates; the urine pH should be monitored and kept at about 7.5 (Arieff and Friedman, 1973). Depending on the gravity of the patient's condition, dialysis may be required. Laxatives may be used to induce catharsis.

Several of the sedative-hypnotics, particularly glutethimide and methaqualone, are highly lipophilic, and consequently these drugs are erratically absorbed and stored in body fats. They are metabolized to active substances that have long half-lives. Excretion via bile results in reabsorption through the enterohepatic circulation. Because of these effects, blood levels of the drug may fluctuate, causing fluctuations in the level of consciousness. It is therefore important to keep patients who have taken overdoses of these drugs under observation for several days.

Benzodiazepines are often metabolized to long-acting active metabolites. Although these drugs produce less respiratory depression than barbiturates, the long-acting metabolites often cause intoxication to last for several days.

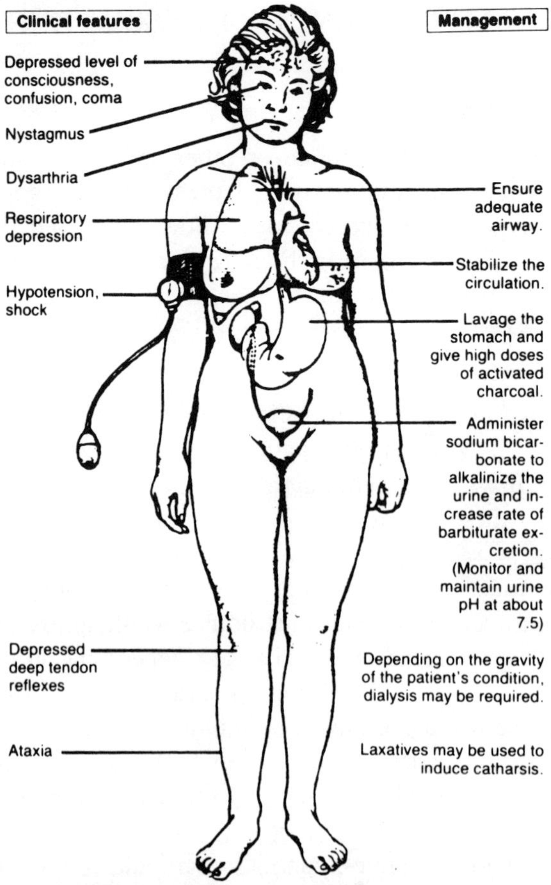

Several of the sedative-hypnotics are lipophilic; consequently, these drugs are erratically absorbed and stored in body fats. Active metabolites often have long half-lives, and excretion via bile results in reabsorption through the enterohepatic circulation. Because of these factors, drug blood levels may fluctuate widely, and patients who have taken such overdoses should be kept under observation for up to several days.

Figure 6.2 Acute intoxication with barbiturates or other sedative-hypnotics: Diagnostic and therapeutic points. Reproduced from *Hospital Medicine,* August 1983, with permission of Hospital Publications, Inc.

Intragastric administration of activated charcoal (100 g) after gastric lavage impedes the absorption of any material not recovered by lavage and remaining in the intestines (Hayden and Comstock, 1975). This treatment reduces reabsorption of the drug through the enterohepatic circulation.

CHRONIC SEDATIVE-HYPNOTIC INTOXICATION

Clinical Findings

Symptoms and signs produced by chronic sedative-hypnotic abuse include confusion, slowing of thought processes, dysarthria, nystagmus, and ataxia. Individuals who are undergoing *withdrawal* develop insomnia, tremulousness, fever, hyperactive deep tendon reflexes, nervousness, tremor, and weakness (Figure 6.3). In addition, generalized seizures may occur, somtimes followed by status epilepticus. As in the case of delirium tremens, confusion and psychotic behavior can be part of any sedative-hypnotic withdrawal.

It is unusual to see patients who are abusing short-acting barbiturates solely. The majority of sedative-hypnotic abusers take one or more benzodiazepines and ethanol, along with barbiturates and other sleeping pills. Since many of the benzodiazepines have long-acting metabolites, the patient may not show any signs of withdrawal for seven to ten days after stopping all drug use.

Treatment

Treatment for withdrawal from barbiturates is identical to that for withdrawal from all sedative-hypnotics, including the minor tranquilizers and alcohol, because all drugs in these categories exhibit cross-tolerance. The first step is to determine objectively an approximate level of drug to which the patient is tolerant, since patients often exaggerate the amount of drug they have been taking. This determination is made by giving oral pentobarbital to the point of drowsiness, dysarthria, and ataxia (Wikler, 1968).

A reasonable starting dose is 200 mg, and an additional 100 mg is administered every hour until the patient is intoxicated (or until a total of 600 mg is reached). Administer the initial dose at 6 P.M. so that the intoxicating dose is achieved about bedtime, which also helps the patient to sleep. Since phentobarbital is a short-acting barbiturate, the patient can usually sleep off the effects without difficulty if, by chance, he or she receives too high a dose.

After the intoxicating dose is determined, the patient is then switched to phenobarbital, 30 mg per 100 mg pentobarbital, and withdrawal is started. The total daily dose is given in three equal amounts.

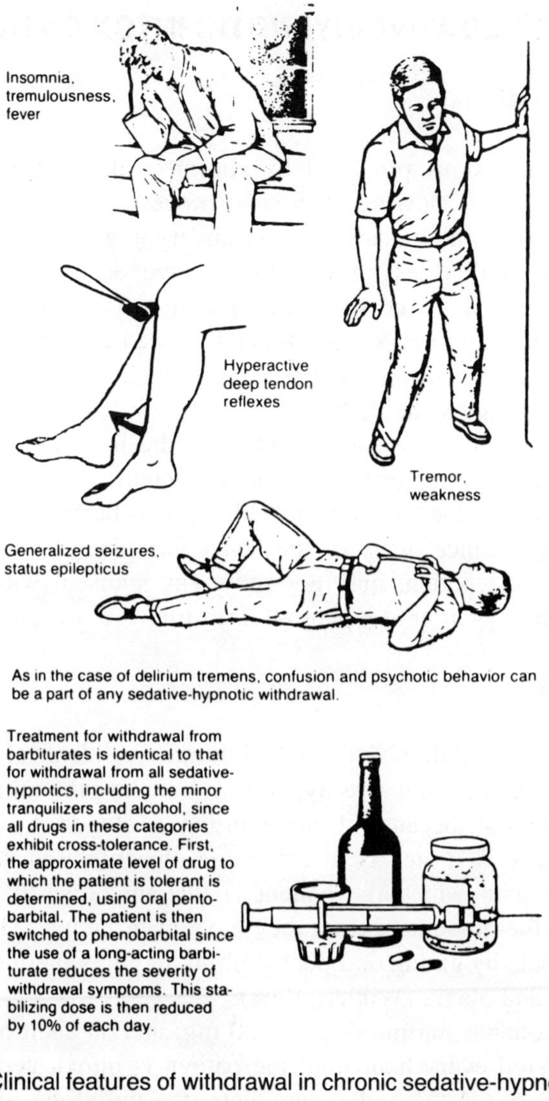

Figure 6.3 Clinical features of withdrawal in chronic sedative-hypnotic abusers. Reproduced from *Hospital Medicine,* August 1983, with permission of Hospital Publications, Inc.

The dose is reduced by 10 percent of the initial starting dose each day. Reductions should be made from the afternoon and morning doses initially, to assist the patient with sleep. The use of a long-acting barbiturate decreases the severity of withdrawal symptoms (Smith and Wesson, 1971), and phenobarbital is chosen in preference to other sedatives with approximately the same half-life, such as diazepam, because patients rarely achieve a "high" from phenobarbital as they do from the other drugs.

STIMULANT INTOXICATION

Clinical Findings

Stimulant intoxication may produce hyperactivity, hyperpyrexia, dilated pupils, tremor, increased pulse and blood pressure, excessive sweating, and a paranoid-type psychotic picture (Figure 6.4). Amphetamine poisoning is the classic example of such findings, but many other stimulants are also widely abused.

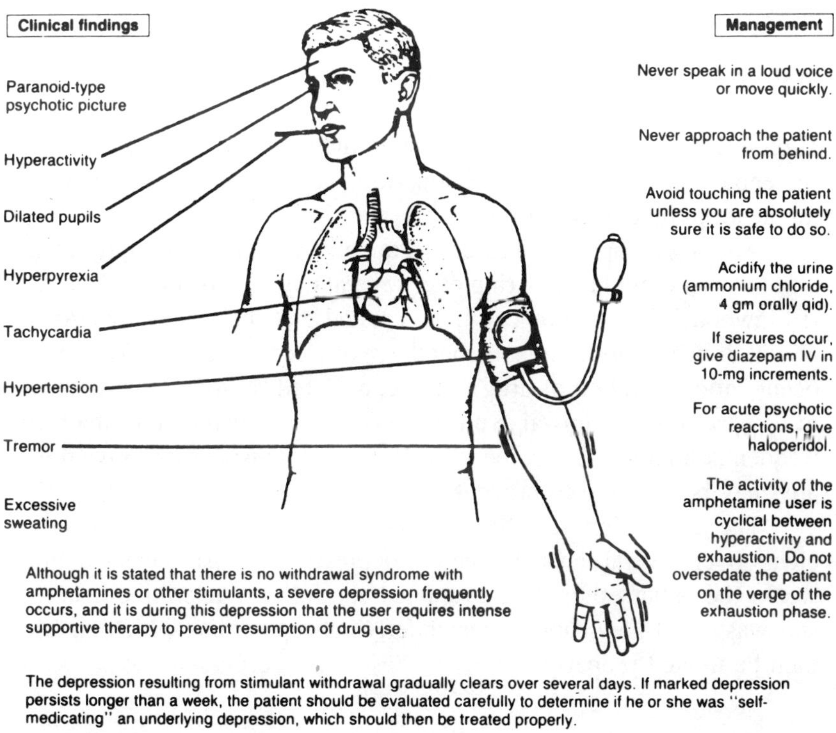

Figure 6.4 Pertinent aspects of stimulant intoxication. Reproduced from *Hospital Medicine,* August 1983, with permission of Hospital Publications, Inc.

In recent years, there has been increased popularity of cocaine, a short-acting local anesthetic with marked stimulant effects. Cocaine is most commonly used by insufflation (snorting), but the drug is also free-based and then smoked, resulting in very rapid attainment of high blood levels—and sometimes extreme paranoid behavior. Free-basing cocaine can also cost several thousand dollars a week; running out of money is the most common reason patients come in for treatment. The long-term medical sequelae of free-basing are not yet known.

Management

It is important to approach the acutely intoxicated stimulant user in a subdued manner: Never speak in a loud voice or move quickly, never approach the patient from behind, and try to avoid touching the patient unless absolutely sure it is safe to do so (which may include the presence of more than one strong, trained assistant).

Treatment of acute stimulant intoxication (assuming no hepatic dysfunction) includes acidification of the urine with ammonium chloride, up to 4 g orally, four times daily (Beckett, Rowland, and Turner, 1965). Diazepam in 10-mg increments may also be administered intravenously if seizures occur. Haloperidol may also be useful in treating the acute psychotic reactions.

Although amphetamines are frequently withdrawn abruptly from chronic users, gradual tapering over several days can be more effective (Ellinwood, 1974). Classically, it is stated that there is no syndrome of withdrawal from stimulants, but the severe depression that frequently occurs after cessation of drug use is considered by some investigators to be part of a withdrawal syndrome. During this depression, the user frequently attempts to resume stimulant use. Intensive supportive therapy may be required to prevent this.

The depression resulting from stimulant withdrawal gradually clears over several days. If marked depression persists longer than a week, the patient should be evaluated carefully to determine if he or she was "self-medicating" an underlying depression, which should then be treated properly.

HALLUCINOGENS

The most commonly used hallucinogens are lysergic acid diethylamide (LSD), mescaline, 2,5-dimethyl-4-methylamphetamine (STP, DOM), psilocybin, methylenedioxyamphetamine (MDA), and dimethyltryptamine (DMT). LSD is used in 99 percent of cases. Hallucinogen abuse dropped off precipitously in the mid- and late 1970s. In the past few years, there has been a slight increase in hallucinogen use on college campuses. However, this is nowhere near the level of use during the late 1960s and early 1970s.

Clinical Findings

Symptoms and signs of hallucinogen intoxication include distortion and intensification of sensory perception (for example, the patient who can "hear" colors or "feel" sounds), dilated pupils, rambling speech, easy suggestibility, nausea, decreased appetite, headaches, dizziness, polyuria, and toxic psychosis (Figure 6.5).

The most significant characteristic of a bad LSD-induced psychedelic state, or "trip," is fear; 99 percent of all bad trips can be handled without medication by a friend, nurse, aide, or physician. It may be difficult at times to distinguish between a bad trip and an acute psychotic reaction, but, with careful observation, this distinction can be made. The hallucinations associated with drug use are predominantly visual, whereas a psychotic reaction is typically associated with auditory hallucinations. A patient under the influence of hallucinogens will report having hallucinations that are interfering with reality; the psychotic patient usually cannot distinguish the hallucinations from reality. Also, a history of recent drug ingestion should lead the physician to suspect a toxic reaction.

Approach to Treatment

When treating a bad trip, it is important to make physical contact with the patient—for example, by taking the patient's hands. This may be the only way that contact can be made with someone who is having very severe hallucinations, but be careful about the patient reacting suddenly or violently to your touch. The physician should continually reassure the patient that adequate medical care is being administered. As in treating any drug overdose, if verbal contact can be made, ascertain what was taken, how much was taken, and how long ago it was taken. In treating a patient in a psychedelic state, this information will provide some idea of the trip's prior and future duration.

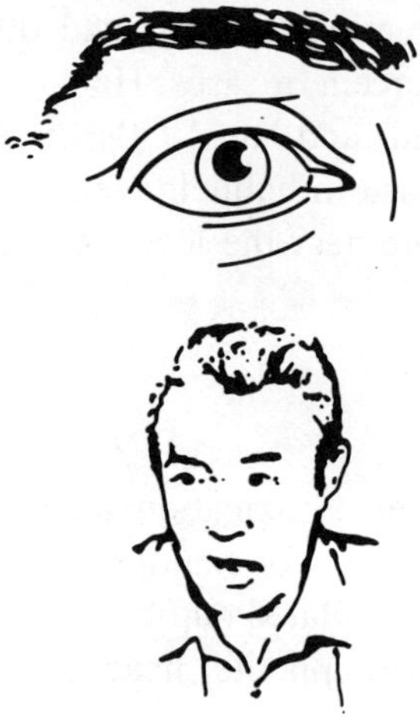

Clinical findings

Headaches, dizziness

Easy suggestability

Distortion and intensification of sensory perception (the patient who "hears" colors, "feels" sounds, for example)

Toxic psychosis

Dilated pupils

Rambling speech

Nausea, anorexia

Polyuria

Basic approach to management

The most significant characteristic of a bad psychedelic experience is fear.

"Bad trip" versus psychotic reaction: Hallucinations associated with a "bad trip" are usually visual; in a psychotic reaction, they are auditory.

It is important to make contact with the patient—verbal if possible, or by taking the patient's hands.

Ascertain what part of the trip the patient is experiencing.

Hallucinogenic reactions are cyclical, with alternating periods of lucidity and intense drug reaction. Early in the trip the cycles increase in frequency; then the reaction peaks and the frequency of the cycles decreases in the latter phase of the trip.

Reassure the patient of the temporary nature of the situation.

Treat the patient in quiet surroundings with soft lighting and possibly a source of music.

Encourage verbalization when the patient has calmed down.

The most commonly used hallucinogens are LSD (more than 99% of cases), mescaline, STP (DOM), psilocybin, MDA, and DMT.

Figure 6.5 Hallucinogens: Important features of abuse and treatment of the acute situation. Reproduced from *Hospital Medicine,* August 1983, with permission of Hospital Publications, Inc.

Reactions to hallucinogenic drugs are cyclical, showing periods of lucidity alternating with periods of intense reaction to the drug. Monitoring the frequency of these cycles can be helpful: If the cycles are frequent, the patient is probably in the early part of a trip and the syndrome has not yet peaked. If the cycles are occurring less often, the syndrome has most likely peaked and is beginning to clear. If this information can be ascertained, the physician should tell the patient what is happening, thereby increasing the patient's confidence in treatment.

Also, try to make contact with the patient during lucid intervals and maintain this contact into the intense periods of drug reaction. Efforts to make contact with the patient during an intense period are generally a waste of time.

The area in which treatment takes place should be quiet (away from large groups of people) and have soft lighting and possibly a source of music to help distract the person. The physician should try to focus the patient's attention on objects in the room, music, or simple tasks, making sure, however, that he or she is not overwhelmed by excessive stimuli. Deep, slow breathing may be helpful as an alternative distraction if a suitably calming or engrossing environment is not available. It may be necessary for the physician to demonstrate such breathing and pace the patient.

If drug treatment is necessary, diazepam 10 mg may be administered orally to reduce the patient's reaction to the hallucinogen. However, drugs should only be administered to a patient who is willing to take them voluntarily. Phenothiazines should not be used in the treatment of an acute reaction to hallucinogens because most street preparations of hallucinogens are impure, and it is impossible to ascertain exactly what drug the person has actually taken (Schnoll and Vogel, 1971). The anticholinergic effects of phenothiazines may seriously potentiate actions of anticholinergic agents that are frequent contaminants in LSD samples.

PHENCYCLIDINE

Phencyclidine has achieved great popularity as a street drug. It is identified by various street names such as "PCP," "peep," "hog," "angel dust," and "krystal." Virtually all tetrahydrocannabinol (THC) that is sold illicitly is actually phencyclidine. Phencyclidine is also frequently sold in mixtures with other drugs (Schnoll, 1980).

The drug can be taken orally or intravenously, smoked, or inhaled. In low-dose intoxication, the patient presents with nystagmus, confusion, ataxia, and sensory impairment. When the drug is taken in moderate doses, the patient presents a catatoniclike picture, staring blankly and not responding to any stimuli. In high doses, the drug produces seizures and severe hypertension. The hypertension should be treated vigorously with diazoxide or nitroprusside because it may cause hypertensive encephalopathy or intracerebral bleeding (Bessen, 1982).

The effects of phencyclidine may last for several days, and while the patient is recovering from the intoxication, levels of consciousness may fluctuate fairly rapidly. The patient may also appear psychotic. Recent studies have demonstrated that the most effective treatment of phencyclidine intoxication is to enhance its urinary excretion by acidifying the urine with ammonium chloride or ascorbic acid. The urine pH should be monitored and kept around 5.5 (Arnow and Done, 1978). The urine should be checked for the presence of phencyclidine to insure that it is being excreted. If psychotic behavior persists, the patient should be treated with haloperidol.

VOLATILES

It was once believed that volatiles were only abused by adolescents who sniff airplane glue. Although this problem persists, especially in indigent areas, new types of volatile abuse have emerged. Factory workers exposed to solvents in industrial processes will sometimes take these home for use in the evening and over weekends (Prockop, 1977). Amyl nitrite "poppers" and butyl nitrite vials have become very popular. Nitrous oxide is also abused.

The most severe consequence from abuse of these substances is hypoxia or anoxia, which may cause death. Many of the solvents are similar to general anesthetics and sensitize the myocardium to catecholamines: Fatal arrhythmias have been reported secondary to solvent abuse. Chronic use by industrial workers has caused peripheral neuropathies; hepatic, renal, and bone marrow damage have been reported. Cases of methemoglobinemia have been reported secondary to butyl nitrite abuse.

Treatment of the short-term effects of these drugs is simply removal of the person from the drug and clearing of the drug through the respiratory system. The chronic complications of abuse usually clear if the person can be kept drug-free.

LONG-TERM TREATMENT

The long-term management of drug abuse is its most important aspect. Although reversal of an acute overdose may be lifesaving, it obviously does not insure that the patient will not return to drug abuse. Definitive treatment is a long process, taking months or years. Addiction is a chronic disorder with remissions and exacerbations. A return to drug use should not be considered a treatment failure, but rather a time to intensify treatment efforts.

Long-term treatment can be a difficult and frustrating process. If you are not willing to take this on, refer the patient to an appropriate treatment center, which is often drug-specific. Formal programs are frequently supplemented by self-help groups. These groups are most often modeled after Alcoholics Anonymous and can be an important part of the rehabilitation process. Narcotics Anonymous (NA), Pills Anonymous (PA), and Families Anonymous (FA) are some of the many groups currently functioning.

The most common treatment for drug abusers is drug-free outpatient counseling. The patient meets with a counselor, either individually or in a group, once a week to discuss problems. This can be supplemented with more intensive (group or individual) psychotherapy.

In recent years, increased importance has been placed on the family in the addict's rehabilitation. If the patient is living with an intact family, they should be included in the treatment process. Employers should also be included, so that the workplace becomes a supportive environment for maintaining a drug-free life-style. The length of time a patient remains in formal treatment will vary, depending on progress.

Medication is sometimes used, such as methadone for narcotic addicts. Some have been weaned from methadone, but others remain on methadone maintenance for many years, enabling them to return to a productive life-style, with employment and a good family life. Although these patients remain dependent on methadone, many refrain from abusing other drugs.

Recently a long-acting narcotic, L-alpha-acetylmethadole (LAAM), has been studied. This drug is similar to methadone but effective for several days, reducing the need for daily visits to the clinic. LAAM is still in experimental testing stages. Naltrexone, a long-acting narcotic antagonist, is also being studied. This drug is not addicting and blocks the effects of narcotics. If the patient should use a narcotic while on naltrexone, the narcotic will have no effect.

Inpatient treatment is available for patients who cannot maintain drug-free status as outpatients. It can be relatively short-term, 21 to 28 days, or long-term, six months to two years. Short-term inpatient care usually takes place in special treatment units in general hospitals or in free-standing facilities. These programs offer intensive counseling and education to the patient who needs to be removed from his or her environment for a period of time.

The longer-term inpatient treatment settings, therapeutic communities, are usually free-standing facilities where patients work toward increased levels of responsibility in the community over several months or years. These programs usually offer group therapy, education, and vocational training. Inpatient treatment should always be followed by outpatient treatment to assist the patient in returning to the outpatient environment.

For patients who need more intensive treatment than can be offered in outpatient care yet cannot take the time off from work or cannot afford inpatient care, evening and weekend programs have been developed. Evening programs offer intensive treatment four or five nights a week for three or four weeks. Weekend programs offer intensive treatment experiences from Friday night until Sunday night. These programs should always be followed up with outpatient care.

Addiction is a difficult disorder to treat. Yet recent studies have shown that remissions can be achieved in from 35 to 60 percent of patients. This variation is based on level of functioning at entry into treatment and the support systems available to the patient. Treating the addict is not a hopeless process, but it is a long and difficult one, as is the treatment of any chronic disorder.

REFERENCES

Arieff, A. I., & Friedman, E. A. (1973), Coma following non-narcotic drug overdosage: Management of 208 adult patients. *Amer. J. Med. Sci.*, 266:405–426.

Arnow, R., & Done, A. K. (1978), Phencyclidine overdose: An emerging concept of management. *J. Amer. Coll. Emerg. Physicians,* 7:56–59.

Beckett, A. H., Rowland, M., & Turner, P. (1965), Influence of the urinary pH on excretion of amphetamines. *Lancet,* 1:303.

Bessen, H. A. (1982), Intracranial hemorrhage associated with phencyclidine abuse. *J. Amer. Med. Assn.*, 248:585–586.

Ellinwood, E. H. (1974), Emergency treatment of acute adverse reactions to CNS stimulants. In: *A Treatment Manual for Acute Drug Abuse Emergencies,* ed. P. Bourne. Rockville, MD: National Clearinghouse for Drug Abuse Information, pp. 63–67.

Fraser, D. W. (1972), Methadone overdose. *J. Amer. Med. Assn.,* 217:1387–1389.

Hayden, J. W., & Comstock, E. G. (1975), Use of activated charcoal in acute poisoning. *Clin. Toxicol.,* 8:515–533.

Kersh, E. S. (1973), Treatment of propoxyphene overdose with naloxone. *Chest,* 63:112–114.

Martin, W. R. (1976), Naloxone. *Ann. Intern Med.,* 85:765–768.

Parker, L. O. (1979), Clinical, circulatory and hematological effects of isobutyl nitrite. In: *Isobutyl Nitrite and Related Compounds,* ed. M. Nickerson. San Francisco: Pharmex Limited, pp. 70–78.

Prockop, L. (1977), Multifocal nervous system damage from volatile hydrocarbon inhalation. *J. Occup. Med.,* 19:139–140.

Schnoll, S. H. (1980a), Patient motivation. *Maryland State Med. J.,* 30:40–43.

——— (1980b), Street PCP scene: Issues on synthesis and contamination. *J. Psyched. Drugs,* 12:229–233.

——— Vogel, W. H. (1971), Analysis of "street drugs." *N. Engl. J. Med.,* 284:781.

Smith, D. E., & Wesson, D. R. (1971), Phenobarbital technique for treatment of barbiturate dependence. *Arch. Gen. Psych.,* 24:56–60.

Wikler, A. (1968), Diagnosis and treatment of drug dependence of the barbiturate type. *Amer. J. Psych.,* 125:758–765.

Commentary

Shirley Y. Hill, Ph.D.

Chapter 6 is a useful and concise reference for physicians and others who must deal with overdoses in the emergency room. Overdose from a variety of drugs, including alcohol, is a challenging problem because the victim often comes into the emergency room in a state in which he cannot accurately, if at all, report which drugs he has ingested. Without reliable informants accompanying the victim, emergency personnel are often confronted with the problem of knowing how to treat the overdose appropriately. The author identifies some of the symptomatology that will aid in correctly identifying the drug the victim has ingested, thereby hastening the process of aggressively treating the overdose.

Once the overdose has been managed acutely the physician is then confronted with how to best aid the victim in obtaining treatment and rehabilitation of the problem that led to the overdose. Too often this step is not carefully considered and appropriate measures are not instituted to prevent reoccurrence. Ideally, the steps should include consultation with substance abuse experts regarding underlying dependence disorders or depressive disorders that may lead to a possible suicide attempt. Those who deal with these victims should be cognizant of the fact that referral to a self-help group such as AA or NA may not be sufficient. Recent studies show that only one in four referrals to AA attend regularly and achieve abstinence (Polich, Armor, and Braiker, 1981). It is important to make a referral to a treatment organization with a good reputation and make follow-up calls to see that the referral actually arrives at the treatment organization. Patients so informed will more often follow through with the suggested referral.

A related issue has to do with the fact that only a small percentage of patients will acknowledge that they have a substance abuse problem. Rather than "seize this opportunity [acknowledgment of substance abuse] and initiate treatment" as Schnoll suggests, I would prefer to see the physician, or other clinician, who routinely sees patients for medical–psychological problems challenge *every* patient who appears to be using alcohol or drugs excessively. One need not label the individual, accusing him of being alcoholic or drug dependent, but rather in a supportive way ask if he would like to decrease the amount of alcohol or drugs he is using. This question, if answered in an affirmative, should be followed by reassurances that changes can be made in the unwanted behavior. A call to substance abuse experts while the patient is in the clinician's office, with an appointment time offered, may be the call that saves his life. These experts should be persons trained to do psychotherapy (preferably licensed therapists). If one views drinking as just one of the many behaviors that one can learn to gain control over, then the possibility for changing other nondrinking behaviors (e.g., marital, interpersonal, or job related) that may be impacting on the likelihood of relapse can also be made through therapy.

References

Polich, J. M., Armor, D. J., & Braiker, H. B. (1981). *The Course of Alcoholism: Four Years After Treatment*. New York: John Wiley.

Annotated Bibliography

Greenblatt, D. J., & Shader, R. I. (1974), Drug abuse and the emergency room physician. *Amer. J. Psych.*, 131:559–562.

This is a still quite instructive paper written by two well-known psychopharmacologists. The authors discuss in detail the emergency treatment modalities of some of the most important drug abuse syndromes seen in the emergency department. They examine the evaluation of the comatose patient and the syndromes of abuse of opiates, sedative hypnotics, amphetamines, hallucinogens, anticholinergics, and alcohol withdrawal. They caution against the use of pharmacotherapy in drug abusers because of the possible compounding of deleterious effects and discuss the need of such agents in overdose and withdrawal. Equally important is the referral of the drug abuser to treatment facilities where more lasting solutions can be undertaken.

Yago, K. B., Pitts, F. N., Burgoyne, R. W., Aniline, O., Yago, L. S., & Pitts, A. F. (1981), The urban epidemic of phencyclidine (PCP) use: Clinical and laboratory evidence from a public psychiatric hospital emergency service. *J. Clin. Psych.*, 42:193–196.

A report on the efficacy of routine blood samples on 145 consecutive patients seen in the Los Angeles County Psychiatric Hospital Emergency Room during a 48-hour weekday period, where the presence of phencyclidine (PCP) was sought. Forty-three percent of the patients showed evidence of PCP. An analysis of the records of these patients revealed a wide variety of psychotic clinical pictures resembling mania, depression, or schizophrenia with relatively few of the supposedly characteristic manifestations of noncomatose PCP intoxication (the latter include nystagmus, hypertension, pyrexia, dissociative states, and hyperreflexia). Ironically, in only half of these cases was PCP (or other drug) intoxication considered. In order for the PCP psychiatric picture to be more fully and precisely defined clinically, access to PCP levels needs to be available.

Biener, L. (1983), Perceptions of patients by emergency room staff: Substance-abusers versus non-substance-abusers. *J. Health & Soc. Behav.*, 24:264–275.

Written from the perspective of the mental health worker, this report provides empirical support for the widely held belief that substance abusers are still strongly disliked by many emergency room staff. The factor most responsible for the negative attitudes is the staff's expectation that the substance abuser is going to behave in an uncooperative manner. While it is realistic to expect that some substance abusers will be hostile or aggressive in the emergency room, this expectation may become a self-fulfilling prophecy.

The results of the study suggest that an important step toward improving treatment of substance abusers in the emergency room (indeed some personality disorders as well) and consequently of improving their chances of accepting referral to long-term treatment, is to help staff members learn effective strategies for dealing with uncooperative patients. This training will also help physicians to recognize their own negative attitudes and how they spread to other staff members.

7

Emergency Treatment of Acute Psychosis, Agitation, and Anxiety

James M. Ellison, M.D.

Psychotic symptoms such as hallucinations, suspiciousness, hyperactivity, hostility, or belligerence may bring a previously nonpsychotic individual to a psychiatric emergency service. Such behaviors may result from functional psychosis or may represent an organic mental disorder secondary to progressive medical illness such as hypoglycemia, hypoxia, alcohol amnestic syndrome, cerebral hemorrhage, or infection of the central nervous system (CNS).

In the emergency treatment of psychosis or agitation the initial step is to rule out such organic illness, along with certain toxic psychoses caused by phencyclidine (PCP) or anticholinergic drugs and withdrawal states such as delirius tremens, since these disorders require specialized interventions in addition to or instead of the treatments discussed below (Anderson and Kuehnle, 1981). Clues to these organic diagnoses are gathered by obtaining a history of medical illnesses or medication use; testing orientation, memory, and alertness; measuring vital signs and observing gait and pupils; and drawing blood for a complete blood count, electrolytes, and glucose. Toxic screens, arterial blood gas measurements, CAT scan, or electroencephalogram may also be indicated if intoxication, hypoxia, cerebral mass or hemorrhage, or seizure disorder are suspected (Ellison, 1984).

During diagnosis evaluation, the clinician should attempt to reduce the patient's psychotic thinking or agitated behavior through non-threatening interview techniques. If these measures fail to reestablish the patient's cognitive or behavioral control, the clinician should consider prompt treatment with medication to alleviate the disturbance. Oral neuroleptics are often chosen for this purpose; they may be high potency (nonsedating) or low potency (sedating) depending on whether sedation would be clinically helpful.

When symptoms are disruptive enough to warrant the somewhat more rapid onset of action obtained with parenteral agents, a high-potency antipsychotic drug such as haloperidol or thiothixene is usually chosen because of the relatively low risk of hypotension or oversedation. An initial dose of 2 to 10 mg of one of these drugs is given as a deltoid or glutal injection; the lower dose range is for patients who are delirious, medically ill, or elderly. Additional injections may be administered every 30 to 60 minutes after reassessment of the patient's mental status and vital signs; several injections are usually sufficient to calm the patient. Some studies have advocated the effectiveness of relatively low total doses (Neborsky, Janowsky, Munson, 1981; Egcobar, Barron, and Kiriakos, 1983). Oral treatment should replace parenteral treatment as soon as feasible (Ayd, 1977).

Unfortunately, the use of high-potency neuroleptics for acute treatment is often complicated by an acute dystonic reaction affecting the patient's tongue, neck, and extraocular or other muscles. Some clinicians attempt to avoid this disagreeable experience by prophylactic treatment with an anticholinergic agent such as benztropine. Less common adverse reactions to treatment include hypotension, cardiac arrhythmias, seizures, and the neuroleptic malignant syndrome, a triad of symptoms consisting of muscular rigidity, fever, and altered mental status that requires the patient's transfer to an intensive care unit for medical treatment.

Two alternative pharmacologic approaches to rapid treatment of acutely psychotic patients have been advocated; they are intravenous benzodiazepines and intramuscular droperidol. In one study diazepam was given intravenously (20 to 35 mg over 3 hours) and proved as therapeutic as haloperidol (30 to 40 mg IV over 3 hours) in relieving severe agitation (Lerner, Liwow, Levitin, 1979). If the patient's agitation is due to intoxication with a CNS depressant, however, a benzodiazepine may be dangerously sedating and should not be used. Paradoxical disinhibition, or an uncharacteristic display of aggressive behavior sometimes seen after treatment with benzodiazepines, is rarely a problem when intravenous doses are administered at these levels.

A recent study found droperidol superior to haloperidol for rapid treatment due to its strong calming effect and low incidence of cardiovascular or extrapyramidal side effects (Resnick and Burton, 1984). This butyrophenone, familiar to anesthesiologists but new to many psychiatrists, is given in an initial intramuscular injection of 5 mg followed as needed by one or two additional injections at 30-minute intervals. Droperidol may be an exciting new tool in emergency psychiatry, but further experience is necessary for a thorough appraisal of its usefulness.

Treatment of Anxiety States

Anxiety states, though often less flagrantly bizarre or destructive than psychosis, cause great distress to patients and may precipitate an emergency room visit. The opportunity to speak openly in a secure environment is sufficiently calming for many individuals, but when further treatment is needed, anti-anxiety drugs can be very effective in alleviating symptoms in appropriately selected patients.

For acute free-floating or situational anxiety, oral benzodiazepines are usually the drug of choice (Shader and Greenblatt, 1981). In choosing a specific agent, the rate of absorption is important, since more rapidly absorbed drugs such as lorazepam and diazepam may provide a more noticeable subjective sense of relief. Several days' supply of lorazepam (for example, 1 mg b.i.d. to q.i.d.) or diazepam (5 mg b.i.d. to q.i.d.) can be safely dispensed to the patient for continuation of treatment, but only when appropriate follow-up care has been scheduled.

When acute anxiety is experienced as a panic attack or is accompanied by very prominent somatic symptoms, the efficacy of propranolol may equal or exceed that of the benzodiazepines in alleviation of these symptoms. Oral doses as low as 10 mg may relieve panic symptoms (Heiser, 1976). Potential acute adverse effects of propranolol include bradycardia, congestive heart failure, hypotension, bronchospasm, and fatigue. Use of propranolol is contraindicated in patients with asthma or Raynaud's phenomenon. In diabetes, propranolol may dangerously mask symptoms of hypoglycemia.

It is important to bear in mind that acute anxiety symptoms sometimes indicate the presence of a potentially progressive organic disorder. Some organic disorders that may present with prominent anxiery include stimulant intoxication, sedative-hypnotic or alcohol withdrawal, cardiac arrhythmia, congestive heart failure, hypoglycemia, CNS infection, delirium, and early states of dementia. A pertinent medical history combined with a limited physical assessment will uncover most such conditions so they can receive more specific medical treatment. Two nonorganic conditions whose nature may be obscured by severe concurrent anxiety are functional depression and psychosis. A careful mental status examination will usually elicit the mood alteration, vegetative signs, or abnormalities of thought process and content associated with these disorders.

In summary, psychopharmacologic agents have important roles in the acute treatment of psychosis or anxiety. Care must be taken not to neglect organic disease manifesting as behavioral symptoms. Acute psychopharmacologic treatment is most successful in conjunction with hospitalization or frequent and consistent outpatient follow-up, psychotherapy, and involvement of helpful members of the patient's social network.

References

Anderson, W. H., & Kuehnle, J. C. (1981), Diagnosis and management of acute psychosis. *N.Eng.J. Med.*, 305:1128–1130.

Ayd, F. J. (1977), Guidelines for using short-acting intramuscular neuroleptics for rapid neuroleptization. *Internat. Drug Ther. Newsletter*, 12:5–12.

Ellison, J. (1984), DSM-III and the diagnosis of organic mental disorders. *Ann. Emerg. Med.*, 13:521–528.

Escobar, J. I., Barron, A., & Kiriakos, R. (1983), A controlled study of neuroleptization with fluphenazine hydrocloride injections. *J. Clin. Psychopharm.*, 3:359–362.

Heiser, J. F. (1976), The treatment of pathological panic states with propranolol. *Amer. J. Psychiat.*, 133:1389–1393.

Lerner, Y., Lwow, E., Levitin, A., et al. (1979), Acute high-dose parenteral haloperidol treatment of psychosis. *Amer. J. Psychiat.* 136:1061–1064.

Neborsky, R., Janowsky, D., Munson, E., et al. (1981), Rapid treatment of acute psychotic symptoms with high- and low-dose haloperidol. *Arch. Gen. Psychiat.* 38:195–199.

Resnick, M., & Burton, B. T. (1984), Droperidol vs haloperidol in the initial management of acutely agitated patients. *J. Clin. Psychiat.*, 45:298–299.

Shader, R. I., & Greenblatt, D. (1981), Benzodiazepine treatment of specific anxiety states. *Psychiat. Ann.* 11:16–20.

Commentary

Benjamin Zimmer, M.D.

Chapter 7 attempts to be a comprehensive review of the phenomenology and pharmacologic treatment of acute psychosis. Particularly useful is the author's historical perspective on the treatment of the acute psychoses. Indeed discussion regarding the development of the diagnosis of specific acute psychoses is presented as well as the pharmacologic interventions and the efficacy of being diagnostically precise when selecting certain agents.

Annotated Bibliography

Adler, G. (1974), Acute psychosis, *N. Eng. J. Med.*, 291:81–83.

This is a quite practical, concise, and yet reasonably thorough paper on the course, differential diagnosis, and management of acute psychosis. The consideration of nonbiological causes of acute psychosis as well as of nonbiological modalities of treatment provide a nice contrast to other articles on a similar topic.

Anderson, W. H., & Kuehnle, J. C. (1974), Strategies for the treatment of acute psychosis. *J. Amer. Med. Assn.*, 229:1884–1889.

This is a thoughtful and practical paper on the management of acute psychiatric behavior. As always, management requires a good differential diagnosis as well as consideration of general medical factors and the need to hospitalize. The use of high-potency antipsychotic chemotherapy needs to be kept in mind. Indeed, the use of such agents may in some case avoid unnecessary hospital admissions.

Ban, T. A., Guy, W., & Wilson, W. H. (1984), Approaches to the management of the acutely psychotic patient. *Psychiat. J. Univ. Ottawa*, 9:36–41.

This paper attempts to be a comprehensive review of the phenomenology and pharmacologic treatment of acute psychosis. Particularly useful is the author's historical perspective on the treatment of the acute psychoses. Indeed, discussion regarding the development of the diagnoses of specific acute psychoses is presented as well as the pharmacologic interventions and the efficacy of being diagnostically precise when selecting certain agents.

8

Hysteria in the Emergency Room

N. Gregory Hamilton, M.D.

In the emergency room, with crowds of people, hurried activity, and a sense of drama, hysterical patients can elicit a pandemonium that resonates with their anxiety, causing it to worsen. Staff and patients alike become frustrated and confused, and the psychiatric consultant is finally called.

As psychiatrists expand their role in emergency room consultation (Nemiah, 1968; Gerson and Basserk, 1980), others will increasingly ask them to assist with the management of acute hysterical episodes. Yet the main body of literature on hysteria is written by and for psychiatrists who manage the long-term, not the acute, manifestations of hysteria. In fact, many psychiatrists have encountered hysteria less frequently in recent years (Chodoff and Lyons, 1958; Merskey and Buhrich, 1975; Nemiah, 1975), though other physicians in neurology, military, and industrial medicine clinics still find such cases (Weintraub, 1968; Chodoff, 1974; Merskey and Trimble, 1979). Some hysterics may also turn to faith-healers for help (Favazza, 1979).

Since the literature on hysteria contains little information on its

This chapter was first published in the *Journal of Operational Psychiatry* (1981), 12:21–23, and it is reprinted by permission.

emergency management, one could turn to the growing work on emergency psychiatry. This literature, however, predominantly deals with psychosis, alcoholism, and depression, which are the most common psychiatric problems seen in emergency rooms (Errera, Wyshak, and Jareck, 1963). And, as Gerson and Basserk (1980) observed in an overview of emergency psychiatry, sufficient discussion of specific management techniques is lacking for most psychiatric disorders.

Considering these circumstances, it may be useful to report the author's experience managing hysteria in the emergency room. Particular emphasis will be placed on the need for rapid diagnosis and a calm, forthright management, often including a present tense interpretation.

THE CASES

During one year (August 1, 1978 through July 31, 1979) representative of his experience, the author saw 2,150 emergency room patients. Of these patients, five (2.3/1000) had acute hysterical reactions of a dramatic nature. Many more patients, of course, may have been found to have somatization disorder had a more detailed review of systems been taken, especially on patients with musculoskeletal pain, abdominal pain, or menstrual irregularities. The emphasis of this communication, however, is the emergency management of hysterical conversion with classic symptoms.

Among the cases reviewed for this report, symptoms mixed and overlapped in combinations of hysterical seizure, blindness, aphonia, involuntary shrieking, astasia-abasia, loss of consciousness, paralysis, and bizarre movement disorders such as serpentine writhing on the floor. All the patients were young women and two of the five dated the onset of their symptoms to their marriage a few days earlier.

Two representative cases will be described in narrative form to emphasize the management.

Case 1

The emergency room doors swung open, and five young men and women led in a 17-year-old bride shouting, "She's blind! She's blind!"

The nurse allowed the husband to stay with the patient and asked the others to be seated in the waiting room while she summoned the physician. When he arrived, the physician found the husband leaning over the patient repetitively reminding her that he was still there. After reassuring the patient that a nurse would stay with her, the physician then asked the patient's husband to talk with him in the hall.

Though reluctant to leave his wife, the husband provided the following history. His wife of three days had moved on the wedding day from her large, poor urban family in Chicago to a remote midwestern town where her husband spent long hours working. The day after arrival, the patient experienced a brief episode of blindness which resolved. Then, on the night of presentation, while sitting with friends who were about to leave the apartment, the patient suddenly and dramatically fell backwards from her chair and shrieked that she was blind. There was no loss of consciousness, unusual movement, incontinence, or complaint of neck pain.

Leaving the husband in the lobby, the physician returned to the patient. As he introduced himself, he put his hand on the patient's wrist to take her pulse and listened to a brief but faltering history. He noticed that her pupils were equal and reactive. Spontaneous extraocular movements were normal as was fundoscopy. Placing his face at the patient's focal point, he stared into her eyes then moved his head laterally. The patient's eyes consistently stayed fixed on the examiner's eyes, demonstrating the intact following reflex despite the patient stating she was still totally blind. Realizing that the optic tracts through and including the optic cortex had to be intact for the patient to follow the gestalt of his face, the physician concluded that the symptom was a conversion phenomenon. Without further ado, he reassured the patient that these kinds of symptoms are transient and he expected her vision to return within a few minutes. Almost immediately, the patient could see and had normal acuity. Only then was the rest of the physical and neurological examination done and found to be normal.

The patient and her husband were relieved to learn that she would not lose her sight and that the understandable stress of a recent separation from her mother and new intimacy with her husband had precipitated her problem. The patient accepted a referral to the psychiatry clinic, with a secondary referral to medicine and ophthalmology "to reassure her that the diagnosis was correct." The actual examination, treatment, and referral were carried out in 20 minutes; and the physician, staff, and patient felt something worthwhile had been accomplished.

Follow-up revealed that the patient came from a family with seven children, and she had been sexually abused by her stepfather in her early teens. The ophthalmologic examination was normal as were her electroencephalogram and skull films, including the sella tursica. The internist also agreed with the emergency room diagnosis.

Case 2

A 33-year-old Oriental woman was seen to run down a road and fling herself into a ditch. As the ambulance attendant wheeled her into the emergency room, he proclaimed, "She had a seizure!"

The patient did not respond to questions, stared straight ahead, and resisted gentle pressure when a nurse attempted to facilitate the examination. This active resistance, rather than the hypotonia of a postictal state, led the examiner to suspect a conversion symptom. Again, he cleared the room of extra people and carried out the examination slowly and calmly while a witness was sought. The physical and neurologic examinations were entirely normal except for aphonia, a trancelike gaze, and astasia-abasia, with groping toward helping personnel yet rejection of assistance to stand. Throughout the examination, the patient was expected to function fully, though she did not, of course, comply with this expectation.

A neighbor who had accompanied the patient informed the physician in another room that the patient had argued with her husband who threatened to beat her. The patient then ran down the street and plunged headlong into a ditch. There was no loss of consciousness, unusual movement, or incontinence. Additionally, it was learned that the patient spoke and understood English well.

Returning to the examining room, the physician sat across from the patient who still appeared dazed. Making deliberate eye-contact, he explained that he realized she was afraid her husband would kill her and that she was furious with him. Perhaps she even feared she might kill him. Furthermore, he guessed that she felt alone and did not know where to turn. She needed help.

The patient, who had not previously spoken, suddenly recovered from her daze and burst into tears. She recovered her speech and balance within a few minutes and agreed to discuss with the nurse and her friend where to spend the night safely. She also accepted a psychiatry referral for herself and her husband the next day. The process took 20 minutes and no hospitalization was needed.

A subsequent review of her records revealed previous treatment for unexplained wrist pain, constipation, abdominal pain, low back pain, menstrual irregularities, and marital discord. Three months after the visit she was still involved in treatment at the mental health center.

DISCUSSION

Those who have experienced hysteria in the emergency room with screaming, thrashing, and crowds of people desperately trying to help will realize the usefulness of a calm and effective approach. Because the simplicity of the above described procedures is somewhat deceptive, the step-by-step management will be described.

First, the physician took control by separating the patient from her family, where the precipitating conflict usually centered; yet he did not leave her isolated. He also separated her from the crowds of helping personnel who were drawn to the patient by assigning a single female nurse to stay with her.

Second, the physician obtained a history from a family member or friend, because the patient could seldom provide an appropriate history until her symptoms resolved.

Third, the physician evaluated the major symptom before doing a detailed neurologic or physical examination. As emphasized by Weintraub (1968), the central issue here is that the symptoms must be inconsistent with known neuroanatomy, physiology, and pathology and must be clearly explained by a conflictual event immediately preceding the onset. A detailed review of systems and complicated examinations or tests are seldom necessary to meet these diagnostic criteria. In fact, a need on the physician's part to doubt his basic medical knowledge defensively may deprive the patient of the treatment she needs and reinforce her symptoms without adding significant information.

Fourth, the physician made contact with the patient by touching her (e.g., taking her pulse) or making eye-contact. This seemingly minor step derived from the separation anxiety apparent in the histories. Because of the sexual implications of touching such patients, this step was performed with a female nurse present.

Fifth, the physician made a commonsense interpretation. This interpretation dealt with the present stresses of separations, new intimacies, or overt hostilities. Early childhood interpretations were avoided in this setting.

Finally, the physician made the appropriate referrals in the presence of the patient and, if possible, the family member who served as a focus of conflict. After referral to psychiatry, the patient was also referred to neurology or medicine and told that such a step was being taken to reassure her that the diagnosis was correct.

CONCLUSION

Acute hysterical conversions of a classic nature do occur and should be treated as psychiatric emergencies. When treatment is instituted promptly, the acute symptoms of hysteria frequently resolve dramatically to the relief of the patient and those around her.

REFERENCES

Chodoff, P. (1974), The diagnosis hysteria: An overview. *Amer. J. Psychiat.*, 131:1073–1078.

——— & Lyons, H. (1958), Hysteria, the hysterical personality, and "hysterical conversation." *Amer. J. Psychiat.*, 114:737–740.

Errera, P., Wyshak, G., & Jarecki, H. (1963), Psychiatric care in a general hospital emergency room. *Arch. Gen. Psychiat.*, 9:105–112.

Favazza, A. R. (1979), Has hysteria decreased? *Amer. J. Psychiat.*, 136:1102.

Gerson, S., & Basserk, E. (1980), Psychiatric emergencies: An overview. *Amer. J. Psychiat.*, 137:1–11.

Merskey, H., & Buhrich, N. A. (1975), Hysteria and organic brain disease. *Brit. J. Med. Psychol.*, 48:359–366.

——— & Trimble, M. (1979), Personality, sexual adjustment, and brain lesions in patients with conversion symptoms. *Amer. J. Psychiat.*, 136:179–182.

Nemiah, J. C. (1968), Help! *Amer. J. Psychiat.*, 124:1698–1699.

——— (1975), Hysterical neurosis, conversion type. In: *Comprehensive Textbook of Psychiatry*, 2nd. ed. eds. A. M. Freedman, H. I. Kaplan, & B. J. Sadock. Baltimore, MD: Williams & Wilkins, p. 1209.

Weintraub, M. J. (1968), *A Clinician's Manual of Hysterical Conversion Reactions*. New York: Interdisciplinary Communications Media.

Commentary

Paul H. Soloff, M.D.

It is a humbling yet reassuring reality that the skillful "laying on of hands" by society's modern healers can still relieve the symbolic expressions of emotional distress. The understanding of conversion phenomena in the annals of psychiatry parallels our professional development from shaman to scientist, from symptom relief through ritual, magic, and suggestion to the exploration and treatment of psychologic and biologic causes. Hamilton's discussion of the treatment of two cases of conversion hysteria in an emergency room setting, divorced as it is from any historical context or discussion of the psychological meaning of the syndrome, its origin, or treatment, leaves one with a ritual for removing the presenting symptom. Given the limitations of the busy emergency room, the physician's response must be rapid and expedient. One is led to believe that magical healing occurs in under 20 minutes! This is both simplistic and deceptive. One must not confuse symptom relief with cure. Hamilton wisely reminds us that each patient "accepted a referral to psychiatry," where, in competent hands, the cause of the conversion may be explored in a more scientific and sophisticated manner, both psychologically and biologically, to prevent repeated visits to the emergency room. This is perhaps his most important point. As for the successful healing by suggestion, one wonders what would be recommended if magic failed. Probably the same prescription, refer to psychiatry!

9

The Borderline Patient in the Emergency Department: An Approach to Evaluation and Management

Richard A. Perlmutter, M.D.

There is a burgeoning of knowledge and literature pertaining to psychotherapy, diagnostic criterion, and inpatient management of borderline patients. Such patients are well known to utilize a disproportionate amount of crisis services (Raphling and Lion, 1970; Schwartz, Weiss, and Miner, 1972) and to be extraordinarily difficult to manage at times of crisis (Schwartz et al., 1972; Groves, 1978; Bassuk and Gerson, 1980). Nonetheless, little has been written applying the knowledge of the borderline syndrome to the management of such patients in emergency settings. This would be an essential application especially since crisis intervention techniques that are so useful for most patients can be inadequate and even dangerous for the borderline. A chronically suicidal subgroup of these patients requires a novel and seemingly counterintuitive approach. Based on current knowledge of the border-

This chapter was first published in *Psychiatric Quarterly* (1982), 54:190–197, and it is reprinted by permission.

line and the clinical observation of many such patients presenting to a psychiatric emergency department (PED) of a university hospital, a dynamically informed approach to crisis management is suggested. It is hoped that this will stimulate awareness, discussion, and research.

DIAGNOSIS

Patients referred to as borderline descriptively meet DSM-III (American Psychiatric Association, 1980) criteria for borderline personality disorder according to at least one emergency department staff member. Structured research interviews were not performed. While nosology is not the focus of this article, research (Gunderson and Kolb, 1978; Soloff and Ulrich, 1981) suggesting the discriminating value of unstable interpersonal relationships and impulsive self-destructive behaviors are relevant as these are also the prominent features of emergency presentations. In addition to descriptive criteria, the genetic and dynamic structures are elucidated throughout the chapter.

In general, this will be a group of patients functioning at a lower level and possessing less ego strength than those discussed in the literature concerned with outpatient psychotherapy of the borderline.

SUICIDE ATTEMPTS AND MUTILATIONS

The vast majority of visits to the PED by borderline patients involve either a self-destructive act that has just been attempted or the threat that one will be attempted soon. Hospital records reveal several prior emergency visits and hospitalizations following an overdose or self-cutting occurring at times of life stress. The life stresses usually are related to an actual or perceived abandonment. The act is designed to prevent a separation from an ambivalently held love object or bring back a lost object. Commonly, one member of a dyad (husband–wife, parent–child) attempts suicide in an attempt to coerce and punish the other member who may be exhausted but enmeshed. After an overdose, one woman shared with PED staff her summation that "Everything would be okay if my boyfriend were available to me 24 hours a day." The act may similarly appear as a manipulation of the therapist and mental health system to gain some gratification such as nurturance, love, drugs, hospitalization.

The patient who presents with a bloody, self-inflicted wound may appear quite unconcerned, much to the horror and perplexity of the emergency staff. In fact, the patient often describes a feeling of relief of tension. One borderline man, a recurrent self-mutilator, told us on a visit after a serious slashing, "You know, I always feel better afterwards." Hence, it is important to note that the self-mutilator may be presenting as self-treated; that is, the immediate intolerable affects have been temporarily relieved. The mutilator presents the wounds to show, and may not be interested in treatment. Suicidal intent, per se, is not necessarily prominent. Awareness of these features is essential when considering recommendations and disposition.

The meaning of an overdose can also vary from highly lethal attempts to die to the more common impulsive attempts to avoid a flood of intolerable affects of rage, despair, emptiness, and deprivation (Buie and Adler, 1972).

THE VISIT TO THE PED

The patient we are discussing uses the PED repeatedly, is well known to the staff, and is a source of frequent discussion. The staff experiences fear and dread when the patient presents. The patient repeatedly uses the PED in a way that can appear to be an abuse of it. The visit of the borderline to the PED is unparalleled in its capacity to elicit feelings of guilt, anger, hate, love, and rejection. This difficult and provocative group of patients suffer intensely and chronically. Their mature defenses fail easily and expose primitive ones that activate desperate attempts to relieve their pain. Primitive defenses like splitting and projection are not just vague theoretical constructs but come alive as the PED worker experiences their force. The staff member learns what it is like to be a screen on which an image is projected. The tendency of borderline patients to invest objects such as the hospital with qualities of their own (Modell, 1963) becomes evident. The hospital can then be viewed as being anywhere from hostile and rejecting, to omnipotent and expected to take care of everything magically. Projective identification and sharing of the symptom may be utilized so smoothly that the patient's intolerable affects are dumped and left behind. The patient leaves angry, but feeling a bit better as targets have been found for the rage. The staff members, however, are left behind feeling anxious, overinvolved, enraged, and perplexed. A dynamic understanding of such transfer of symptoms does not prevent the feelings but can decrease judgment distortions regarding disposition plans.

The borderline patient who is in ongoing psychotherapy and presents to the PED brings special considerations. Subtle splitting mechanisms, if not recognized, soon have the interviewer demeaning the patient's therapist as not adequate or skillful enough. The therapist is blamed for the patient's decompensation and need to visit the PED.

Skodal and colleagues (Skodal, Kass, and Charles, 1979) have looked descriptively at patients in psychotherapy who present to a PED. They see the prototype as a borderline who discusses the ongoing relationship in terms that are either hypercritical or idealizing. We underscore their conclusion that "the crisis of a patient in treatment, who presents to an emergency room service, cannot be understood out of the context of problems in ongoing psychotherapy" (p. 595). For example, the patient's sense of self as a cohesive, constant entity is fragile and can break down under circumstances like a therapist's absence. Such perceived abandonments lead to a panic expressed as rage, emptiness, destructiveness, or transient psychosis.

It is essential for the emergency psychiatrist to become an expert in how to consult to therapy relationships, and even more delicately, how to include issues of inexperience, transference, and countertransference. A most difficult issue is the awareness that a therapist has become destructively enmeshed with a borderline patient. It is the staff of the emergency department that becomes most crucially aware that certain therapists in the community have extreme difficulty with these patients. They require careful consultation with elements of supervision, support, and confrontation.

THE FAMILY

When the family accompanies the patient, a unique opportunity for learning is possible. For an understanding of the borderline patient nothing is comparable to observing and experiencing the family's transactions with each other and with the PED staff. The observations provide valuable assistance in formulating a treatment plan or disposition. If the patient is in psychotherapy, these observations can be quite useful for the primary therapist, who often has no primary data on the family.

For the chronically acting-out adolescent borderline, the opportunity to interview the family conjointly may quickly reveal the repetitive dangerous threats of abandonment that precede the destructive acts, the so-called "retaliatory withdrawal of supplies" (Shapiro, 1978). It may also highlight the parental inability to set the limits for which the adolescent is asking. In such cases, the emergency room therapist's recommendation that the family be included in the treatment plan can be helpful, sometimes lifesaving.

There is no single description of the family of the borderline either in practice or in the literature. Some families in crisis situations appear free of gross psychopathology and appear appropriately distressed and mobilized by the borderline patient's crisis. Other families rank among the most disturbed that are seen, and members may be highly provocative and even violent.

When a multigenerational unit presents, a wide range of dynamics and interactions are observed. Certain features, however, are demonstrated repeatedly and deserve comment. Most often the family patterns reveal the rewarding of regressed, symbiotic behavior and the punishment of autonomy. The parents may be distraught over their child's crisis but can be observed to reinforce the asking for help via mutilation, overdose, or brief psychosis. The parents are brought closer to the child by failures and are panicked by moves toward success or health. Their own unresolved conflicts over autonomy (Masterson, 1976; Shapiro, 1978) haunt the interview room. Hence we observe that peculiar phenomenon that goes beyond masochism; the offspring's pain and self-destructive behavior become linked with a feeling of relative family closeness (or at least the temporary cessation of the threat to abandon).

> A 37-year-old borderline woman presented to our emergency department with her mother. She was a frequent visitor to our emergency department, inpatient services, outpatient services, and day treatment program. She had suicidal ideation chronically, but had been more stable in her functioning in recent months. The experience of the psychiatric staff who interacted with the mother made the presence of a borderline personality organization in the daughter eminently understandable. Mother had been calling the daughter repeatedly, telling her that the daughter was sick

> and needed to be in the hospital. This persisted in the PED and mother angrily accosted the staff: "Why did you tell my daughter she was not sick and was an intelligent human being. She is sick and has been for 20 years."
>
> Mother had moved into a two-bedroom apartment so daughter could move in with her. She explained this: "My daughter needs to go to day care during the day and come back with me at night. She needs to be with me." Her projective mechanisms were evident but even more revealing was the use of the term "day care," to refer to her 37-year-old daughter's time spent in the day treatment program.

It is also worthwhile to emphasize that the borderline is not a passive victim of parental psychopathology. The effects are complexly interactive and the devastating influence of the borderline member's behaviors on other family members is all too evident.

AN APPROACH

Knowledge of these dynamics and patterns can help the clinician formulate interventions aimed at reinforcing more adaptive functioning. For the chronically suicidal patient, emphasis is placed on the ultimate responsibility and control that the patient has over the decision to live or die.

The approach must be coordinated with any ongoing treatment relationships. The periodically overwhelming demands of the borderline can be shared with the PED in a way that mitigates the therapist's isolation, frustration, or loss of perspective. In this way, relationships that are viable and useful can be preserved through repeated crises.

When it becomes evident that a patient repeatedly seen in PED exhibits a borderline personality disorder, we suggest a meeting of the primary therapist (or other agency) with a PED staff member to develop a protocol for future visits. This allows coordination of the crisis management with the therapist's overall style and strategy. Some specific points to be included are (1) when the therapist should be contacted, (2) when admission is essential, (3) would admission to a general hospital psychiatry unit or the state hospital be of more benefit, (4) what confrontations and psychologic interventions might be most useful during the visit, (5) what are the family/social supports, and (6) suggestions for handling self-destructive, acting-out, or threatening behavior, especially the "upping of the ante" (i.e., "if you don't admit me, I'll kill myself").

It is useful to have enough dynamic understanding to identify and explore the precipitants that lead to crisis in a particular patient. For those patients who mutilate or overdose in avoidance of intolerable affects, it is useful to have enough insight into this to interpret and confront in a way that allows the patient to control the impulse (Buie and Adler, 1972). Patients may be supported for their decision to visit the PED instead of acting on destructive impulses and can be encouraged as part of the protocol to do so whenever the urge to cut or overdose becomes strong. The emphasis is shifted from the PED assuming responsibility for destructive impulses to helping with the pains and problems of living so the patient can increase control.

The question of when to admit is complex. Gerson's work (Gerson, 1979) indicates that a poor therapist/patient relationship in the emergency department increases frequency of admission, implying that the tendency is to repeatedly hospitalize the borderline. For the borderline, however, hospitalization may hold a long-term danger. It may represent a rewarding of regressive, self-destructive behavior with nurturance and suspension of responsibility. While there may be some short-term benefit or at least therapist comfort, the risk of future suicide attempts or completion may be increased (Schwartz, 1979). The hospital system, then, is found responding in the binding, regressive manner described above for the borderline family.

The protocol should therefore include informing the patient that PED visits may be encouraged but will usually not end in admission. It can be shared with the patient that staff can understand the intense pain and need for relief but they will resist the pull from the patient and family to do something that in the long run will be more harmful.

While we are striving for a more reasoned approach than repeated hospitalizations of chronically suicidal people, clinical judgment must prevail. Admission may still be indicated if it is part of a rational therapeutic or diagnostic plan, if the patient is psychotic, if the intent to die is imminent and acute, if the patient can mobilize no resources, or if the PED approach does not help in control of the impulses. The point is that the clinician must balance the possible gains from admission or other interventions against the easily overlooked risk.

There is less hesitation to admit if the hospital units have expertise in inpatient treatment of the borderline. This includes awareness of its "double-edged" properties and hazards (Friedman, 1969). Ideally the admitting staff can contract with the patient before leaving the PED that the stay be brief, focused, and goal oriented (Wishnie, 1975; Adler, 1977; Sadavoy, Silver, and Book, 1979). The contract may include contingencies for discharge or transfer to a state hospital if regressive behavior increases (Friedman, 1969).

A PED staff that has experience with such patients and protocols develops expertise. The staff becomes alert to primitive defenses and is less likely to be controlled by them. Powerful interpersonal maneuvers such as splitting, attempts to get rejected, transferring the pain, and "upping the ante" are rendered less destructive by a staff familiar with them.

For the patient in crisis, the PED can be viewed as an auxiliary ego working to reward impulse control and decrease acting out of intolerable affects. This is done, in part, by strategically harnessing the drive for human contact. The approach aims to bolster overwhelmed defenses by a blend of reality testing, confrontation, clarification, and support.

COMMENTS

Emergency room psychiatrists are familiar with the anxious dilemma of the patient who presents with something like "I will kill myself if you don't admit me." One implication of this chapter is that hospitalization can and sometimes should be avoided. From the vantage of the traditional suicide prevention principles this, may appear unethical or counterintuitive (Clements, Sider, and Perlmutter, 1982), especially since the patient is likely to demonstrate a capacity for self-destructive behavior. Such principles of vigorous intervention and protection remain essential for the vast majority of acutely suicidal people but have a high risk–benefit ratio for the borderline. The knowledge of this unique subgroup of chronic patients, then, is the basis for the clinical and ethical justification for designing alternate, more comprehensive interventions.

The frequency of repeated visits to the PED is due to several factors. Defense mechanisms such as splitting predispose them to consultations outside any ongoing psychotherapeutic relationship (Skodal et al., 1979). Other defenses including projection, avoidance by action

(Bulie and Adler, 1972), and an inability to delay make it more likely that the setting for such consultations is an emergency room. Raphling and Lion's (1970) descriptive study of borderline repeaters points out how the deficits in object relations and intimacy predispose to difficult long-term treatment relationships and frequent use of the more impersonal PEDs. Intense interpersonal anxiety compels them to seek services that preserve distance. In addition, tremendous demand for immediate relief attracts patients to a service that offers 24-hour availability.

It may be argued that encouraging repeated use of such service fosters the PED becoming a transitional object with all the attributions of regression and magical protection that this implies. We view such an approach as an attempt to engage the patient at a level that can be achieved, and this may include an ability to hold transitional objects. It is the holding of transitional objects and the use of words that we try to substitute for impulsive actions. If the therapist or PED staff can declare themselves as helping but not on the side of regression, this may advance the capacity to relate.

Theoretically, it is useful here to recall the borderline pathology as rooted in failure to negotiate successfully the rapprochement subphase of separation–individuation (Mahler, 1974). Successful psychotherapy involves providing the patient with an experience of closeness that allows for separateness and therefore partially heals the earlier deficits. The popularity and potential usefulness of emergency services for borderline patients in crises may also be viewed in this context. The PED can be conceptualized as offering some of the "emotional refueling" that is needed in the practicing subphase. Most important in applying theory to practice is the need for the therapist and emergency service to maintain that "quiet availability" that allows the patient to give up gestures for words as the main mode of communication. Such quiet availability is the basis for an approach that encourages frequent visits and the use of words to replace self-destructive acts. And while the PED is available, the patient retains responsibility for life–death decisions. The hospital emergency department then functions in a way that supports efforts aimed at helping the patient attain a healthier adaptation to adult life. The challenge is to provide the patient with a small corner of the world that is neither engulfing nor abandoning.

REFERENCES

Adler, G. (1977), Hospital management of borderline patients and its relation to psychotherapy. In: *Borderline Personality Disorders*, ed. P. Hartocollis. New York: International Universities Press.

Bassuk, E., & Gerson, S. (1980), Chronic crisis patients: A discrete clinical group. *Amer. J. Psychiat.*, 137:1513–1517.

Buie, D. H., & Adler, G. (1972), The uses of confrontation with borderline patients. *Internat. J. Psychoanal. Psychother.*, 1:90–108.

Clements, C. D., Sider, R. C., & Perlmutter, R. A. (1982), The ethics of suicide: Act and intervention. In: *Science and Morality: New Directions in Bioethics*, eds. D. Teichler-Zallen, T. Land, & C. D. Clements. Lexington, MA: D.C. Heath (Lexington Books).

Friedman, H. J. (1969), Some problems of inpatient management with borderline patients. *Amer. J. Psychiat.*, 126:299–304.

Gerson, S. (1979), Determinants of psychiatric emergency room disposition. *Diss. Abs. Internat. Bull.*, 39/11:5551-B.

Groves, J. E. (1978), Taking care of the hateful patient. *New Eng. J. Med.*, 298:883–887.

Gunderson, J. G., & Kolb, J. E. (1978), Discriminating features of borderline patients. *Amer. J. Psychiat.*, 124:792–796.

Mahler, M. S. (1974), Symbiosis and individuation, the psychological birth of the human infant. *The Psychoanalytic Study of the Child*, 29. New Haven, CT: Yale University Press.

Masterson, J. F. (1976), *Psychotherapy of the Borderline Adult*. New York: Brunner/Mazel.

Modell, A. H. (1963), Primitive object relationships and the predisposition to schizophrenia. *Internat. J. Psycho-anal.*, 44:282–292.

Raphling, D. L., & Lion, J. (1970), Patients with repeated admissions to a psychiatric emergency service. *Comm. Men. Health J.*, 6:313–318.

Sadavoy, J., Silver, D., & Book, H. E. (1979), Negative response of the borderline to inpatient treatment. *Amer. J. Psychother.*, 33:404–417.

Schwartz, D. A. (1979), The suicidal character. *Psychiat. Quart.*, 51:64–70.

——— Weiss, A. T., & Miner, J. M. (1972), Community psychiatry and emergency service. *Amer. J. Psychiat.*, 129:710–715.

Shapiro, E. R. (1978), The psychodynamics and developmental psychology of the borderline patient: A review of the literature. *Amer. J. Psychiat.*, 124:1305–1315.

Skodal, A. E., Kass, F., & Charles, E. (1979), Crisis in psychotherapy: Principles of the emergency consultation and intervention. *Amer. J. Orthopsychiat.*, 49:585–597.

Soloff, P. H., & Ulrich, R. F. (1981), Diagnostic interview for borderline patients, a replication study. *Arch. Gen. Psychiat.*, 38:686–692.

Wishnie, H. A. (1975), Inpatient therapy with borderline patients. In: *Borderline States in Psychiatry*, ed. J. Mack. New York: Grune & Stratton.

Commentary

Paul H. Soloff, M.D.

The role of the emergency department in care of patients with borderline disorder is a blend of support and structure, of concern and confrontation. Borderline patients present a bewildering array of complaints in the emergency department, both overt and implied, in their affective, schizotypal, and impulsive behavioral symptoms. Their affect is most often angry, their behavior argumentative, manipulative, demanding, and inappropriate to the setting. They insist that the hospital assume responsibility for their actions, decisions, and even—in the case of suicidal threat—their very lives. The high drama of their presentation, interpersonal appeal, and emotional immaturity are very seductive, drawing on the needs of individual care givers for involvement as players in a stimulating game of "rescue" or "punishment." Perlmutter defines clearly these psychodynamic interactions, which help explain both patient and staff behavior in the emergency room setting. His emphasis lies with increasing the insight of the staff into the patients' problems and presentation. Unfortunately, insight is never enough. The emergency room visit must be kept in perspective—as a very brief moment in a long history of instability. The meaning of the patient's behavior can be thoroughly understood only in the context of an ongoing therapy. The function of the emergency department should be limited to assessment of behavior. Supportively, but firmly, staff should obtain history needed to place the patient's behaviors in context, including a history of recent interpersonal events, perceived rejections, or changes in therapy. Risk of suicide should be assessed in the context of previous history, with a decision on hospitalization dependent on degree of genuine risk and availability of community support. Above all, the emergency department should be a piece of clear reality in the patient's otherwise uncertain and distorted perception of the world. The response of staff should be reasoned and consistent. Strong and effective limits should be placed on inappropriate behavior. When staff become excessively preoccupied by their psychodynamic role in a patient's therapy, they lose effectiveness in confrontation and limit setting that the borderline patient so often needs. The emergency department is truly "transitional" in that the patient's regressed behavior may stop here with the help of strict behavioral limits and support. To Perlmutter's psychodynamic perspective, one must add clear behavioral limits or run the risk of rewarding regression and encouraging "chronicity." The work of therapy lies elsewhere.

Annotated Bibliography

Looney, J. G., & Gunderson, E. K. (1978), Transient situational disturbances: Course and outcome. *Amer. J. Psychiat.*, 135:660–663.

This short paper examines the validity and usefulness of the DSM-III diagnostic category of transient situational disturbance in 2,078 naval personnel seen in an emergency room. The condition was found to be less severe and disabling than major psychiatric disorders in terms of chronicity, length of hospitalization, and disposition, and its outcome in terms of rehospitalization rates and work effectiveness also was relatively favorable. However, a substantial proportion of these patients, when reevaluated at a three-year follow-up, manifested personality disorder problems. The authors suggest that clearer criteria are needed to define situational disturbances operationally and to identify patients with underlying personality disorders.

Clayton, P. J., Herjanic, J., Murphy, G. E., & Woodruff, R. (1974), Mourning and depression: Their similarities and differences. *Canad. Psychiat. Assn. J.*, 19:309–312.

This paper, written by well-known investigators of bereavement, attempts to differentiate this condition from major depression. Two groups, patients with primary depressive illness and bereaved people, were compared. The depressive group seemed to have more symptoms and to seek help more frequently than the bereaved one. Because of their considerable overlap in symptomatology the two groups could not be differentiated satisfactorily for research purposes. For research purposes if the symptoms of depression occur only after the death of a near relative, the subjects should not be included in the group diagnosed as suffering from primary affective disorder. Interestingly enough, DSM-III contains as an exclusion the diagnostic criterion for major depression, the inference that the clinical manifestations are due to uncomplicated bereavement.

Singh, B., & Raphael, B. (1981), Postdisaster morbidity of the bereaved. A possible role for preventive psychiatry? *J. Nerv. Ment. Dis.*, 169:203–212.

The organization and implementation of a primary prevention program for the bereaved relatives of the Granville disaster is described in this paper. It utilized what was currently known about the process of bereavement in an attempt to facilitate that pertinent assistance was available to those who needed or could accept it. The exigencies of the situation, however, meant that help had to be organized and implemented on the spur of the moment. The analysis of the program outcome indicated that while bereavement counseling following a disaster may be helpful, the patterns of resolving grief may not be as standard as we think. Bereavement seems to be highly individual and related to factors such as age, relationship with the deceased (with parents most at risk for high morbidity), and basic emotional and cognitive style of the person involved.

Krupnick, J. L., & Horowitz, M. J. (1980), Stress response syndromes. *Arch. Gen. Psychiat.*, 38:428–435.

A look at recurrent themes in the case material of 30 psychotherapy patients treated for posttraumatic stress disorder after bereavement or personal injury. Rage at the source of the trauma figured prominently in both bereavement and personal injury cases. The themes found to be most prominent in bereavement cases included sadness over the loss and discomfort over discovered personal vulnerability. In the personal and injury cases, fear of a repetition of the event and feelings of responsibility emerged most frequently.

10

Trends in Suicidal Behavior and Its Management

R. D. Goldney, M.D., and P. W. Burvill, M.D.

> Since tea has been in fashion, even suicide has been more familiar amongst us than in times past.
>
> Jonas Hanway (1712–1786)

Fluctuating rates of suicidal behavior inevitably evoke statements regarding causality, and just as the social reformer Jonas Hanway (quoted by Muir [1976]) felt compelled to incriminate tea as contributing to an increase in suicide in the eighteenth century, even in the latter part of the twentieth century we are not free from sweeping assertions as to the genesis of suicidal behavior and its optimum management.

In reviewing the literature it is apparent that there has been a marked increase in research into such behavior in recent years. This has been documented by Farberow (1976) who noted that over 300 publications per year were appearing in the early 1970s, more than double the average number published in each of the preceding 13 years, and vastly more than the 2,100 items documented between 1897 and 1957 by the American National Clearinghouse for Mental Health In-

This chapter was first published in *Australian and New Zealand Journal of Psychiatry* (1980), 14:1–15, and it is reprinted by permission.

formation. However, in an examination of this literature, it is necessary to pay heed to the acerbic criticism of Kahne (1966), who claimed that the monotonous regularity with which the same types of data were reported, and the same stereotyped conclusions inferred from information organized in a fashion whose methodological error had long since been demonstrated, was only too rarely broken by original ventures beyond the conventional. Furthermore, he was of the opinion that most of the literature did not even qualify as research in the sense of deliberate hypothesis testing or careful evaluation of the theoretical alternatives implicit in a specific set of events. While not all recent work is free from such criticism, it appears that there have been developments in our understanding of suicidal behavior and its management which bear scrutiny.

Before pursuing these changing trends, it is perhaps pertinent to comment upon the very words "suicidal behavior," as they may provoke comment from some who would prefer to focus on either suicide or attempted suicide, regarding each as separate entities with different determinants. While Stengel (1960) is frequently referred to as having delineated two patterns of behavior, the fact that he also emphasized that there was overlap between them is sometimes disregarded. Furthermore, more recent reviews have suggested that it is possible to extrapolate from findings of attempted suicide to completed suicide (Lester, 1970a; Lester, Beck, and Mitchell, 1979), and Ottoson (1979) has concluded "that they are expressions of a common suicidal process." While not all would agree with Lester and Ottoson, there do appear to be grounds for considering them together in a review of this nature, although cognizance of the differences will also be made.

CHANGING RATES OF SUICIDAL BEHAVIOR

There have been marked fluctuations in the rates of suicide and attempted suicide in various countries. Sainsbury, Baert, and Jenkins (1979) reported that of the European countries, only Greece, Scotland, England, and Wales had recorded falls in suicide rate from 1961–1963 to 1972–1974, whereas it had increased in 15 other countries, including increases of over 30 percent in Denmark, Hungary, Ireland, the Netherlands, and Poland. The decrease had been most marked in England and Wales, where the fall had been a substantial 36 percent. There have also been fluctuations in the Australian figures. Thus the rates for 1977 of 16.0 and 6.2 per 100,000, respectively, for men and women represent a fall from the peak figures of 18.8 and 10.8 per 100,000 for 1965, but are of the same order as those recorded in 1955 of 15.1 and 5.4 per 100,000.

Kreitman (1979) pointed out that in recent years, throughout those parts of the world where reliable suicide data are available, there has been observed a fall in rates among the elderly in many countries, an increase among younger people, and a rise among females. In Australia, since 1971 the suicide rate has fallen most markedly in those aged 60 years and older, whereas it has been steadily rising among males aged 15–29 years (Burvill, 1980). Kreitman (1976) has raised the possibility that the increase in the younger males might be a relatively new phenomenon related to the illicit drug subculture among the young. However, another possibility is that it might be related to heavier alcohol consumption of younger males in recent years, since there is firm evidence of an association between alcoholism and heavy drinking, on the one hand, and suicide on the other.

One of the most universal findings of suicidal data throughout the world has been the increasing rate in females (Kreitman, 1979). It is very tempting to interpret this phenomenon as being due to the increasing emphasis on women's rights in the past two decades. This is a move that, no matter what the long-term benefits may be, in the short term has placed many women in situations of ambiguity, uncertainty, and conflict. French and Bryce (1978) have attempted to relate this to female aggression and anomic suicide. However, suicide is a very complex phenomenon with very many possible interacting causative variables, and as Kreitman (1979) has pointed out, we do not yet have a scientifically defensible model.

Rates for attempted suicide have increased dramatically in the last three decades, such that in Britain admissions for suicidal behavior to medical wards of general hospitals have become second in frequency only to those for coronary heart disease (Hetzel, 1974). Weissman (1974) reviewed the epidemiology of suicide attempts from 1960 to 1971 and reported wide variations in increase, up to a thirtyfold increase noted by Stanley (1969) between 1947 and 1968 in Ashton-under-Lyne in England. Australia has not been spared this worldwide trend. Thus Mills, Williams, Sale, Perkin, and Henderson (1974) reported a 58 percent increase of hospital treated cases of attempted suicide between 1968 and 1972 in Hobart, and Burvill (1975) noted an increase of approximately 100 percent in the number of attempted suicides admitted to the hospital in Perth over the 10–11 year period of 1961–1971–1972. Weissman and her colleagues (Wexler, Weissman, and Kasl, 1978) have recently reviewed further studies and observed: "When the international literature was brought up to date, no substantial changes in the trends observed in 1970 were noted . . . the high rates reported previously have been maintained." However, there is some evidence to suggest that the rate of attempted suicide may have peaked. Thus Holding, Buglass, Duffy, and Kreitman (1977) reported from Edinburgh that the attempted suicide rate for men had fallen, and that the rate for women, although still increasing, was leveling off. More recently, Koller and Slaghuis (1978) from Hobart noted a decline and leveling out of rates for both men and women, as have Burvill, Hobbs, and Armstrong (1980a) since 1974 in Perth.

Such fluctuations of the incidence of behaviors which tend to arouse mixed feelings in those who have contact, be it therapeutic or otherwise, have not unexpectedly produced a diversity of explanatory hypotheses. These hypotheses can be broadly considered under four main categories: first, the questioning of the statistics; second, the effect of social change; third, changes in the availability of method; and fourth, the provision of intervening services.

VALIDITY OF STATISTICS

Researchers agree that suicide is underreported, although estimates of the extent vary (Ovenstone, 1973). Dublin (1963) suggested one-third. Seager and Flood (1965) estimated that possible suicides among deaths reported as accidents, misadventure, or open verdicts might be as many as 50 percent of those actually returned as suicide. Important sources of underreporting lie in the method of ascertaining and recording suicide as well as in the religious and social attitudes of some countries.

The very low rate of suicide in Ireland has been critically examined by several workers. McCarthy and Walsh (1975) concluded that the discrepancy between official and "true" suicide rates was greater than in Scotland and in England and Wales, as religious and social attitudes tended to make coroners reluctant to return a suicide verdict. Furthermore, Barraclough (1978) demonstrated that the incidence of suicide in England and Wales in 1968–1970 was only twice as high as that in Eire, and not four times as stated in the official statistics. It is of note that the suicide rate of Irish immigrants to Australia, consisting of an unknown mixture of people born in both Eire and Northern Ireland, was found to be approximately the same as immigrants from Scotland and from England and Wales (Burvill, 1973).

Douglas (1967) cogently argued that since international comparisons of suicide rates were based on official statistics, which were of doubtful validity, the sociological theories developed to explain the alleged differences were meaningless. Ruzicka (1976) also considered them to be of doubtful value. Brooke and Atkinson (1974) exchanged samples of suicides from several centers in England and Denmark, and concluded that differences in ascertainment were probably too great to allow international comparisons to be made. However, Ross and Kreitman (1975) argued that the samples of cases used in their study were small, nonrandom, and selected to allow for possible differences of opinion, so that it was not possible to gauge how representative they were of countries from which they were drawn.

Sainsbury and Barraclough (1968) concluded that national and international statistics were sufficiently reliable to be of scientific value, although they need to be interpreted critically. They made the point that, although suicide was almost certainly underreported, for the purpose of most epidemiological studies the absolute rate was not needed. McCarthy and Walsh (1975) have argued that, if the extent of suicide underreporting in countries was known and appropriate adjustments were made to official figures, useful and meaningful comparisons would be possible. Brugha and Walsh (1978) maintained that there was a constancy in the degree of underreporting in any one country, and hence changes in statistics accurately reflected changes in the true rate.

To date there have been no studies of differential reporting of suicide between the various states of Australia apart from a working paper that ascertained differences in attitudes of practice of the various state coroners (Oliver, 1971). Oliver considered that the majority of unreported cases were classified as accidental death, with certain categories lending themselves to hiding suicide more than others. Poisoning with drugs was one, and others included death by gas and firearms, and possibly some cases of drowning and falling from heights.

The problem of what constitutes attempted suicide has been addressed by many authors, and has produced a plethora of terms, including "pseudocide" (Lennard-Jones and Asher, 1959),"self-poisoning" (Kessel, 1966), "parasuicide" (Kreitman, Philip, Greer, and Bagley, 1969), "acute poisoning" (Lawson and Mitchell, 1972a), "deliberate self-injury" (Jacobson and Tribe, 1972), "self-injury" (*Lancet,* 1974), "non-fatal deliberate self-harm" (Morgan, Pocock, and Pottle, 1975), and most recently "propetia" (Seager, 1978). Fortunately, for ease of comparison of studies, such terms do not obscure the fact that clinicians appear to be relatively consistent in what constitutes a subject for inclusion in reports. However, it should be noted that many studies contain extremely heterogeneous groups of patients, and broad conclusions drawn from such samples may not be applicable to other clinical populations.

No Australian study has tried to determine the number of attempted suicides who are treated by their general practitioner, or some other agency, without going to a hospital. Kennedy and Kreitman (1973) in a prospective study of general practitioners, found that hospital studies in Edinburgh underestimated the frequency of attempted suicide by at least 30 percent. Workers in London, Ontario, a town of 200,000 inhabitants went a step further. Information from all kinds of hospitals, nursing homes, doctors, welfare agencies, and the county jail gave a recorded rate of attempted suicide of 730 per 100,000 per year and an estimated rate of 1,433—a staggering 1 in 70 of the population each year (*Lancet,* 1971). Several Australian studies have included patients admitted to private hospitals. Edwards and Whitlock (1968) found seven such cases in Brisbane in 12 months, Henderson, Eastwood, and Montgomery (1972) two in Hobart in 12 months, and Burvill (1975) none in Perth in two years. It is suspected that, although the number going to private hospitals may be small, those who do so receive a different diagnostic designation.

While difficulties in assessing the reliability of the statistics of suicidal behavior are readily apparent, most modern researchers have sufficient confidence in such statistics to justify continued research in this area. However, until shortcomings in their derivation can be minimized, caution is urged in the interpretation of epidemiological or sociodemographic theories based on such data.

SOCIAL FACTORS

In a historical review, Rosen (1971) presented data that demonstrated that suicide has been regarded in quite diverse ways at different periods of time. He suggested that when suicide was examined in relation to changing social conditions, value systems, institutions, and ideologies different formulations of suicidal behavior became apparent. Thus it is of interest to reflect that it was not until the nineteenth century that sociological and medical explanations of suicide emerged.

Recent sociological theories have been well summarized by Lester (1972). Many of these (Powell, 1958; Gibbs and Martin, 1964; Ginsberg, 1966; Johnson, 1979) appear to derive directly from the hypotheses of Durkheim (1952), and merely provide a different way of viewing or reformulating the concept of "anomie." It is doubtful if any of these sociological theories advance our understanding of suicide beyond that provided by Durkheim. In contrast to these, Henry and Short (1954) employed the frustration-aggression hypothesis developed by Dollard, Miller, Doob, Mowrer, and Sears (1939) as their basic framework. Their conclusion was that suicide and homicide were acts of aggression, undifferentiated with respect to their common source in frustration generated by business cycles. Douglas (1967) rejected the validity and reliability of official statistics on suicide and the deductive-hypothetical approach. Instead he sought to identify the "meanings" of suicidal behavior. Bagley (1972) has suggested that suicide rates may be related to an authoritarian or clearly defined social structure. These theories are concerned only with suicide, but Wilkins (1967) has pointed out that there is no reason why a sociological theory of suicide should not also be germane to attempted suicide.

Lester (1972) discussed cultural differences in suicidal behaviors, and asserted that the task of explaining diverse cultural differences was difficult as our knowledge of the determinants of suicide was rudimentary. He put forward the view that it was likely that the determinants of suicide in individuals were similar to those behind cultural differences in suicide. If this were so, then he felt that the cultural investigation of suicide would have less general interest than the psychological and sociological investigations.

It is generally accepted that the rate of suicide is positively correlated with a wide variety of social factors such as loneliness, isolation, being single, widowed, or separated, divorce, alcoholism, urban rather than rural residence, being white rather than black (in the United States), and being in the upper social class. Other factors are less well established, and differences exist between different centers. Thus McCulloch, Philip, and Carstairs (1967) in Edinburgh, reported positive correlations with the density of population, the degree of overcrowding, the divorce rate, juvenile delinquency, and attempted suicide. He found no such correlation with the incidence of infant mortality and stillbirth, migrant and senior citizen status, rent arrears, subpoenas, and road fatalities. Comparable studies have been conducted by Sainsbury (1955) in London, Chuaqui, Lemkau, Legarreta, and Contreras (1966) in Santiago, Chile, Maris (1969) in Chicago, and Lester (1970b) in Buffalo, New York. The results of these studies conflict; for example, population density and overcrowding were found to correlate positively with suicide by McCulloch et al., and Chuaqui et al., but not by Sainsbury or Lester. Lester (1972) listed three possible explanations for these conflicts: the inconsistencies could mean the associations were unreliable and that there was probably no association between the variables; they could indicate that the associations were weak and so not found in every case; or they could indicate that the cities of Edinburgh, London, Santiago, Chicago, and Buffalo were very different and that suicidal behavior was differently determined in each. Unfortunately, there appears to be no satisfactory way at present of distinguishing between these alternatives.

One explanation of these inconsistencies could be that suicidal behavior is not a single entity. For example, Bagley and Jacobson (1976) tested a hypothesis in Brighton, England that three types of suicide ("old and handicapped," "sociopathic," and "depressed") would vary in prevalence across ecologically defined urban areas. The hypothesis was supported with respect to the old and handicapped suicide, which predominated in middle-class areas with established residents of middle-class status, and with respect to sociopathic suicide, which predominated in central areas with high social pathology of all kinds and poor housing conditions.

The features characterizing those who attempt suicide have also been extensively reported, and Weissman (1974) noted that there was a general consensus that such persons were likely to be younger women, more often separated and/or divorced, more frequently in the lower socioeconomic groups, living in a city, excessively hostile and depressed with personality disturbances, and that they would have used alcohol and had a recent interpersonal conflict before their attempt. These findings are by no means invariable, and individual studies require critical analysis with regard to sampling and assessment procedures. The constraints of this review preclude a detailed examination of these factors, but there are two additional social issues that are particularly relevant to the current Australasian scene and warrant close scrutiny. These are the factors of migration and unemployment.

Migration

The possibility that migration may have an effect on the suicide rate has long been assumed. For example, Pfister-Ammende (1955) found among just over 5,000 refugees in Switzerland a suicide rate 5.4 times that of the Swiss population, whereas no suicide was recorded among 3,000 repatriates, and Yap (1958) showed that the suicide rate for post-World War II immigrants to Hong Kong was four times that of the population comprising prewar immigrants and persons born in Hong Kong. In the United States, Dublin (1963) noted that the suicide rate among foreign born males was twice that of the total United States male rate. Whitlock (1971) found the suicide rates of immigrants to Australia to be substantially higher than those prevailing in their countries of origin and among the Australian-born population. However, he cautioned that the results were based on comparatively small numbers of suicides in minority population groups, and that his results might well have been different had they been based on larger populations.

There are more striking differences when individual migrant groups are considered. Thus Burvill (1973) found a ninefold difference between the highest and lowest suicide rates of the 15 most populous European immigrant groups in Australia. Those immigrant groups with high rates in Australia came from European countries with high rates, and vice versa. Immigrants from four countries, Italy, Greece, Malta, and the Netherlands, each had suicide rates in 1962–1966 substantially lower than the Australian born. Subsequently Burvill, Woodings, Stenhouse, and McCall (1980) have found low rates for the years 1962–1971 also in immigrants from India/Pakistan, all other Asian countries, and in those from the United Arab Republic. Available published data show that these countries all have lower suicide rates than Australia. There were also marked differences in methods of suicide used by the various immigrant groups, although recent evidence suggests that the longer immigrants are in Australia, the more likely they are to adopt methods of suicide chosen by native-born Australians (Burvill, 1973; Burvill et al., 1980).

There are conflicting findings with regard to the importance of migration and attempted suicide. Thus, while Gold (1965) reported attempted suicide rates for migrants twice those expected in northeast Tasmania, Buckle, Linnane, and McConaghy (1965) found no difference in rates between migrants and nonmigrants in Melbourne, and Krupinski and Stoller (1965), also in Melbourne, reported a higher incidence of attempted suicide in non-British immigrants than among British and Australian born. On the basis of their own work and a review of earlier Australian studies, Edwards and Whitlock (1968) concluded that immigration was not a significant cause of attempted suicide, although they did report a significantly lower rate in immigrants from the United Kingdom. More recent reports have continued the debate. Ewing et al. (quoted by Burvill [1973]) found a higher incidence among immigrants than Australian born in Perth, and Burvill (1975) also in Perth, using data standardized for age (an essential prerequisite for studies of this type), reported almost identical rates for immigrant and Australian-born women, but an excess rate for immigrant men. He also pointed out large variations in attempted suicide rates between different immigrant groups. Such a finding has also been reported in Birmingham by Burke (1976a,b,c) who noted a higher rate among Irish immigrants compared with the native born, both in Ireland and in Britain. By contrast, he found lower rates of attempted suicide among Asian (Bangladesh, India, and Pakistan) and West Indies immigrants.

Burvill, Hobbs, and Armstrong (1980) are currently analyzing further attempted suicide data in Perth, and preliminary results indicate statistically significant lower rates in immigrants from Italy, Greece, the Netherlands, India, Pakistan, and other Asian countries.

Such findings illustrate the complexity of this area, and the comment of Murphy (1977), although not made specifically with regard to suicidal behavior, is particularly germane: "[I]t should be clear that generalizing about the mental health of migrants without specifying the cultural origins, the conditions of migration and the type of disorder being referred to is likely to be both misleading and unhelpful, being a carry-over of the old 'we' and 'they' attitude."

Unemployment

Difficulty in evaluating conflicting reports is also evident in considering the effect of unemployment on suicidal behavior. In an early study, McMahon, Johnson, and Pugh (1963) demonstrated a close correlation between the suicide rate for males in the 45–54 year age group and the total unemployment rates over the years 1930–1955 in the United States. However, Maris (1969) and Lester (1970c) were unable to confirm this in studies in Chicago and Pennsylvania respectively, and in fact reported a negative association between suicide and unemployment rates. There have been several studies that have demonstrated that those who are unemployed are disproportionately represented among those who commit suicide (Sainsbury, 1955; Ovenstone, 1973; Morris, Kovacs, Beck, and Wolffe, 1974), but a causal relationship cannot be assumed. High suicide rates during the depression years of the 1930s, a time of major unemployment, have been well documented. However, in Australia, the 1960s were a time of economic prosperity and full employment, yet male suicide rates rose to levels comparable with those of the 1930s, and the corresponding female rates were, by far, the highest recorded in this century (Burvill et al., 1980). By contrast, there has been a progressive fall in suicide rates during the 1970s, the latter years of which have had unemployment rates second only to the 1930s.

Unemployment and suicidal behavior is a particularly emotive area, and conclusions must be drawn with great caution. Indeed, the comment of Kreitman (1979) in a paper appropriately titled "Preventive Enthusiasm and Scientific Caution," is most pertinent: "Studies which combine elegant epidemiology with crude journalism do a great deal of harm, and represent one of the barriers to further understanding."

The Interpersonal Environment

Although sociological issues undoubtedly influence suicide and attempted suicide, it must be emphasized that many of the factors alluded to are merely correlated with such behavior, and causality should not necessarily be inferred. Furthermore, many of these broad issues do not readily lend themselves to experimental manipulation, and there now appears to be a trend in the literature toward focusing down on the actual circumstances preceding suicidal behavior. Thus Paykel, Prusoff, and Myers (1975), found "a strong and immediate relationship between suicide attempts and life events," Cochrane and Robertson (1975) reported that such patients had experienced far more unpleasant life changing events in the year preceding the act than had controls; Wilson (1971) noted evidence for a serious disruption of interpersonal relationship between young people attempting suicide and key personnel in their immediate environment; and Adam, Bianchi, Hawker, Nairn, Sandford, and Scarr (1978) reported "a high percentage of all subjects were found to have had a family life rated as unstable to chaotic and an even greater number were experiencing serious difficulties in their current interpersonal relationships."

These findings suggest that at the time of crisis prior to their suicide attempt, subjects perceive themselves as having insufficient or inadequate supports to cope with their changing environment.

While such findings may appear self-evident to the clinician, it may not be until hypotheses regarding the nature of interpersonal relationships can be critically evaluated that intervention on a scientific basis can be offered. Indeed, the work of Henderson, Byrne, Duncan-Jones, Adcock, Scott, and Steele (1978) in Canberra, who have developed an interview schedule for social interaction that allows quantification of the amount and adequacy of social relationships, may well prove to be of value in this area.

AVAILABILITY OF METHOD

Opinion is divided in the literature as to whether elimination of a method of suicide results in a drop in overall suicide rates. Stengel (1969) cited evidence from Switzerland that suggested that as one method of suicide was eliminated another method was soon substituted. By contrast Kreitman (1976) wondered if, for some, the scenario of suicide specified the use of a particular method, and that if this were not available actual suicide then became less likely. The *International Classification of Diseases* (ICD) included railroads as a suicidal method from 1940 to 1950. The elimination of this method from the ICD categories of suicide after 1950 was presumably due to a worldwide reduction in reporting of this method of suicide. It is difficult to be convinced that there was a reduced availability of railway engines dating from 1951. Similarly the use of cutting and piercing instruments formed 18 percent of all male suicides in Australia in the early part of this century, but rapidly dropped after the 1930s (Burvill, 1980). There has been no shortage of opportunity for using this method since then.

Inspection of the methods of suicide in different countries suggest that tradition, or some other social or cultural factor, determines suicide method as much as availability of method. Thus hanging has long been, by far, the most commonly used method of male suicide in most European countries, in contrast to the almost equal use of domestic gas (until the 1960s) and overdosage in British males, and of shooting in American, Australian, and Canadian males.

Coal Gas

The most frequently cited example of suicide rates dropping with the elimination of a commonly used method is that of the reduction in the number of suicides in the United Kingdom being attributed to the conversion of domestic gas from a toxic to a nontoxic form (Hassall and Trethowan, 1972; Kreitman, 1976). Such a relationship has also been reported in Australia (Snowden, 1979). However, this view has recently been challenged by Sainsbury et al. (1979) who reported that "the widely advocated claim that the decline in the suicide rate in England and Wales is due to the removal of the method of killing oneself by coal gas poisoning is tested by the detailed studies in England and in the Netherlands that show that this hypothesis cannot be upheld." Such a challenge appears to be based on the continued increase in suicide rate in the Netherlands despite the detoxification of their gas. In the absence of published data, such a refutation must be considered extremely carefully. One must remember that poisoning by coal gas represented a major proportion of the deaths by suicide in the United Kingdom, whereas it has never been so in the Netherlands, where suicide by hanging has been predominant. Thus the disappearance of coal gas suicides from the Netherlands figures would have minimal effect on the overall suicide rate. Indeed, Kreitman (1979) remains of the opinion that at present there does not appear to be published data to refute the impact of detoxified gas on the suicide rates of those countries in which death by coal gas contributed significantly to the suicide rate.

It is of interest to note that those who survive jumping from the Golden Gate Bridge (a very small number) do not attempt suicide by alternative methods (Rosen, 1975), and the proponents of the coal gas story would similarly suggest that those who may have suicided by gas do not choose other methods. However, the number of such survivors is very small, and it may be unwise to extrapolate from this special group to those who may have used toxic gas had it been available. Furthermore, Burvill (1980) has demonstrated that in Australia, for males but not females, suicide rates from poisoning from nondomestic gas (in practice, carbon monoxide poisoning from motor vehicle exhausts) rose sharply from the mid-1960s to 1977, in proportion to the dramatic drop in suicide from domestic gas. This suggests that Australian males substituted one form of gas poisoning for another when the latter became unavailable, and the coal gas debate does not appear to be conclusively resolved.

Prescribed Drugs

An increase in the availability of prescribed sedative drugs has been cited as contributing to the increased rate of suicide and attempted suicide in the 1960s (Hetzel, 1971). By contrast, Gibbs (1972), who was employed in the pharmaceutical industry, vigorously refuted this suggestion. Kreitman (1977) reported that there was no difference in the proportion of subjects attempting suicide by using prescribed as compared to nonprescribed drugs from 1962 to 1972 in Edinburgh, and concluded that this "militates against the often cited opinion that the increase in parasuicide is largely the consequence of more liberal prescribing by doctors."

What can more confidently be asserted is that changing prescribing patterns influence the type of drugs ingested in suicide and attempted suicide. Whereas barbiturates were used predominantly in the 1960s, now the benzodiazepine class of drug is most commonly ingested in attempted suicide. The tricyclic antidepressants have also assumed an increasing role, and their use is now comparable to that of the barbiturates (Proudfoot and Park, 1978). The correlation of suicide rates with barbiturate prescribing was noted by Oliver and Hetzel (1972), although Whitlock (1975) has suggested that suicide may not simply have been related to the ready availability of those drugs, but to "a sharp increase in barbiturate dependence, a condition known to be associated with a high frequency of attempted suicide." Limitation on the prescription of barbiturates may have been responsible for a fall in suicide by barbiturates, but equally it is possible that the advent of the safer benzodiazepine drugs may have been used for those patients previously prescribed barbiturates.

It is also pertinent to note the suggestion by Edwards and Whitlock (1968) that the packaging of individual drugs in cellophane or tinfoil may have had an effect on those persons whose suicidal behavior appears to have been impulsively determined.

While one may have firmly held beliefs regarding the effects of the prescription and nature of drugs in influencing suicidal behavior it is again evident that the determining of causal links is very difficult.

Firearms

The use of firearms deserves mention as this represents the most common method of male suicide in Canada and the United States (Stengel, 1969). In Australia the age standardized rate of male suicide from firearms and explosives has remained fairly constant, except for a drop during World War II, in spite of marked fluctuations in the rates of other methods (Burvill, 1980). Except at the peak of suicide rates from overdosages in the mid-1960s, the use of firearms and explosives has always been the most common male suicide method in Australia, and in rural areas, in Western Australia at least, this method of suicide comprises up to 44 percent of all male suicides (Burvill, 1970). By contrast it has never been a very common form of suicide in the United Kingdom. These differences between the United States, Canada, Australia, and the United Kingdom are probably related to different licensing laws and general use and availability of guns in society.

The use of firearms in suicide also appears to be associated with their concurrent use for murder. In Canada no less than 10 percent of suicides follow murder, thus investing this problem with even greater significance (Sim, 1979). While a complete ban on the use of firearms would be unrealistic, there does appear to be a case for a greater degree of control than at present.

A recent hypothesis may throw light on the apparent contradictions of some of the foregoing studies. Farmer (quoted by Kreitman [1979]) has suggested that three clusters of suicide methods can be identified: first, those involving violent methods such as shooting, hanging, and the like, all of which appear to be closely interrelated; second, deaths due to domestic gas; and third, the large group due to drugs. He claimed that each of these groups seems to pursue a partially independent course over time, such that if one declines there is no automatic compensation by an increase in other groups. This hypothesis would be consistent with Whitlock's (1975) opinion that curtailing the availability of "easy" methods of suicide (domestic gas, hypnotics, and sedatives) does not inevitably lead to greater use of other methods.

It is thus apparent that although certain general assumptions can be made about the availability and choice of method used in suicidal behavior, scientific studies confirming such assumptions appear either to be lacking or in some doubt. Whether reduction in availability of a common method of suicide provides a legitimate avenue of suicide prevention is also currently in some doubt.

EFFECT OF INTERVENTION

It may appear somewhat specious to speculate on the possibility that improved treatment facilities may have influenced the rate of suicidal behavior when attempted suicide has increased throughout the world, and suicide has similarly increased in all but a handful of countries. However, a number of clinical studies have demonstrated the importance of psychiatric illness and social problems in association with both suicide (Robins, Murphy, Wilkinson, Gassner, and Kayes, 1959; Barraclough, Bunch, Nelson, and Sainsbury, 1974; Kraft and Babigian, 1976; Chynoweth, Tonge, and Armstrong, 1980) and attempted suicide (Weissman, 1974; Kreitman, 1977), thus suggesting that intervention should influence the rate of suicidal behavior.

Primary Intervention

The prevention of such behavior should ideally be considered as one of primary prevention, aimed at averting a first suicidal act by focusing therapeutic measures on those most at risk. While it is evident that a number of studies have delineated sociodemographic factors correlated with suicidal behavior, it is again noted that causality cannot be assumed. Furthermore, while these factors may be of use in assessing individual patients, they do not necessarily lend themselves to experimental manipulation in order to ascertain the effectiveness of intervention programs. Thus, it is not unexpected that there is a paucity of reports of the primary prevention of suicidal behavior.

Certainly there have been speculative comments such as those of Parnell and Skottowe (1957) that "the number of suicides at Oxford University has dropped since widespread public and private discussions brought better recognition of this problem," and of Koller and Slaghuis (1978) that the attempted suicide rate in Hobart had declined because "public attitudes have become increasingly hardened and intolerant of attempted suicide." However, when one seeks hard data, it is germane that Kreitman (1977) reported: "there does not appear to be in the literature any report of a service specifically set up with the aim of prevention of parasuicide."

Although not designed in order to reduce the rate of suicidal behavior, there are several studies that allow such an evaluation. Walk (1967) has provided a detailed analysis of the effect of the comprehensive community psychiatry service provided at Chichester in England. This service has been described in detail by Morrissey (1966), and is generally regarded as being a pioneer in the field of the community provision of psychiatric care. Walk concluded that although there appeared to be no effect on the overall suicide rate of the area, "it may have protected some elderly patients from suicide."

Nielsen and Videbach (1973) reported no difference in the suicide rate on the Danish island of Samsø following the introduction of a community psychiatry service. It should be noted that this service, in contrast to that in Chichester, comprised only a visiting psychiatrist, who was able to make hospital, outpatient, and home consultations at least once a week.

A further report of a comprehensive community based service is provided by Ebie and his colleagues (Ebie, Hicks, Lythe, and Short, 1970; Ebie, 1971) from Edinburgh. A Health, Welfare, and Advice Centre was established in the Craigmillar ward of Edinburgh, an area comprised of a predominantly lower socioeconomic group, with numerous social problems and a high rate of attempted suicide when compared to other areas of the city. A wide range of social agencies was represented, with at least one being constantly available, and contact with the police and citizens' organizations was said to be excellent. Although the center appeared to attract persons considered at risk for attempting suicide, the actual rate remained relatively constant over the next two years. This constancy of attempted suicide rates could be construed as a favorable outcome when compared to the increasing rates of other Edinburgh wards, but insufficient data were available for a definitive statement to be made, and Kreitman (1977) noted that "the safest conclusion would appear to be one of 'not proven.' "

The role of telephone counseling organizations, such as the Samaritans, has received serious consideration as to whether they influence suicidal behavior. The work of Bagley (1968) has been influential in suggesting that such organizations are associated with a reduction in the suicide rate. He demonstrated that the suicide rate in 15 towns in England and Wales with Samaritan Suicide Prevention Schemes was significantly less than that of matched control towns. Other studies from Los Angeles (Litman and Farberow, 1969) and Vienna (Ringel, 1969), although lacking adequate control populations, appeared to support this view. However, Lester (1974) and Bridge, Potkins, Zung, and Soldo (1977) in the United States, and Barraclough and his colleagues (Barraclough, Jennings, and Moss, 1977; Jennings, Barraclough, and Moss, 1978) in England have not supported these earlier findings. The most cogent rebuttal of the role of the Samaritans in reducing the suicide rate is presented by Jennings et al. (1978). They selected control towns on the basis of a greater number of ecological variables and predictors of suicide rate than did Bagley (1968). Thus they were able to compare the suicide rates of towns with Samaritan schemes with four sets of control towns: 15 towns matched for Bagley's original towns; 23 pairs from all England and Wales county boroughs; 33 matched on suicide rates before the opening of the Samaritans; and 35 towns matched on the percentage of single-person households, a variable which correlates well with the suicide rate. They found no significant difference between the Samaritan and control towns, and concluded "our findings seriously undermine the scientific case for the Samaritan's effectiveness in reducing the suicide rate."

Also pertinent to the role of such organizations is the study of Holding (1974) which reported the effects of a BBC program based on the Samaritans' work entitled "The Befrienders," which ran for ten weeks at peak viewing time on Saturday evenings. While the number of calls to the Samaritan organization increased dramatically, neither the rate for suicide nor attempted suicide was affected.

While carefully controlled studies suggest that such organizations may not influence the rate of suicidal behavior, such results cannot be used to assert that they do not play an important role in the alleviation of stress in those who call.

Secondary Intervention

It is well documented that a significant proportion of those who engage in suicidal behavior have previously done so. Thus for the Edinburgh Regional Poisoning Treatment Centre 40 percent of patients have a previous history of attempted suicide, and 19 percent can be anticipated to repeat their act within the ensuing year (Chowdhury, Hicks, and Kreitman, 1973). Australian figures are lower, with Edwards and Whitlock (1968) noting that 32 percent of men and 38 percent of women attempters had previously done so, and that 5 percent would repeat their attempt within a year. Koller and Slaghuis (1978) reported even lower figures of previous attempts of 22.2, 23.5, and 13.8 percent for those who attempted suicide in the years 1973, 1975, and 1977 respectively.

Assessment

There have been conflicting views as to the value of specialized treatment centers for such patients. Kennedy (1972) suggested that fewer patients treated at the Edinburgh Regional Poisoning Treatment Centre repeated their attempt, but Lawson and Mitchell (1972b) presented data that suggested that comparable results could be obtained by using a general medical unit with visiting psychiatrists. There are also differing opinions as to who should initially assess these patients.

Since the recommendation of the British Ministry of Health (1968) that all persons who attempt suicide have psychiatric assessment, this has been the accepted practice (ideally), certainly in Britain, Australia, and New Zealand. However, recently this view has been challenged (Gardner, Hanka, O'Brien, Page, and Rees, 1977, Gardner, Hanka, Mountford, O'Brien, and Roberts, 1978; Blake and Mitchell, 1978; Blake and Bramble, 1979; Newson-Smith and Hirsch, 1979) and it appears important to examine these reports in some detail.

Gardner and his colleagues presented data that demonstrated that "junior doctors and nurses" on a medical team were as effective as psychiatrists in evaluating suicidal risk, and identifying patients requiring psychiatric or social work management. However, it is of note that initially they felt "junior doctors . . . did not know how to undertake the psychological and social evaluation of self-poisoned patients" and, therefore, a teaching program designed to assist in the evaluation of such subjects was instituted for the reported study. Indeed, it is partly because of this special teaching program that Hill (1978) and Enoch and Copeland (1978) have urged caution before disregarding the Ministry of Health Guidelines.

Blake and Bramble (1979), contrary to Gardner and his colleagues, expressed confidence in the assessment of these patients by junior doctors. They reported considerable agreement between junior doctors and psychiatrists in the allocation of patients to either admission to psychiatric hospital, psychiatric outpatient appointment, referral to the social services department, or to take no further action. However, the junior doctor participants in this study, although receiving no special instructions, had to complete a questionnaire regarding their management before routine psychiatric assessment, and it is difficult to avoid considering the possibility that such a procedure may have enhanced their clinical assessment.

Blake and Mitchell (1978), in a study of patients who had attempted suicide in Nottingham, reported a considerable variation in management between ten psychiatric teams. Although the percentage of patients referred on for psychiatric hospital admission varied only between 12 and 24 percent, there were marked differences between the teams in the percentage of subjects where no further action was taken. Thus one team recommended no further action for 51 percent of subjects, and another, no further action for only 4 percent, whereas the average was for no further action in 31 percent of subjects. For these reasons, and the fact that 51 percent of patients actually did not receive continuing care (through either not being considered in need of it, or by nonattendance), they suggested that "the time has come to re-examine the widely held assumption that every overdose is a cry for skilled psychiatric help." While one can agree that all assumptions should be periodically challenged, it would appear that some of their reasoning extends beyond the data presented. Thus reference is made to "psychiatric and vocational scheme trainees" being mostly foreign medical graduates, such that linguistic and cultural barriers may have impaired their assessment, and also to their belief that "they do not have sufficient experience either in psychiatry or in general medicine to convince the medical ward team that the consultation has added to their own appraisal of the problem.'' While it is possible that their results are not unique to Nottingham, such findings should be replicated before drawing far-reaching conclusions.

Newson-Smith and Hirsch (1979) reported a study which demonstrated that social workers could ''safely and reliably'' assess patients who had attempted suicide. However, they were ''more cautious'' than psychiatrists in that they excluded mental illness less often. On the basis of their findings they suggested that social workers could provide the initial assessment of such patients, although ''it would be necessary for a psychiatrist to be available for consultations about urgent problems.''

Kennedy and Oswald (1979) have made comment on the findings of Gardner et al. (1977, 1978) and Newson-Smith and Hirsch (1979). They noted that the psychiatrists in those studies referred twice as many patients for both inpatient and outpatient follow-up than were so referred at the Edinburgh Regional Poisoning Treatment Centre, and suggested that this may be due to the fact that ''psychiatric services for parasuicides in these other centers largely depend on junior psychiatrists, who share out the work and have other commitments, and therefore diluted experience and supervision.'' They further suggested that the specialized unit in Edinburgh may, therefore, in fact, be more efficient than those other centers against which the junior doctors and social workers had been compared.

Clearly, as in the other areas of suicidal behavior discussed, it is a complex matter and has yet to be resolved. For the present time, it would appear to be in the patient's best interest to be assessed by the most experienced psychiatric clinician available.

Management

It was not until 1971 that Greer and Bagley demonstrated that psychiatric intervention was associated with a significant reduction in subsequent suicidal behavior. Since that time there have been a number of studies designed to determine whether improved follow-up management would result in a further reduction of such behavior. Chowdhury et al. (1973) in Edinburgh provided an intensive after care service for persons who had repeated suicide attempts. It comprised a full-time psychiatrist and psychiatric social worker, and two part-time social workers, and allowed for the provision of domiciliary visits and a 24-

hour emergency service, as well as outpatient clinics. They precluded 42 of 197 subjects because of their high risk of repetition (based on a prediction of further suicidal behavior scale developed by Buglass and McCulloch [1970]), and allocated the other patients to either their treatment program or to the conventional care offered by other unit staff. After six months there was no difference between the treatment and control groups with regard to repeated suicide attempts, there being 24 and 23 percent respectively. However, there was a significant improvement, which was most marked for women, in the social circumstances of the treated group when compared with the controls.

Ettlinger (1975) reported disappointing results from Stockholm. Six hundred and seventy patients treated in the years 1964–1966 were offered extensive follow-up care at the time of their suicide attempt, at one month, six months, and one year. The outcome of these patients was compared to that of 681 patients admitted to the same ward under the same circumstances in the preceding three years, before prolonged and intensive follow-up was available. She found the number of suicides and repeated suicide attempts to be similar for the two groups in a follow-up of 5–6 years. In addition, after 3–4 years, the outcome in the two groups was similar with regard to registered sickness, criminality, abuse of alcohol, and social assistance.

The report of Termansen and Bywater (1975) from Vancouver is noteworthy as it offered no treatment, apart from that given by emergency room staff, to one group of patients. A second group was assessed in the emergency room by a mental health worker and followed by that person with direct contact; the third was assessed by a mental health worker, but then followed by a crisis center volunteer by telephone only; and the fourth was assessed by a mental health worker, but no follow-up was made. All were assessed after 12 weeks, and the group with the direct contact were reported to have a greater degree of improvement with respect to a variety of measures of "role impairment," and less repeated attempts.

These findings are gratifying, but should be regarded with some caution. Of the original 280 patients, only 202 participated, and of these only 128 could be evaluated after the short period of 12 weeks. It may also be pertinent that the assessment of outcome was performed by the same mental health worker who had had the continuing contact. Furthermore, such contact was quite intensive, the minimum being "daily for week 1, every two days for week 2, twice a week for weeks

3 and 4, once a week for weeks 5 to 8, and every two weeks for weeks 9 to 12.''

Welu (1977) reported the results of a ''special outreach program'' employed in Pittsburgh. Suicide attempters were allocated on the basis of a table of random numbers to either the routine existing service or the experimental program. Members of the team saw patients as soon as possible after discharge, in their homes, and then each week, or at least biweekly, during the follow-up period. Subjects were assessed after 4 months, and ''the experimental group showed a statistically significant reduction in suicide reattempts and excessive use of alcohol.'' It is of interest to reflect that there were 63 subjects who received the special program, and that the team consisted of four registered nurses, three social workers, and two community workers.

An evaluation of the effect of a social work service for patients who had attempted suicide has been reported by Gibbons, Butler, Urwin, and Gibbons (1978) in Southampton, U.K. They allocated patients to either a social work follow-up, which comprised a mean number of 10 interviews in the patient's home, or to routine treatment, which included general practice and psychiatric referral. However, it must be noted that 139 of 539 initially assessed patients were excluded from the study, either because they had a severe psychiatric illness requiring immediate treatment, they were thought to be an immediate suicide risk, or they were already in treatment with another psychiatrist or social worker. Thus Gibbons and his colleagues acknowledge that their sample ''represents relatively lower-risk self-poisoners.''

Assessment after one year demonstrated no difference between the groups in the proportion of repeated suicide attempts (about 14 percent), and both groups had improved significantly on measures of depressed mood and of social problems. However, those patients who had social work follow-up ''showed more change in social problems and were more satisfied with the service they had received.''

Notwithstanding the methodological difficulties in these reports they appear to stand as landmarks in attempts to provide controlled studies of the effectiveness of psychosocial intervention for those who have attempted suicide. It is of note that the two studies that reported less subsequent suicidal behavior had the briefest follow-up periods. It is also of note that although social change was effected in four of the five reports, the ratio of therapists to patient and the degree of contact provided would tax most general hospital social and psychiatric departments to the utmost.

A quite different approach was recently reported by Montgomery, Montgomery, Rani, Roy, Shaw, and McAuley (1979).They selected patients with a history of two or more previous episodes of suicidal behavior, and excluded subjects with "overt schizophrenia or depression." Thus 37 patients were randomly allocated in a double blind placebo-controlled trial to receive either 20 mg intramuscular flupenthixol decanoate or placebo. Thirty patients completed a six-month trial, and it is of note that even by the end of the second month there was a significant difference between the groups, and that after six months only 3 of 14 patients who had flupenthixol had repeated their suicidal behavior, whereas 12 of the 17 who had placebo had done so, a highly significant difference. It would appear that this is the only report of a prophylactic benefit from any drug in the prevention of repeated suicidal behavior, and as such it warrants not only the closest scrutiny, but also replication in other centers.

Such a finding, with a carefully selected group of patients, is a salutary vindication of the comment by Henderson and Williams (1974), who in support of distinguishing a typology of suicidal behavior observed: "since it is not a unitary phenomenon . . . a single preventive measure is therefore unlikely to have widespread success." Such a comment and such research indicates the need to further distinguish specific subgroups. However, it cannot then be assumed that such a delineation of particular groups at risk will necessarily be of practical value in all instances. For example, Chowdhury et al. (1973) and Gibbons et al. (1978) were able to identify patients most at risk for repeating suicide attempts, but the fact that 56 percent of the Edinburgh high-risk group repeated within six months and 36 percent of the Southampton sample did so within one year suggests that although psychiatric and social services were apparently available and used by the most disturbed patients, at the very least such services did not prevent further suicidal behavior.

Other categorizations of attempted suicide have been proposed in the last 15 years (Dorpat and Boswell, 1963; Shneidman, 1966; Patel, 1974; Kiev, 1976; Henderson, Hartigan, Davidson, Lance, Duncan-Jones, Koller, Ritchie, McAuley, Williams, and Slaghuis, 1977), but although each appears to have heuristic value, they do not appear to have been systematically evaluated in the clinical setting.

Depression

The clinician does not have a body of data that unequivocally points toward one treatment program, but must rely on his clinical judgment with individual patients. It is thus important to focus on depression, the condition most likely to be encountered in those who have attempted suicide, and which is of major importance in those who actually suicide. The difficulties in the area of psychiatric diagnosis and the nosology of depression tend to obscure its importance in suicidal behavior. It is generally diagnosed in 35–80 percent of those who have attempted suicide (Weissman, 1974), but it has also been argued that all those who attempt suicide manifest some degree of depressive affect, and that it is "legitimate to try to measure this in every case" (Birtchnell and Alarcon, 1971). It is of interest that when standardized measures of depression are employed, higher rates of depression are recorded than when rates are derived from clinical assessment alone (Weissman and Myers, 1978). Thus patients who have attempted suicide have been demonstrated to have depression comparable to that of other psychiatric patients undergoing treatment (Birtchnell and Alarcon, 1971; Weissman, Fox, and Klerman, 1973; El Gaaly, 1974; Goldney, 1978).

It is also pertinent to note that there appears to be no difference in the degree of depression between those whose suicide attempt has been medically life threatening, and those whose attempt has produced minimal physical effect (Pallis and Birtchnell, 1977; Goldney, 1979a). Furthermore, additional work, which awaits replication, indicates that even in that subgroup of patients most prone to attempting suicide, women aged 18–30, as many as one-third may have the biological features of depression which are generally considered to respond to antidepressant medication (Goldney, 1979a).

The optimum management of the depressive component of those who have attempted suicide is another area in which differences of opinion exist, and in which sweeping statements are sometimes made. Thus Birtchnell (1975) has gone so far as to say that "treatment of depressive symptoms *per se* is undesirable and may even be dangerous," and Hale (1977) has noted "one might venture to question whether one should ever prescribe psychotropic medication for the under 40s (apart of course from the neuroleptics)."

Such views appear to be unnecessarily restrictive, especially when the work of Weissman, Kasl, and Klerman (1976) and Weissman, Prusoff, Dimascio, Neu, Goklaney, and Klerman (1979), investigating the use of psychotherapy and antidepressant medication, either alone or in combination is considered. In reporting the outcome of "non-bipolar, non-psychotic, acute primary major depression" they reported that "the combination treatment of psychotherapy and pharmacotherapy was more effective than either treatment alone and delayed the onset of symptomatic failure." Although these results were not for subjects who had specifically attempted suicide, it would be unexpected if they were totally irrelevant to such patients.

It is also pertinent to consider the suggestion of Barraclough (1972) that 15 to 20 percent of suicides in Britain could be prevented if lithium prophylaxis for recurrent depressive illnesses were effectively employed. Finally, it should be noted that a large number of medically prescribed drugs have been claimed to cause depression in some patients. Whitlock (1977) has provided a list of some 50 drugs (no doubt this list is now longer), and has pointed out that: "putting it bluntly, we can do a lot to prevent suicide if we make use of the medical facts associated with the behaviour."

CONCLUSION

The outcome of such a discursive examination of recent trends in suicidal behavior and its management is satisfying neither to the reviewers, nor to the reader. It is apparent that far-reaching conclusions have sometimes been reached, more on the basis of firmly held belief than by scientific enquiry, but it is equally apparent that scientific testing of some hypotheses will prove to be difficult given the ethical considerations involved and the nature of the problem. Although the complexity of suicidal behavior has long been recognized (Stengel, 1960), it bears reiteration, and one can only but agree with the comment of Kreitman (1979) "that we know less than we usually imagine."

While it is possible that broad public health measures such as the provision of community supports, the restriction of certain drugs and their packaging, and legislation regarding the availability of firearms may have an effect on the rate of suicidal behavior, there is an increasing body of data that can be applied in the clinical situation. Thus there is now evidence that intervention following attempted suicide is associated with an improvement in social outcome, and possibly less repeated suicide attempts. However, the intensity of this intervention is such that few hospital departments could offer this service at the present time. Difficult decisions will have to be made in the future allocation of limited health resources, as it would appear that it is only by a marked increase in the follow-up care of these patients that a measurable impact can be made both in terms of a reduction in the frequency of repeated suicidal behavior, and an improvement in their social well being.

It should also be emphasized that in the majority of those who commit suicide, and in no less than one-third of those who attempt suicide (Kreitman, 1977), psychiatric illness is present, most commonly depression. Given that a large proportion of these patients have had recent contact with a medical practitioner, it appears, as has been pointed out previously (Barraclough, 1972; Whitlock, 1977; Goldney, 1979b), that the medical profession is in a unique situation to modify these events by optimally applying that knowledge which is already available.

REFERENCES

Adam, K., Bianchi, G., Hawker, F., Nairn, L., Sandford, M., & Scarr, G. (1978), Interpersonal factors in suicide attempts. A pilot study in Christchurch. *Austral. & N.Z. J. Psychiat.*, 12:59–63.

Bagley, C. (1968), The evaluation of a suicide prevention scheme by an ecological method. *Soc. Sci. & Med.*, 2:1–14.

——— (1972), Authoritarianism, status integration and suicide. *Sociol.*, 6:395–404.

——— Jacobson, S. (1976), Ecological variation of three types of suicide. *Psycholog. Med.*, 6:423–427.

Barraclough, B. (1972), Suicide prevention, recurrent affective disorder and lithium. *Brit. J. Psychiat.*, 121:391–392.

——— (1978), The different incidence of suicide in Eire and England and Wales. *Brit. J. Psychiat.*, 132:36–38.

——— Bunch, J., Nelson, B., & Sainsbury, P. (1974), A hundred cases of suicide: Clinical aspects. *Brit. J. Psychiat.*, 125:355–373.

——— Jennings, C., & Moss, J. R. (1977), Suicide prevention by the Samaritans: A controlled study of effectiveness. *Lancet*, 2:868–870.

Barter, J. T., Swaback, D. O., & Todd, D. (1968), Adolescent suicidal attempts: A follow-up study of hospitalized patients. *Arch. Gen. Psychiat.*, 29:523–527.

Birtchnell, J. (1975), The special place of psychotherapy in the treatment of attempted suicide, and the special type of psychotherapy required. *Psychother. & Psychosom.*, 25:3–6.

——— Alarcon, J. (1971), Depression and attempted suicide: A study of 91 cases seen in a casualty department. *Brit. J. Psychiat.*, 118:289–296.

Blake, D. R., & Bramble, M. G. (1979), Self-poisoning—Psychiatric assessment by junior staff. *Brit. Med. J.*, 1:1763.

——— Mitchell, J. R. A. (1978), Self-poisoning. Management of patients in Nottingham, 1976. *Brit. Med. J.*, 1:1021–1035.

Bridge, T. P., Potkin, S. G., Zung, W. W. K., & Soldo, B. J. (1977), Suicide preventive centres. *J. Nerv. & Ment. Dis.*, 164:18–24.

British Ministry of Health (1968), *Hospital Treatment and Acute Poisoning*. London: Her Majesty's Stationery Office.

Brooke, E. M., & Atkinson, M. (1974), Ascertainment of deaths from suicide. In: *Suicide and Attempted Suicide*, ed. E. M. Brooke. Public Health Paper 58. Geneva: World Health Organization.

Brugha, T., & Walsh, D. (1978), Suicide, past and present—The temporal constancy of under-reporting. *Brit. J. Psychiat.*, 132:171–179.

Buckle, R. C., Linnane, J., & McConaghy, N. (1965), Attempted suicide presenting at Alfred Hospital, Melbourne. *Med. J. Austral.*, 1:754–758.

Buglass, D., & McCulloch, J. W. (1970), Further suicidal behaviour: The development and validation of predictive scales. *Brit. J. Psychiat.*, 116:483–492.

Burke, A. W. (1976a), Attempted suicide among Asian immigrants in Birmingham. *Brit. J. Psychiat.*, 128:528–533.

——— (1976b), Attempted suicide among the Irish-born population in Birmingham. *Brit. J. Psychiat.*, 128:534–537.

——— (1976c), Socio-cultural determinants of attempted suicide among West Indians in Birmingham. Ethnic origin and immigrant status. *Brit. J. Psychiat.*, 129:261–266.

Burvill, P. W. (1970), Methods of suicide in Western Australia. *Med. J. Austral.*, 2:411–414.

——— (1973), Immigration and mental disease. *Austral. & N.Z. J. Psychiat.*, 7:155–162.

——— (1975), Attempted suicide in the Perth statistical division, 1971–1972. *Austral. & N.Z. J. Psychiat.*, 9:273.

——— (1980), Suicide in Australia, 1901–1977.

——— Hobbs, M., & Armstrong, B. (1980), Attempted suicide in immigrants in Perth, Western Australia, 1969–1977.

——— McCall, M. G., Stenhouse, N. S., & Reid, T. A. (1972), Deaths from suicide, motor vehicle accidents and all forms of violent death among migrants in Australia, 1962–1966. *Acta Psychiat. Scand.*, 49:28–50.

——— Woodings, T., Stenhouse, N. S., & McCall, M. G. (1980), Differential suicide rates in immigrants in Australia, 1962–1971.

Chowdhury, N., Hicks, R. C., & Kreitman, N. (1973), Evaluation of an after-care service for parasuicide (attempted suicide) patients. *Soc. Psychiat.*, 8:67–81.

Chuaqui, C., Lemkau, P. V., Legarreta, A., & Contreras, M. A. (1966), Suicide in Santiago, Chile. *Pub. Health Rep.*, 81:1109–1117.

Chynoweth, R., Tonge, J., & Armstrong, J. (1980), Suicide in Brisbane: A retrospective psychosocial study. *Austral. & N.Z. J. Psychiat.*, 14(1):37–45.

Cochrane, R., & Robertson, A. (1975), Stress in the lives of parasuicides. *Soc. Psychiat.*, 10:161–171.

Dollard, J., Miller, N. E., Doob, L. W., Mowrer, O. H., & Sears, R. R. (1939), *Frustration and Aggression*. New Haven, CT: Institute of Human Relations, Yale University.

Dorpat, T. L., & Boswell, J. W. (1963), An evaluation of suicidal intent in suicide attempts. *Comprehen. Psychiat.*, 4:117–125.

Douglas, J. (1967), *The Social Meaning of Suicide*. Princeton, NJ: Princeton University Press.

Dublin, L. (1963), *Suicide*. New York: Ronald Press.

Durkheim, E. (1952), *Suicide: A Study in Sociology*. London: Routledge & Kegan Paul.

Ebie, J. C. (1971), Features of psychiatric relevance at an experimental multidisciplinary social casework centre in Edinburgh. *Soc. Psychiat.*, 6:122–128.

——— Hicks, R. C., Lythe, G. J., & Short, R. (1970), An integrated approach to a community's health & social problems. *Health Bull.*, 28:35–41.

Edwards, J. E., & Whitlock, F. A. (1968), Suicide and attempted suicide in Brisbane 1 & 2. *Med. J. Austral.*, 1:932–938, 989–995.

El Gaaly, A. A. (1974), Social dysfunction in depressives and attempted suicides. *Acta Psychiat. Scand.*, 50:341–345.

Enoch, M. D., & Copeland, J. R. M. (1978), Psychological evaluation in cases of self-poisoning. *Brit. Med. J.*, 1:300.

Ettlinger, R. (1975), Evaluation of suicide prevention after attempted suicide. *Acta Psychiat. Scand.*, Suppl., 160:5–125.

Farberow, N. L. (1976), Research in suicide, 1971–1973, a review. In: *Suicide Research,* eds. K. Achte & J. Lonnquist. *Psychiat. Fenn. Suppl.*

French, I., & Bryce, F. O. (1978), Suicide and female aggression: A contemporary analysis of anomic suicide. *J. Clin. Psychiat.*, 39:761–765.

Gardner, R., Hanka, R., O'Brien, V. C., Page, A. J. F., & Rees, R. (1977), Psychological and social evaluation in cases of deliberate self-poisoning admitted to a general hospital. *Brit. Med. J.*, 2:1567–1570.

——— ——— Mountford, P. M., O'Brien, V. C., & Roberts, S. J. (1978), Consultation-liaison scheme for self-poisoned patients in a general hospital. *Brit. Med. J.*, 2:1392–1394.

Gibbons, J. S., Butler, J., Urwin, P., & Gibbons, J. L. (1978), Evaluation of a social work service for self-poisoning patients. *Brit. J. Psychiat.*, 133:111–118.

Gibbs, J., & Martin, W. (1964), *Status Integration and Suicide: A Study in Sociology*. Oregon: University of Oregon Press.

Gibbs, W. T. (1972), Rise and fall in suicide rates in Australia: Relation to sedative availability. *Med. J. Austral.*, 2:1149–1150.

Ginsberg, R. B. (1966), Anomie and aspirations. *Dissert. Abs.*, 27A:3945–3946.

Gold, N. (1965), Suicide and attempted suicide in northeastern Tasmania. *Med. J. Austral.*, 2:361–364.

Goldney, R. (1978), Attempted suicide. Programmes of management and the depressive component. In: *Psychiatry in the General Hospital,* ed. I. Pilowsky.

Proceedings of the Geigy Psychiatry Symposium, Adelaide, 21–22, April 1977, pp. 65–69.

Goldney, R. D. (1979a), Attempted suicide: Correlates of lethality. MD Thesis, University of Adelaide.

——— (1979b), Medical responsibility in murder and suicide. *Med. J. Austral.* 1:50–51.

Greer, S., & Bagley, C. (1971), Effect of psychiatric intervention in attempted suicide: A controlled study. *Brit. Med. J.*, 1:310–312.

Hale, R. (1977), The suicidal risk. *J. Internat. Med. Res.*, 5 Suppl., 4:92–98.

Hassall, C., & Trethowan, W. H. (1972), Suicide in Birmingham. *Brit. Med. J.*, 1:717–718.

Henderson, A. S., Eastwood, M. R., & Montgomery, I. M. (1972), Self-poisoning in Edinburgh and Hobart: A comparison. *Soc. Psychiat.*, 7:30–35.

——— Hartigan, J., Davidson, J., Lance, G. N., Duncan-Jones, P., Koller, K. M., Ritchie, K., McAuley, H., Williams, C. L., & Slaghuis, W. (1977), A typology of parasuicide. *Brit. J. Psychiat.*, 131:631–641.

Henderson, S., Byrne, D. G., Duncan-Jones, P., Adcock, S., Scott, R., & Steele, G. P. (1978), Social bonds in the epidemiology of neurosis: A preliminary communication. *Brit. J. Psychiat.*, 121:463–466.

——— Williams, C. I. (1974), On the prevention of parasuicide. *Austral. & N.Z. J. Psychiat.*, 8:237–240.

Henry, S., & Short, J. (1954), *Suicide and Homicide*. Glencoe, IL: Free Press.

Hetzel, B. (1971), The epidemiology of suicidal behaviour in Australia. *Austral. & N.Z. J. Psychiat.*, 5:146–166.

——— (1974), *Health and Australian Society*. Ringwood, Victoria: Penguin.

Hill, D. (1978), Psychological evaluation in cases of self-poisoning. *Brit. Med. J.*, 1:362.

Holding, T. (1974), The B.B.C. "Befrienders" series and its effects. *Brit. J. Psychiat.*, 124:470–472.

Holding, T. A., Buglass, D., Duffy, J. C., & Kreitman, N. (1977). Parasuicide in Edinburgh—A seven year review 1968–1974. *Brit. J. Psychiat.*, 130:534–543.

Jacobson, S., & Tribe, P. (1972), Deliberate self-injury (attempted suicide) in patients admitted to hospitals in mid-Sussex. *Brit. J. Psychiat.*, 121:379–386.

Jennings, C., Barraclough, B. M., & Moss, J. R. (1978), Have the Samaritans lowered the suicide rate? A controlled study. *Psycholog. Med.*, 8:413–422.

Johnson, K. K. (1979), Durkheim revisited. Why do women kill themselves? *Suicide & Life Threat. Behav.*, 9:145–153.

Kahne, M. J. (1966), Suicide research. *Internat. J. Soc. Psychiat.*, 12:177–186.

Kennedy, P. (1972), Efficacy of a regional poisoning treatment centre in preventing further suicidal behaviour. *Brit. Med. J.*, 4:244–257.

——— Kreitman, N. (1973), An epidemiological survey of parasuicide (attempted suicide) in general practice. *Brit. J. Psychiat.*, 123:23–34.

——— Oswald, I. (1979), Cheaper care of parasuicides. *Brit. J. Psychiat.*, 135:92.

Kessell, N. (1966), The respectability of self-poisoning and the fashion of survival. *J. Psychosom. Res.*, 10:29–36.

Kiev, A. (1976), Cluster analysis profile of suicide attempters. *Amer. J. Psychiat.*, 133:150–151.

Koller, K., & Slaghuis, W. (1978), Suicide attempts, 1973–1977—Urban. Hobart. A further five-year follow-up reporting a decline. *Austral. & N.Z. J. Psychiat.*, 12:169–173.

Kraft, D. P., & Babigian, H. M. (1976), Suicide by persons with and without psychiatric contacts. *Arch. Gen. Psychiat.*, 33:109–215.

Kreitman, N. (1976), The coal gas story. *Brit. J. Prevent. & Soc. Med.*, 30:86–93.

——— (1977), *Parasuicide*. London: John Wiley.

——— (1979), Preventive enthusiasm and scientific caution. Paper presented at the 10th International Congress for Suicide Prevention and Crisis Intervention, Ottawa, June 17 20.

——— Philip, A. E., Greer, S., & Bagley, C. R. (1969), Parasuicide. *Brit. J. Psychiat.*, 114:746–747.

Krupinski, J., & Stoller, A. (1965), Psychiatric disturbance in attempted and completed suicide in Victoria during 1963. *Med. J. Austral.*, 1:773–778.

Lancet (1971), Suicide—A world problem. Lancet, 1:1411.

——— (1974), Self-injury. Lancet, 1:936–937.

Lawson, A. A. H., & Mitchell, I. (1972a), Patients with acute poisoning seen in a general medical unit (1960–1971). *Brit. Med. J.*, 4:153–156.

——— ——— (1972b), Poisoning treatment centres. *Brit. Med. J.*, 4:790.

Lennard-Jones, J. E., & Asher, R. C. (1959), Why do they do it? A study of pseudocide. *Lancet,* 1:1136–1140.

Lester, D. (1970a), Relation between attempted suicide and completed suicide. *Psycholog. Rep.*, 17:719–722.

——— (1970b), Social disorganization and completed suicide. *Soc. Psychiat.*, 5:175–176.

——— (1970c), Suicide and unemployment. *Arch. Environ. Health*, 20:277–278.

——— (1972), *Why People Kill Themselves*. Springfield, IL: Charles C. Thomas.

——— (1974), Effect of suicide prevention centers on suicide rates in the U.S. *Health Serv. Rep.*, 89:37–39.

——— Beck, A. T., & Mitchell, B. (1979), Extrapolation from attempted suicides to completed suicides: A test. *J. Abnorm. Psychol.*, 88:78–80.

Litman, R. E., & Farberow, N. L. (1969), Evaluating the effectiveness of suicide prevention. In: *Proceedings of the Fifth International Conference for Suicide Prevention*, London, pp. 136–250.

MacMahon, B., Johnson, S., & Pugh, T. F. (1963), Relation of suicide rates to social conditions. *Pub. Health Rep.*, 4:285–291.

McCarthy, P. D., & Walsh, D. (1975), Suicide in Dublin: 1. The underreporting of suicide and the consequences for national statistics. *Brit. J. Psychiat.*, 126:301–308.

McCulloch, J. W., Philip, A. E., & Carstairs, G. M. (1967), The ecology of suicidal behaviour. *Brit. J. Psychiat.*, 112:313–319.

Maris, R. W. (1969), *Social Forces in Urban Suicide*. Homewood, IL: Dorsey Press.

Mills, J., Williams, C., Sale, I., Perkin, G., & Henderson, S. (1974), The epidemiology of self-poisoning in Hobart, 1968–1972. *Austral. & N.Z. J. Psychiat.*, 8:167–172.

Montgomery, S. A., Montgomery, D. B., Rani, S. J., Roy, D. H., Shaw, P. M., & McAuley, R. (1979), Maintenance therapy in repeat suicidal behaviours: A placebo controlled trial. In: *Proceedings of the 10th International Congress for Suicide Prevention and Crisis Intervention,* Ottawa, pp. 221–229.

Morgan, H. G., Pocock, H., & Pottle, S. (1975), The urban distribution of nonfatal deliberate self-harm. *Brit. J. Psychiat.*, 126:319–328.

Morris, J. B., Kovacs, M., Beck, A. T., & Wolffe, A. (1974), Notes toward an epidemiology of urban suicide. *Comprehen. Psychiat.*, 15:537–547.

Morrissey, J. D. (1966), The Chichester and District Psychiatric Service. *Milbank Memorial Fund Quart.*, 44:(1) part 1:28–36.

Muir, F. (1796), *The Frank Muir Book: An Irreverent Comparison to Social History*. London: Heinemann, 1976.

Murphy, H. B. M. (1977), Migration, culture and mental health. *Psycholog. Med.*, 7:566–684.

Newson-Smith, J. G. B., & Hirsch, S. R. (1979), A comparison of social workers and psychiatrists in evaluating parasuicide. *Brit. J. Psychiat.*, 134:335–342.

Nielsen, J., & Videbach, T. (1973), Suicide frequency before and after introduction of community psychiatry in a Danish island. *Brit. J. Psychiat.*, 123:35–39.

Oliver, R. G. (1971), Comments on the differences in rates of reported suicide between States of Australia. Melbourne, Australia: Dept. of Social and Preventive Medicine, Monash University, mimeo.

——— Hetzel, B. S. (1972), The rise and fall of suicide rates in Australia: Relation to sedative availability. *Med. J. Austral.*, 1:919–923.

Ottoson, J. O. (1979), The suicidal patient—Can the psychiatrist prevent his suicide? In: *Origin, Prevention and Treatment of Affective Disorders*, eds. M. Schou & E. Stromgren. London: Academic Press.

Ovenstone, I. M. K. (1973), Spectrum of suicidal behaviours in Edinburgh, *Brit. J. Soc. & Prevent. Med.*, 27:27–35.

Pallis, D. J., & Birtchnell, J. (1977), Seriousness of suicide attempts in relation to personality. *Brit. J. Psychiat.*, 130:253–259.

Parnell, R. W., & Skottowe, I. (1957), Towards preventing suicide. *Lancet*, 1:106–208.

Patel, N. S. (1974), A study on suicide. *Med., Sci. & Law*, 14:129–136.

Paykel, E. S., Prusoff, B. A., & Myers, J. K. (1975), Suicide attempts and recent life events. *Arch. Gen. Psychiat.*, 32:327–333.

Pfister-Ammende, M. (1955), Symptomatology: Treatment and prognosis of mental disorders among refugees and repatriates in Switzerland. In: *Displaced Persons*, ed. H. B. M. Murphy. Paris: UNESCO.

Powell, E. H. (1958), Occupation, status and suicide: Towards a redefinition of anomie. *Amer. Sociolog. Rev.*, 23:131–139.

Proudfoot, A. T., & Park, J. (1978), Changing pattern of drugs used for self-poisoning. *Brit. Med. J.*, 1:90–93.

Ringel, E. (1969), An international survey: Central and S. Europe. In: *Proceedings of the Fifth International Conference for Suicide Prevention*, London, pp. 11–14.

Robins, E., Murphy, G. E., Wilkinson, R. H., Gassner, S., & Kayes, J. (1959), Some clinical considerations in the prevention of suicide based on a study of 134 successful suicides. *Amer. J. Pub. Health,* 49:888–899.

Rosen, G. (1971), History in the study of suicide. *Psycholog. Med.,* 1:267–285.

——— (1975), Suicide survivors: A follow-up study of persons who survived jumping from the Golden Gate and S.F.–Oakland Bay bridges. *West. J. Med.,* 122:289–294.

Ross, O., & Kreitman, N. (1975), A further investigation of differences in the suicide rates of England and Wales and of Scotland. *Brit. J. Psychiat.,* 127:575–582.

Ruzicka, L. T. (1976), Suicide, 1950–1971. In: *World Health Statistics Report,* 29:396–413. Geneva: World Health Organization.

Sainsbury, P. (1955), *Suicide in London.* London: Chapman & Hall.

——— Baert, A., & Jenkins, J. (1979), Suicide trends in Europe: A study of the decline in suicide in England and Wales and the increase elsewhere. In: *Proceedings of the 10th International Congress for Suicide Prevention and Crisis Intervention,* Ottawa, pp. 365–366.

——— Barraclough, B. (1968), Differences between suicide rates. *Nature,* 226:1252.

Seager, C. P. (1978), What's in a name? Attempted suicide. *Brit. J. Pschiat.,* 132:206–207.

——— Flood, R. A. (1965), Suicide in Bristol. *Brit. J. Psychiat.,* 111:919–932.

Shneidman, E. S. (1966), Orientations towards death: A vital aspect of the study of lives. *Internat. J. Psychiat.,* 21:167–100.

Sim, M. (1979), Gun control and suicide. In: *Proceedings of the 10th International Congress for Suicide Prevention and Crisis Intervention,* Ottawa, pp. 187–189.

Snowden, J. (1979), Suicide in Australia: A comparison with suicide in England and Wales. *Austral. & N.Z. J. Psychiat.,* 13:301–306.

Stanley, W. J. (1969), Attempted suicide and suicidal gestures. *Brit. J. Prevent. & Soc. Med.,* 23:190–195.

Stengel, E. (1960), The complexity of motivation to suicidal attempts. *J. Ment. Sci.,* 106:1388–1393.

——— (1969), *Suicide and Attempted Suicide,* rev. ed. Harmondsworth, U.K.: Penguin.

Termansen, P., & Bywater, C. (1975), S.A.F.E.R.: A follow-up service for attempted suicide in Vancouver. *Canad. Psychiat. Assn. J.,* 20:29–34.

Walk, D. (1967), Suicide and community care. *Brit. J. Psychiat.,* 113:1381–1391.

Weissman, M. M. (1974), The epidemiology of suicide attempts, 1960 to 1971. *Arch. Gen. Psychiat.,* 30:737–746.

——— Fox, K., & Klerman, G. L. (1973), Hostility and depression associated with suicide attempts. *Amer. J. Psychiat.,* 130:450–455.

——— Kasl, S. V., & Klerman, G. L. (1976), Follow-up of depressed women after maintenance treatment. *Amer. J. Psychiat.,* 33:757–760.

——— Myers, J. K. (1978), Rates and risks of depressive symptoms in a U.S. urban community. *Acta Psychiat. Scand.,* 57:219–231.

——— Prusoff, B. A., Dimascio, A., Neu, C., Goklaney, M., & Klerman, G. (1979), The efficacy of drugs and psychotherapy in the treatment of acute depressive episodes. *Amer. J. Psychiat.,* 126:555–558.

Welu, T. C. (1977), A follow-up program for suicide attempters: Evaluation of effectiveness. *Suicide & Life-Threatening Behav.*, 7:17–30.

Wexler, L., Weissman, M. M., & Kasl, S. V. (1978), Suicide attempts, 1970–1975: Updating a U.S. study and comparisons with international trends. *Brit. J. Psychiat.*, 132:180–185.

Whitlock, F. A. (1971), Migration and suicide. *Med. J. Austral.*, 2:840–848.

——— (1975), Suicide in Brisbane, 1956 to 1973. The drug-death epidemic. *Med. J. Austral.*, 1:737–743.

——— (1977), Psychiatric epidemiology: Its uses and limitations. *Austral. & N.Z. J. Psychiat.*, 11:9–18.

Wilkins, J. (1967), Suicidal behaviour. *Amer. Sociolog. Rev.*, 32:286–298.

Wilson, K. W. (1971), *Sociological Factors in Attempted Suicide*. Unpublished thesis. Western Australian Institute of Technology, Bentley.

Yap, P. M. (1958), Suicide in Hong Kong. *J. Ment. Sci.*, 104:166–301.

Commentary

David Brent, M.D.

Goldney and Burvill begin by noting the overlap between those who attempt and those who complete suicide. In fact, while these two groups are relatively distinct, those who attempt suicide are at high risk to reattempt and/or to complete suicide, probably at a rate equivalent to patients with affective disorders.

The authors also comment on the validity of suicide statistics as a basis of international comparisons; interpretations based on such data are quite prone to "ecological fallacies." The increase in the suicide rate among adolescents and young adults does appear to be robust and a finding common to a large proportion of Western nations. While the etiology of this upward trend is unknown, the increase does correspond to a time when there has been an increased rate of alcohol and drug abuse among the young. Some data to support this hypothesis comes from an increase in the proportion of suicides in patients who were intoxicated noted in two metropolitan areas (Brent and Perper, 1985; Ford, Rushforth, Rushforth, Hirsch, and Adelson, 1979).

The role of the availability of method in "producing" suicides is also discussed. While the rate of suicide in Britain declined as a close correlate to the detoxification of domestic gas, this effect lasted about 10 years, and recently, suicide victims have been turning to vehicular exhaust as a method of suicide and the rate has again been rising (McClure, 1984). Other methods of restricting the access of lethal means for suicide that were mentioned included—packaging of drugs to discourage impulsive overdose, more restrictive prescribing practices, and stricter gun control laws. (There is evidence that among suicide attempters that the medical lethality of their attempts among impulsive attempters is more dependent on the availability of a lethal agent [Brent, 1983]; therefore, such restriction would be most helpful in preventing suicides among those who are impulsive.)

A review of treatment and prevention programs to deal with suicide attempters and those considered at high risk for suicide yielded little in the way of support of a particular approach over any other. However, among those who already have a diagnosable psychiatric disorder, treatment of their DSM-III (1980) Axis I diagnosis may do a lot to reduce the risk of suicide—particularly in those with alcohol and drug problems and affective disorders. Whereas the availability of specific agents to treat depression may theoretically avert suicide, there is evidence that medication, compared to ECT is much less effective in dampening the propensity to continue suicidal behavior (Avery and Winokur, 1978). However, for a suicidal patient with unipolar affective disorder, there is some evidence to favor psychosocial treatment over medication, particularly if cognitive therapy is employed (Kovacs, Rush, Beck, and Hollon, 1981; Rush, Beck, Kovacs, and Hollon, 1977).

The following were Goldney and Burvill's main points in terms of the management of suicidal patients:

1. The importance of the social environment in monitoring and supporting (or stressing) a suicidal individual.
2. The role of specific disorders in suicide—such as alcohol and/or drug abuse, and depression.
3. Treatment should focus both on the life context, but in addition should be disorder-specific.
4. Given the evidence on the role of the availability of lethal agents in "producing suicides," prescriptions of tricyclic and antidepressants to suicidal patients should only be given in small amounts. In addition, firearms should be removed from the house of a potentially suicidal individual.

REFERENCES

Avery, D., & Winokur, G. (1978), Suicide, attempted suicide, and relapse rates in depression. *Arch. Gen. Psychiat.*, 35:749–753.

Brent, D. A. (1983), Correlates of the medical lethality of suicide attempts in children and adolescents. Paper presented at the 30th Annual Scientific Meeting of the American Academy of Child Psychiatry, San Francisco, CA.

——— Perper J. A. (1985), Suicide among youth aged 10–19 in Allegheny County, PA: Temporal trends, 1960–1983. Paper presented at the 32nd Scientific Meeting of the American Academy of Child Psychiatry, San Antonio, TX.

Ford, A. B., Rushforth, N. B., Rushforth, N., Hirsch, C., & Adelson, L. (1979), Violent death in a metropolitan county. II. Changing patterns in suicide (1959–1974). *Amer. J. Pub. Health*, 69:459–464.

Kovacs, M., Rush, J., Beck, A., & Hollon, A. (1981), Depressed outpatients treated with cognitive therapy or pharmacotherapy. A one-year follow-up. *Arch. Gen. Psychiat.*, 38:33–39.

McClure, G. (1984), Trends in suicide rate for England and Wales 1975–1980. *Brit. J. Psychiat.*, 144:119–126.

Rush, A., Beck, A., Kovacs, M., & Hollon, S. (1977), Comparative efficacy of cognitive therapy and pharmacotherapy of depressed patients. *Cog. Ther. Res.*, 1:17–37.

Commentary

Duane G. Spiker, M.D.

Suicide is fortunately a relatively rare event with an incidence of approximately 1–2 percent per year in depressed patients. However, by the very nature of rare events, it is difficult to pick out accurately the subjects who will subsequently commit suicide. When dealing with rare events one needs to understand two concepts—sensitivity and specificity. Sensitivity is basically the rate of true positives, that is, what percentage of patients who you predict will do something actually do it. Specificity is just the reverse: the rate of true negatives. For a detailed explanation of these concepts, the interested reader should consider Galen and Gambino (1975).

The inherent problem can be seen by giving an example. In a one-year follow-up study with over 1,200 subjects, Pallis, Gibbons, and Pierce (1984) have presented sensitivity and specificity of three different scales used to predict suicide. Although there are some differences between the scales and also some variation with follow-up time, a reasonable estimate of sensitivity is approximately 80 percent and of specificity 75 percent. Now, let us assume that we evaluate 1,000 patients and that 20 of them will commit suicide in one year after our evaluation. Thus, we would accurately predict 16 of the 20 actual suicides. However, we also predicted that an additional 245 patients would commit suicide who actually didn't. Thus, we over-predicted suicide to actual suicide by about a 15:1 ratio (245:16) and failed to predict four actual suicides.

What, then, is the busy clinician to do? There are probably two groups of patients who should be hospitalized when they present for mental health care. These are older males who communicate suicide intent and have the diagnosis of either depression or alcoholism. These patients are probably at the highest risk for completed suicide (Robins, 1984) and we have reasonably effective treatments for them. For the other patients, one must make a decision based on clinical judgment and Goldney and Burvill's chapter provides a good discussion of relevant factors. Alternatively, one may want to use one of the two suicide prediction scales which have been reasonably well studied (Beck, Schuyler, and Herman, 1974; Pallis, Gibbons, and Pierce, 1984).

References

Beck, A. T., Schuyler, D., & Herman, I. (1974), Development of suicidal intent scales. In: *The Prediction of Suicide*, eds. A. T. Beck, H. L. Resnick, and D. J. Lettieri. Bowie, MD: Charles Press, pp. 45–56.

Galen, R. S., & Gambino, S. R. (1975), *Beyond Normality: The Predictive Value and Efficiency of Medical Diagnosis*. New York: John Wiley.

Pallis, D. J., Gibbons, J. S., & Pierce, D. W. (1984), Estimating suicide risk among attempted suicides. II. Efficiency of predictive scales after the attempt. *Brit. J. Psychiat.*, 144:139–148.

Robins, E. (1984), Psychiatric emergencies. In: *Comprehensive Textbook of Psychiatry*, Vol. 2, 4th ed., eds. H. I. Kaplan & B. J. Sadock. Baltimore, MD: Williams & Wilkins.

Annotated Bibliography

Frederick, C. J. (1977), Current trends in suicidal behavior in the United States. *Amer. J. Psychother.*, 77:172–200.

A thorough review of the literature on suicidal behavior as well as by age, geographic area, race, occupation, seasons of the year, and time and methods of suicide during the first 75 years of this century in the United States. The above makes this paper quite a classic and of high interest for anyone who treats suicidal patients.

Morrison, J. R. (1982), Suicide in a psychiatric practice population. *J. Clin. Psych.*, 43:348–352.

A practical and demographically rich paper to help mental health evaluators decide on suicidal risk. It presents data from adult psychiatry private practice. Noteworthy is the author's comment that despite strongly suggestive data from numerous studies, clinicians must resist the false sense of security that some diagnoses seem to offer.

Hillard, J. R., Ramm, D., Zung, W. W., & Holland, J. M. (1983), Suicide in psychiatric emergency room. *Amer. J. Psychiat.*, 140:459–462.

Important demographic data is presented in this paper in which attention is focused on a particular emergency room. Of particular importance are the authors' comments on the need for intensive follow-up of the suicidal patient. They report that suicide immediately following release appears to be very rare in a well-functioning emergency room.

Paykel, E. S., Hallowell, C., Dressler, D. M., Shapiro, D. L., & Weissman, M. M. (1974), Treatment of suicide attempters. *Arch. Gen. Psychiat.*, 31:487–491.

A still timely article that looks at suicidal attempters, their disposition, and treatment. As in other similar papers, the issue of noncompliance with follow-up referrals and the need to be more attuned to this problem is raised. Interesting is the fact that in this particular study, half of the patients were immediately admitted to an inpatient facility.

Kricgfcr, G. (1978), Common errors in the treatment of suicidal patients. *J. Colin. Psych.*, 39:649–651.

This is an outstanding report that elucidates errors of omission and commission made by mental health professionals and paraprofessionals. These errors include (1) failure to use appropriate therapy when indicated; (2) staff attitude that the case was hopeless and would inevitably end in suicide; (3) failure to properly assess a patient's communication; (4) an intrastaff failure to communicate clearly; and (5) returning the patient to the same social system in which suicidal attempts had occurred.

Rynearson, E. K. (1981), Suicide internalized: An existential sequestrum. *Amer. J. Psychiat.*, 138:84–86.

Based on the author's own experience of being a survivor of his wife's suicide, this paper presents a thoughtful and readable report on suicidal bereavement. This experience seems to involve more than the personalized reaction to the death of another, as the bereaved appears to be left with the cognitive and emotional dilemma of death as a chosen option for existence. Rynearson depicts a pointed existential dilemma when he writes "unlike my wife, I would remain committed to existence as a chosen direction towards self-affirmation while simultaneously focusing on her chosen direction toward nonexistence and self-annihilation."

Motto, J. A. (1979), The psychopathology of suicide: A clinical model approach. *Amer. J. Psychiat.*, 136:516–520.

The author is a well-known contributor to the suicide literature, and this paper continues to have relevance to the assessment of suicidal behavior. Two models, a broad one, "males under forty," and a specific one, "stable with forced change" represent the author's attempt to understand those patients at risk who complete the act of suicide.

——— Heilbron, D. C., & Juster, R. P. (1985), Development of a clinical instrument to estimate suicide risk. *Amer. J. Psychiat.*, 142:680–686.

This paper takes advantage of years of suicidality assessment experience. Its authors present the development of a clinical instrument to estimate suicide risk within two years of its administration.

11

Prediction Research and the Emergency Commitment of Dangerous Mentally Ill Persons: A Reconsideration

John Monahan, Ph.D.

Rarely have research data been as quickly or universally accepted by the scholarly community as those supporting the proposition that mental health professionals are highly inaccurate in predicting violent behavior. Since Dershowitz's conclusion in an influential 1969 article that "for every correct psychiatric prediction of violence, there are numerous erroneous predictions" (p. 47), psychiatrists, psychologists, and lawyers have increasingly come to accept the gross inaccuracy of the prediction of violence as a scientifically established fact (Diamond, 1974; Ennis and Litwack, 1974; Stone, 1975; Geis and Monahan, 1976; Miller, 1976). Indeed, it appears as though the only people who still believe that accurate predictions of violence are possible are those mental health professionals who make their living at such tasks and

This chapter was first published in the *American Journal of Psychiatry* (1978), 135:198–201, and it is reprinted by permission.

the courts that base proceedings for institutionalization on predictive judgments. Even there, the tide appears to be turning.

The conclusion that psychiatrists and psychologists "have absolutely no expertise in predicting violent behavior" (Ennis and Litwack, 1974, p. 734) has led some to call for the abolition of all forms of preventive intervention that are predicated on a clinical prediction of future violence (Monahan, 1973; Roth, Dayley, and Lerner, 1973; Diamond, 1974).

The purpose of this paper is twofold. It will propose that a careful reading of the prediction research reported to date does not support the unqualified conclusion that the accurate prediction of violence is impossible under all circumstances or that psychiatrists, psychologists, and others will invariably overpredict its occurrence by several orders of magnitude. Further, it will suggest that there are theoretical reasons why one could expect that one set of circumstances—those which typically apply in the *short-term emergency commitment* of mentally ill persons predicted to be imminently violent—may be exempt from the systematic inaccuracy found in the current research. Since, at the time of this writing, there are no data on the accuracy of predictions made in emergency situations, the debate on emergency commitment must proceed on theoretical rather than empirical grounds until such time as relevant data are available. If this argument has merit, then proposals for "the abolition of involuntary mental hospitalization in any form—long-term or emergency" (Roth et al., 1973, p. 445) cannot legitimately adduce the existing prediction data in their support, and the empirical basis for emergency commitment is an open question rather than the dead issue many presume it to be.

RESEARCH ON THE PREDICTION OF VIOLENCE

The basis for the lack of confidence in the ability of psychiatrists and psychologists to predict violence is a large and growing body of research dramatically demonstrating that when a group of prisoners or mental patients who have been predicted to be violent are nonetheless released into the community, the majority, frequently the vast majority, do not commit the violent behavior expected of them (Kozol, Boucher, and Garofalo, 1972; Wenk, Robison, and Smith, 1972; State of Maryland, 1973; Steadman and Cocozza, 1974, 1976; Thornberry and Jacoby, 1974; Cocozza and Steadman, 1976). The persistence of this finding is itself remarkable: no study has ever found prediction to be more accurate than inaccurate. As I have noted previously, ''The literature has been consistent on this point ever since Pinel took the chains off the supposedly dangerous mental patients at La Bicêtre in 1792, and the resulting lack of violence gave lie to the psychiatric predictions which had justified their restraint'' (Monahan, 1976, p. 21).

While the major studies of the prediction of violence differ from each other in many respects, most (Kozol et al., 1972; State of Maryland, 1973; Steadman and Cocozza, 1974; Thornberry and Jacoby, 1974; Cocozza and Steadman, 1976) conform to the following methodological pattern:

1. Individuals were institutionalized. Institutionalization could have been on the basis of a criminal or juvenile arrest, conviction, or determination that an individual was a ''mentally ill offender,'' ''defective delinquent,'' or ''incompetent to stand trial.''
2. In the institution, predictions were made that a group of these individuals would be violent if released into the community. It is important to note that it was these predictions, made in the institution (jail, prison, or hospital), that were being tested in the research and not the predictions that may have occasioned the original institutionalization.
3. The group predicted to be violent if released into the community was in fact released into the community. This often occurred by virtue of a judicial order or parole board action. A natural experiment was thereby created.
4. The group predicted to be violent was monitored for a number of years in the community as to its actual performance of violent behavior. This was accomplished by checking police and (occasionally) mental health records.
5. Low frequencies of violent behavior were recorded, thereby revealing the inaccuracy of the predictions. No violent behavior was noted on the community records of 54–99 percent of the persons who had been predicted to be violent. Other studies (e.g., Steadman and Cocozza, 1976) compared groups

predicted to be dangerous and those predicted not to be dangerous and found no differences.

What was tested in these studies? The most reasonable interpretation is that they tested predictions *made in an institution* of violence *to occur in the open community*. Persons who, for whatever reason, had been institutionalized for a substantial period of time (a mean of 15 years in one study [Steadman and Cocozza, 1974] and not less than several months in any other) were predicted to engage in violent behavior if released into the open community. They were eventually released and most were not violent.

While it is true that some studies (Steadman and Cocozza, 1976) included violence in the hospital as part of their criteria, the fact that "potentially violent" patients were likely to be medicated makes it unclear whether a lack of violence in the hospital reflects predictive inaccuracy or simply the pharmacological suppression of violent tendencies.

Rather than demonstrating that all forms of violence prediction are "doomed" (as I have previously stated [Monahan (1976)], a more discerning reading of the existing research suggests that it demonstrates the invalidity only of predictions made in one context that an individual will be violent in another, very different context. The *context of prediction* in the existing research is a closed institution in which the individual has resided for a significant period of time (several months to several decades). The *context of validation* is the open community.

There is an enormous body of research that would lead one to expect that the correlation between behavior predicted in one context and observed in another would be low (Mischel, 1968, 1973; Bowers, 1973; Bem and Allen, 1974). Since Hartshorne and May's (1928) finding that the assessment of "moral character" was specific to the context in which it was measured (Hartshorne and May, 1928), scores of investigations have reluctantly concluded that the cross-situational consistency of any type of behavior rarely exceeds the "sound barrier" (Arthur, 1971) of a .40 correlation coefficient. As Mischel (1968) noted,

> Findings demonstrating the specificity of the interactions between persons and situations constrain how broadly we can generalize from

> an individual's behavior in any one situation to his reactions under different conditions. . . . Predictive validity tends to decrease as the gap increases between the behavior sampled on the prediction measure and the behavior that is being predicted [p. 323].

It is precisely this "gap" that exists in the current research on violence prediction. The jails, prisons, and mental hospitals in which predictions are made differ in obvious ways from the open community situations that are the truest test of predictive validity. This point is underscored by the fact that institutional performance has little effect on postinstitutional (community) behavior (Steadman and Cocozza, 1974). It is exacerbated by the fact that substantial time periods intervene between the point when the institutional prediction is made and the community validation is undertaken, and/or between the most recent exposure to the community context in which the prediction will be validated and the point at which the institutional prediction is made. In the former case, there is too much opportunity for the individual or the environment to change in unknown ways before the prediction is tested. In the latter case, the information on how the person behaves in the open community is made obsolete by the unknown changes that have occurred since he or she was institutionalized.

As Mischel (1968) noted, "The assessor who tries to predict the future without detailed information about the exact environmental conditions influencing the individual's criterion behavior may be more engaged in the process of hoping than of predicting" (p. 140). It is the relative absence of current knowledge about the "exact environmental conditions" that are operating in the community context in which the individual will be functioning that relegates long-term institutional predictions to the realm of whimsy.

To be sure, these are not the only reasons why violence has been inaccurately predicted under the circumstances investigated (Monahan, 1976). However, they may help to account for the degree of inaccuracy that has been observed and may serve to differentiate the type of prediction that has been tested and found wanting from another type that has yet to be investigated; that is, the prediction of imminent violence typically made in the short-term emergency commitment of the mentally ill.

PREDICTION OF VIOLENCE IN THE EMERGENCY SETTING

In emergency commitment, a person residing in the open community is brought to the attention of a mental health professional, usually by a family member, friend, neighbor, or police officer, for a determination of whether he or she is mentally ill and a prediction of whether he or she will engage in violent behavior in the immediate future. A positive diagnosis and prediction results in the short-term "emergency" confinement of the person in a mental health facility.

Note the following differences between emergency commitment of this type and the kinds of prediction investigated in the research discussed earlier. In emergency commitment:

1. The context of prediction is the same as the context of validation. A prediction is being made in the open community that a person will be violent in that same context. Often a prediction is made in a room in a home that the person will soon be violent in the same room.
2. The time between the point of prediction and the validation period is very short. Frequently the prediction is that the person will be violent in a matter of minutes or hours.
3. Since the prediction is being made in the same context in which it will be validated, there is little time intervening between the most recent exposure to the context of validation and the point of prediction. The prediction is made immediately after observing how the person behaves in the context in which the prediction would be validated. The information available to the predictor is thus fresh and current.

In emergency commitment, unlike the legal procedures studied in the current research, there is a small situational and temporal "gap" between the behavior used as a predictor and the outcome that is being predicted. One is directly sampling actions (e.g., threatening words and gestures) that are "as similar as possible to the behavior used on the criterion measure" (Mischel, 1968, p. 323), for example, fulfilled threats. In violence as in other areas, it is potentially true that "predictions about individual behavior can be generated accurately from knowledge of the environments in which the behavior occurs" (Mischel, 1968, p. 164).

DISCUSSION

Given the above factors, it would appear that there is a qualitative difference between predictions of violence made in the community for the purpose of short-term emergency commitment and those reported for longer term institutionalized patients and prisoners. Research on the abysmal failure to predict violence accurately in the latter situation cannot reasonably be extrapolated to a similar conclusion in short-term emergency commitment cases.

The validity of the existing body of research on violence prediction, or many of the policy implications that have legitimately been drawn from it (Fagin, 1976; Monahan and Cummings, 1976; Heller and Monahan, 1977; Shah, 1977), are not at issue. There is no question that long-term predictions of violence, or predictions from institutional to community settings, are grossly inaccurate. I am merely restricting the range of predictive decision-making situations to which the currently available research can reasonably be said to apply.

I know of no data substantively relevant to the question of predictive accuracy in emergency commitment situations. The empirical question, therefore, is an open one. It is not capable of being resolved by recourse to the currently existing body of research on violence prediction. There are theoretical considerations, discussed above, which suggest that predictions made under the conditions that typically apply in emergency commitment situations *should* be better than those made in the institutional settings studied to date. But whether they are in fact better and, if so, how much better is not now known.

There is no a priori reason to assume that psychiatrists or psychologists would be any better at prediction in emergency situations than other observers or participants (e.g., a police officer or a potential victim). The unresolved question is whether they would be equally accurate or equally inaccurate (see Steadman and Cocozza, 1976). Undoubtedly, there will be some degree of overprediction in predictive judgment of any sort. In emergency commitment situations, some protagonists will be bluffing in their actions or, for whatever reason, will decline to carry through with their threatened violent behavior. Some predictors will rely upon illusory correlations or take extraneous factors, such as a belief that treatment would be beneficial, into account in making their predictions (Monahan and Cummings, 1975).

Indeed, it is difficult to conceive of a design for a study that ethically could put predictions in emergency situations to the test, since the situations are defined as "emergency" ones presumably in need of immediate and decisive action. Could one ethically decline to intervene in a random half of the cases in which a mental health professional has both diagnosed mental illness and predicted imminent violence and return the next day for a body-count validation, as has been suggested (Dix, 1976)? Lacking any research data (Monahan, 1977a), one is left with only prudent judgment with which to assess the accuracy of short-term predictions of violence in emergency commitment situations.

If research should bear out the theoretical position argued here and reveal emergency predictions to be more valid than those previously studied, what relevance would this have for the legal process in emergency commitment? By the point at which a full hearing is held on the issue of dangerousness (two weeks after initial confinement, according to *Lessard v. Schmidt* [1972] standards), the "emergency" nature of the prediction may well have dissipated (Monahan, 1977b). Enough time may have elapsed and the psychological context may have changed sufficiently that the pattern of overpredictive inaccuracy, repeatedly demonstrated by Steadman and others, may have set in. While the position argued here would offer no solace to the psychiatrist or psychologist confronted with predicting dangerousness for the purpose of prolonged institutionalization, it would be relevant to justifying the initial "emergency" period of confinement, that is, the two-week period before the full hearing. Predictive accuracy may end at approximately the same time that full legal protection begins. If so, the emergency commitment of those diagnosed as mentally ill and predicted to be dangerous may be limited on both empirical and legal grounds to a brief period.

REFERENCES

Arthur, R. (1971), Success is predictable. *Milit. Med.*, 136:539–545.

Bem, D., & Allen, A. (1974), On predicting some of the people some of the time: The search for cross-situational consistencies in behavior. *Psychol. Rev.*, 81:506–520.

Bowers, K. (1973), Situationism in psychology: An analysis and a critique. *Psychol. Rev.*, 80:307–326.

Cocozza, J., & Steadman, H. (1976), The failure of psychiatric predictions of dangerousness: Clear and convincing evidence. *Rutgers Law Rev.*, 29:1048–1101.

Dershowitz, A. (1969), Psychiatrists' power in civil commitment. *Psychology Today*, 2:43–47.

Diamond, B. (1974), The psychiatric prediction of dangerousness. *Univ. Pennsylvania Law Rev.*, 123:439–452.

Dix, G. (1976), "Civil" commitment of the mentally ill and the need for data on the prediction of dangerousness. *Amer. Behav. Scient.*, 19:318–334.

Ennis, B., & Litwack, T. (1974), Psychiatry and the presumption of expertise: Flipping coins in the courtroom. *Calif. Law Rev.*, 62:694–752.

Fagin, A. (1976), The policy implications of predictive decision-making: "Likelihood" and "dangerousness" in civil commitment proceedings. *Pub. Pol.*, 24:491–528.

Geis, G., & Monahan, J. (1976), The social ecology of violence. In: *Moral Development and Behavior*, ed. T. Lickona. New York: Holt, Rinehart & Winston, pp. 342–356.

Hartshorne, H., & May, M. A. (1928), *Studies in the Nature of Character*, Vol. 1. New York: Macmillan.

Heller, K., & Monahan, J. (1977), *Psychology and Community Change*. Homewood, IL: Dorsey Press.

Kozol, H., Boucher, R., & Garofalo, R. (1972), The diagnosis and treatment of dangerousness. *Crime & Delinquency*, 18:371–392.

Lessard *v*. Schmidt, 349 F Supp 1079 (ED Wis 1972).

Maryland, State of, Department of Public Safety and Correctional Services (1973), Maryland's Defective Delinquency Statute—A Progress Report. Baltimore, MD: State of Maryland.

Miller, K. (1976), *Managing Madness: The Case Against Civil Commitment*. New York: Free Press.

Mischel, W. (1968), *Personality and Assessment*. New York: John Wiley.

——— (1973), Toward a cognitive social learning reconceptualization of personality. *Psychol. Rev.*, 80:252–283.

Monahan, J. (1973), The psychiatrization of criminal behavior. *Hosp. Comm. Psych.*, 24:105–107.

——— (1976), The Prevention of Violence. In: *Community Mental Health and the Criminal Justice System*, ed. J. Monahan. New York: Pergamon Press, pp. 13–34.

——— (1977a), Strategies for an empirical analysis of the prediction of violence in emergency civil commitment. *Law & Hum. Behav.*, 1:363.

——— (1977b), Empirical analyses of civil commitment: Critique and context. *Law & Soc. Rev.*, 11:619–628.

——— Cummings, L. (1975), The prediction of violence as a function of its perceived consequences. *J. Crim. Justice*, 2:239–242.

——— ——— (1976), Social policy implications of the inability to predict violence. *J. Soc. Issues*, 31:153–164.

Roth, R., Dayley, M., & Lerner, J. (1973), Into the abyss: Psychiatric reliability and emergency commitment statutes. *Santa Clara Lawyer*, 13:400–446.

Shah, S. (1977), Dangerousness: Some definitional, conceptual, and public policy issues. In: *Perspectives in Law and Psychology,* ed. B. Sales. New York: Plenum Press, pp. 91–119.

Steadman, H., & Cocozza, J. (1974), *Careers of the Criminally Insane: Excessive Social Control of Deviance.* Lexington, MA: Lexington Books.

——— ——— (1976), A natural experiment in the psychiatric prediction of dangerousness, unpublished.

Stone, A. (1975), *Mental Health and Law: A System in Transition.* Rockville, MD: National Institute of Mental Health.

Thornberry, T., & Jacoby, J. (1974), The uses of discretion in a maximum security mental hospital: The Dixon case. Paper presented at the 26th annual meeting of the American Society of Criminology, Chicago, IL.

Wenk, E., Robison, J., & Smith, G. (1972), Can violence be predicted? *Crime & Delinquency,* 18:393–402.

Commentary

Jeffrey L. Geller, M.D., M.P.H., and Loren H. Roth, M.D., M.P.H.

Chapter 11 can be seen as a midpoint in the evolution of the author's thinking about the prediction of violent behavior. Monahan's early position (1976) was that "efforts by mental health professionals to prophesy the perpetrators of violence appear to be doomed" (p. 29). In the (1978) paper reprinted here, Monahan indicates that prior research on the prediction of violence concerned institutionalized individuals thought to be violent if released, who, when released, demonstrated low frequencies of violent behavior. Such research indicates that prediction of violence made within an institutional context but applied to a community context could not be reliably done. If violence in this community is what concerns us, then prediction of dangerousness should be studied within the context of imminent violence in emergency settings.

Following the foundation laid out in chapter 11, Monahan (1981) has advocated the inclusion of actuarial correlates and environmental factors in the clinical prediction of violent behavior. The former include: age, sex, race, socioeconomic status and employment stability, opiate or alcohol use, and a history of prior violence. The latter include family, peer, and job environments, and the availability of victims, weapons, and alcohol. In the context of these factors, Monahan (1981) has developed a clinical examination for predicting violent behavior.

Monahan is critical of earlier, overzealous acceptance of what he calls first generation research of violence; these studies, though valid, should not be generalized to all settings or individuals. In a later paper, Monahan (1984) has noted that second generation research is more likely than earlier works to recognize the limits of our knowledge, to provide a "guarded optimism" about predicting accuracy, and to examine the task of violence prediction from a relative rather than an absolute moral–political position.

Since, as Monahan implies in chapter 11, the perfect experiment can never be done—randomly discharging from the emergency setting 50 percent of those predicted to be imminently dangerous on the basis of their mental illness, and monitoring their subsequent violent behavior—the practitioner needs to take what is known and make his best clinical judgment. Because predictions in the emergency room are very "short range," they are best viewed as interventions requiring ongoing reassessment and modification; prediction and treatment in the emergency room are necessarily intertwined.

What Monahan has done is expand the horizon of our knowledge about violence prediction and inform us that our task, while difficult, may be less of a conundrum than we once believed.

References

Monahan, J. (1976). The prevention of violence. In: *Community Mental Health and the Criminal Justice System*, ed. J. Monahan. New York: Pergamon Press.

——— (1981), *Predicting Violent Behavior*. Beverly Hills, CA: Sage Publications.

——— (1984), The prediction of violent behavior: Toward a second generation of theory and policy. *Amer. J. Psychiat.*, 141:10–15.

12

EVALUATING AND MANAGING THE VIOLENT PATIENT

William R. Dubin, M.D.

INTRODUCTION

The violent patient poses one of the most difficult treatment problems in emergency medicine. Generally these patients are brought in by family or police for treatment against their will. They can be verbally abusive and physically threatening. Furthermore, mismanagement of the violent patient can result in physical harm to staff and destruction of property. Although it is difficult to predict an individual's long-range potential for violence, a proper initial assessment can lead to an accurate prediction of the patient's potential for violence over a brief time period (not longer than one hour).

The most effective management of the violent patient is preventive management. The crux of successful prevention depends on recognizing early the clues that indicate a high probability of violence and responding in a manner that will defuse the potential violence. This

This chapter was first published in *Annals of Emergency Medicine* (1981), 10:481–484, and it is reprinted by permission.

chapter outlines the procedures followed in the Thomas Jefferson Hospital Crisis Service, Philadelphia for evaluating and managing potentially violent patients. Violence is defined as verbally threatening and/or assaultive behavior.

PREDICTION OF VIOLENCE

Diagnostic Clues

Diagnosis can be a helpful clue in assessing a patient's potential for violence. Frequently the diagnosis is immediately self-evident, such as in cases of delirium, psychosis, or alcohol/drug intoxications and withdrawals. Fortunately sudden, unexpected attacks are rare, and violence occurs only after a period of mounting frustration and tension in the patient. Thus the physician has time during the interview to make a tentative diagnosis that alerts him to a patient's potential for violence. In the absence of a firm diagnosis, other clues must be relied upon. The diagnostic groups of patients with a propensity for violence include the following:

1. *Drug or alcohol intoxication* (Lion, Bach-y-Rita, and Ervin, 1969; Eaton, Stetten, and Kitchen, 1971; Bach-y-Rita, Lion, and Clement, 1971; Tauson, 1971; Leroy and Hartocollis, 1976; Hackett, 1977; Cohen, 1979)—Patients who are intoxicated from alcohol or drugs, especially amphetamines, LSD, or phencyclidine, have a much greater potential for violence than do ordinary patients.

2. *Drug or alcohol withdrawal* (Rockwell, 1972; Hackett, 1977; Cohen, 1979)—Patients in withdrawal often attempt to manipulate staff to obtain drugs to alleviate their withdrawal symptoms. When they are refused drugs by medical personnel, they often become threatening and abusive. Patients experiencing delirium tremens can be the most assaultive patients seen in an emergency department.

3. *Acute organic brain syndrome (delirium)* (Lion, 1968; Tauson, 1971; MacDonald, 1971; Rockwell, 1972; Hackett, 1977)—The potential for violence in these patients may be overlooked by the medical staff, who often become preoccupied with the medical problem of the patient.

4. *Acute psychosis* (MacDonald, 1971; Tauson, 1971; Madden, Lion, and Penna, 1976; Hackett, 1977)—This includes patients with

acute schizophrenic episodes and patients who are acutely manic. It has been our experience that manic patients are more dangerous because staff members tend to gain a false sense of security from the manic's expansive mood and good humor. However, manics can become quite violent when demands are placed on them.

5. *Paranoid character* (Kalogerakis, 1971; Tauson, 1971; Rockwell, 1972; Hackett, 1977)—Paranoid characters pose a potential for violence, especially when the examiner begins to probe for dynamic information despite the patient's resistance and warning to leave him alone. After repeated questioning and a period of increasing tension and turmoil, the patient may explode and attack.

6. *Borderline personality* (Lion et al., 1969; Madden et al., 1976)—Generally these patients can become violent when they perceive the staff is rejecting them after their demands have not been met, or if they are intoxicated with alcohol or drugs.

7. *Antisocial personality* (MacDonald, 1971; Tauson, 1971; Lion, 1975)—Violence in these patients is generally associated with drug intoxication or withdrawal.

Other diagnostic categories are potentially violent, including temporal lobe epilepsy (Lion et al., 1968; Bach-y-Rita et al., 1971; Lion, 1972; Rockwell, 1972), passive-aggressive personality (MacDonald, 1971; Lion, 1975), and pathological intoxication (Lion et al., 1969; Lion, 1972; Cohen, 1979). We, however, have not found these diagnostic categories to be as much of a problem because patients with temporal lobe epilepsy or pathological intoxication are brought to the emergency department after the assaultive behavior has occurred, and thus are automatically managed as violent patients.

Behavioral Clues

The critical element in assessing a patient's potential for violence is the behavioral clues. The best guide to behavioral clues has been formulated by Hackett (1977) and includes the following:

1. *Posture*—Observe how the patient is sitting during the interview. If the patient is sitting tensely on the edge of the chair or is gripping the arm rests, the interviewer should be cautious and alert to the fact that increased tension often precedes violent behavior.

2. *Speech*—The speech of the patient can be a clue to his degree of agitation. Is he talking in a calm voice, or is his voice loud and

strident? Is the patient verbally threatening? The louder, more strident the patient's voice, the greater the potential for violence.

3. *Motor activity*—Perhaps the most important and most ignored sign of impending violence is the patient's motor activity. The patient who is unable to sit still and who paces around the examining room or in the halls poses the most serious threat of violence. This behavior, in combination with the above-mentioned diagnostic categories, is a psychiatric emergency that demands immediate intervention.

Past History

A past history of violent behavior is another important clue to predicting violence. If the patient states that he has attacked people before and he now feels like he wants to attack someone, the interviewer should assume the patient will act on his feelings, and psychiatric intervention should be initiated. At times there is a tendency to overlook verbal threats of violence, but in view of a history of violence, a verbal threat is a serious prognostic sign.

MANAGEMENT OF THE VIOLENT PATIENT

General Treatment

When a violent or potentially violent patient is first interviewed, it is helpful to interview the patient alone because he may feel overwhelmed and threatened by staff; this sense of vulnerability may further agitate him (Lion, 1972). However, when the interviewer feels uneasy and anxious or is unsure of how the patient is going to respond, the interviewer should ask police, security, or family to remain nearby in the hall so that if the patient becomes violent, the additional personnel will be close enough to help control him. All patients should be interviewed with the interviewer between the patient and the door. If the interviewer thinks the patient poses an extremely high potential for violence, he should consider interviewing him with the door open or in the hall with security personnel present (Hackett, 1977).

Treatment personnel should not approach patients suddenly or rapidly (DiBella, 1979). The interviewer should allow some physical distance to remain between himself and the patient. Especially with psychotic patients, the closer the interviewer moves to the patient, the more likely it is that he will increase the patient's anxiety level (Kalogerakis, 1971). A useful guideline is to stay at least an arm's length away (Rockwell, 1972).

Placement of patients in the emergency department setting can also have an effect on their potential for violence. A patient should not be placed near other disturbed patients who are provocative (Kalogerakis, 1971). Neither should he be left alone (Lion, 1972; Lion, Levenberg, and Strange, 1972), for this could be interpreted as rejection or could allow him to hurt himself while unobserved. If possible, he should be placed in a quiet area of the emergency department where the environmental stimulation is minimal, but where he can be readily observed and evaluated by the staff. Placing a patient in an area where there is frequent patient and staff traffic, or where he must contend with the constant noise of police sirens, may provoke a potentially violent patient who is feeling frightened and overwhelmed.

Specific Management

The most effective treatment approach is to talk to the patient. A direct, calm inquiry as to what is going on or "how can we help you?" will greatly alleviate anxiety. Most often the patient is relieved to have someone to talk with whom he feels is going to help him (Rockwell, 1972). The interviewer should try to encourage the patient to express his feelings verbally (Lion, 1972). Only after the patient shows some degree of relaxation and rapport with the examiner should the current illness be discussed. The interviewer should conduct himself in a manner that conveys to the patient an expectation of appropriate behavior (Stewart, 1978). It is important to convey to a patient that violence is not acceptable, and that his lack of control will be dealt with by the staff's firm control (Lion et al., 1968; DiBella, 1979). A helpful comment might be, "I'm going to stop you from losing control." The staff should also acknowledge that the patient can do harm; for example, "Look, you can really hurt someone with that chair" (Lion et al., 1972). When a patient is loud and belligerent, the technique of talking softly will frequently result in him lowering his voice. Staff members, however, frequently let their fantasies about the threatening patient interfere in a way that further provokes anxiety and tension in the patient. A patient can detect a staff member's anxiety, and this often leads to an exacerbation of the patient's agitation and culminates in violent behavior (Lion et al., 1968, 1972; Adler and Shapiro, 1973; Whitman, Armao, and Dent, 1976). It is important not to force the issue of talking with a patient if a staff member feels particularly anxious or out of control.

If talking does not defuse the situation, then offer the patient something to eat or drink. Frequently, offering food before the interview attenuates the patient's anxiety and serves to demonstrate the interviewer's genuine interest. Based on our experience, a combination of talk and food will generally defuse the vast majority of potentially violent situations.

If talk and food do not attenuate the patient's tension, then medication is recommended. The interviewer should remark that he can see the patient is upset and nervous and that he would like to offer him some medication. Medication should be used to decrease a patient's tension and anxiety. The relief it brings is usually welcomed by the patient (Lion et al., 1968, 1972). However, "Effective management does not involve rendering the patient helpless and physically inert, but rather helps him to modulate his own aggressiveness" (Lion, 1975). In the patient who is paranoid and reluctant to talk to the interviewer, the psychiatrist could comment that he knows the patient is having thoughts and feelings that are upsetting, and if he takes medication this will help him feel a little more relaxed.

Although studies (Donlon, Hopkin, and Tupin, 1979) indicate that rapid tranquilization can be achieved with intramuscular medication, we prefer instead to offer the patients a concentrate in orange juice. The patients are generally much more receptive to this and we have found tranquilization to be as rapid as with intramuscular injection.

Generally tablets and capsules have too long an absorption time to exert an immediate effect. The literature (Anderson and Kuehnle, 1974; Mason and Granacher, 1976; Dolon et al., 1979; Appleton and Daris, 1980) on rapid tranquilization suggests a dosage range that is empirically determined by the size, age, and weight of the patient; for example, smaller, frailer, older patients would receive doses at the lower end of the dose range. Recommended doses include Navane, 10–15 mg; Stelazine, 10–15 mg; Haldol, 5–10 mg; Serentil, 25–50 mg—sedating drug; and Thorazine, 50–75 mg—sedating drug. All drugs are given every 30 minutes in concentrate or intramuscularly until tranquilization is achieved.

The goal of rapid tranquilization is to reduce the tension, anxiety, and hyperactivity of the patient. Rapid tranquilization, however, will not diminish hallucinations and delusions, which require a longer period of appropriate neuroleptic treatment.

Using the medication in the lower dosage range, we have found one to three doses is generally sufficient to induce tranquilization without sedation. We are aware that the recommended doses do not correlate well if compared in terms of relative potency. However, these doses have been found empirically to be the most effective when used in concentrate for rapid tranquilization, and the discrepancy in potency is now under further study. Most patients seem to be concerned that they will become too sedated and should be reassured that all attempts will be made to avoid "knocking them out." In the paranoid patient a larger initial dose (the equivalent of two doses) might be given if there is concern about future compliance during the interview.

If the physician is having difficulty establishing rapport with the patient, it is often helpful to seek help from someone who seems to have had some positive interaction with the patient. This might be a security guard, a family member, or a secretary. This person should talk with the patient under the supervision of the physician, and once the patient is calm he should be encouraged to take medication. If this fails and the threat of violence still exists, the next strategy is to call in security guards.

When calling the security guards, the interviewer should use a code name. If the patient hears one staff member telling another to call security or the police, this will often incite him to violence. We refer to security as "Dr. Armstrong" and this allows them to be called without agitating the patient. When security personnel arrive they should not immediately rush into the patient's room; instead, a staff member should meet the security guards and place them so they can be seen by the patient. Their presence will reassure the patient that if he gets out of control there are enough personnel to restrain him. It is crucial for the patient to feel there are enough staff to prevent him from losing control and harming himself or others (Lion et al., 1968, 1972; Lion and Pasternak, 1971; Stewart, 1978). The reassurance of seeing the security guards will frequently defuse the tension the patient is experiencing.

The security guards are a critical part of the management team. In our experience, successful management of violent patients depends on the staff's confidence in the security personnel and, conversely, the security personnel's confidence in staff. When security guards are needed, the treating staff should spend a few minutes briefing the guards on the patient's problem and how they will be able to help in treatment. The physician should clearly spell out their role. Frequently security personnel are frightened and unsure of what they should do, and the communication between the treating staff and security will not only serve an educational function, but will also serve to improve their cooperation (Lion, 1972). When possible it is beneficial to have permanent security guards in the emergency department because they will develop an expertise in managing patients that is difficult to develop on a part-time basis. It is also useful to have frequent in-service training for security personnel in which they are taught rudimentary patient management.

If none of the above interventions is successful and the patient's agitation reaches a point at which restraints are necessary, security is asked to restrain the patient. Once the decision is made to restrain, it should be acted upon immediately without staff debate of the issue. Physical restraints can be humane and effective (Lion, 1975). Negotiating with the patient is generally futile. Staff members should not interfere with the security force while they are restraining a patient. For maximum safety five people should be used when restraining a patient: one for each limb and one to help hold the patient's head to keep him from biting (Hackett, 1977). If the patient is swinging a chair or some other weapon, distracting the patient by throwing a blanket over him or by approaching him with a light mattress will help protect the staff while subduing the patient (Stewart, 1978). The presence of one or two nurses talking to the patient while the security guards restrain him often calms him and renders him more compliant. Once the patient is in restraints, however, this is a psychiatric emergency, and all attempts by the staff are aimed at getting the patient out of restraints. This usually involves rapid tranquilization and supportive therapy.

Physical restraints are usually necessary when the patient remains agitated and noncompliant; for example, when he will not take medication, sit down, go into the interview room—the patient "cannot be talked to, reasoned with, persuaded, contained, delayed or denied . . ."

(Lion, 1975). Restraints may be needed to protect the patient and the staff.

The legalities involved in restraining patients are complex because each state has its own mental health laws that determine under what conditions patients may be restrained and treated against their will. Further complicating the issue is the fact that laws governing restraints and treatment by psychiatric personnel differ from laws governing restraints and treatment by nonpsychiatric personnel. Each physician, however, is strongly advised to become aware of the state laws governing therapeutic restraint and treatment in patients who refuse it. Further discussion of these legal issues is beyond the scope of this chapter.

If a patient has a weapon, the interviewer has the right to refuse to examine him until he either surrenders the weapon or allows security guards to search him and remove it. If the patient surrenders the weapon, the interviewer should have the patient place it on the table or floor. In normal circumstances, the interviewer should never take a weapon directly from the patient (Hackett, 1977). The patient may instinctively pull the trigger or lunge at the interviewer.

A final problem that frequently occurs in the emergency department is disruptive, violent behavior by a nonpatient (e.g., a friend or family member who accompanies the patient to the emergency department). To our knowledge, there is no literature that addresses this problem. Our policy is to have security personnel handle the disruptive, violent nonpatients. When this occurs, emergency department staff members view the situation as a civil rather than a medical problem. In some instances, after confronting hospital security, the nonpatient will request to see a psychiatrist or emergency physician. In this case the nonpatient then becomes a patient.

CONCLUSION

A careful assessment of the patient's behavior, coupled with appropriate diagnostic clues, can give an interviewer a reliable means of predicting the imminence of violence in a given patient. The key elements in defusing a patient's potential for violence center on the willingness of the interviewer to talk with the patient in a firm, empathetic manner. When used judiciously, medication and restraints are important adjuncts in helping to control violent or potentially violent patients. The goal of the treatment should be to provide patients with a setting that will facilitate a release of tension while conveying to the patient a sense of security and safety.

REFERENCES

Adler, G., & Shapiro, L. N. (1973), Some difficulties in the treatment of the aggressive acting out patient. *Amer. J. Psychother.*, 27:548–556.

Anderson, W. H., & Kuehnle, J. C. (1974), Strategies for treatment of acute psychosis. *J. Amer. Med. Assn.*, 229:1884–1889.

Appleton, W. S., & Daris, J. M. (1980), *Practical Clinical Psychopharmacology*, 2nd ed. Baltimore, MD: Williams & Wilkins, p. 29.

Bach-y-Rita, G., Lion, J. R., & Clement, C. E. (1971), Episodic dyscontrol: A study of 130 violent patients. *Amer. J. Psychiat.*, 127:1473–1478.

Cohen, S. (1979), Aggression: The role of drugs. *Drug Abuse & Alcoh. Newsletter*, 8:1–4.

DiBella, G. A. (1979), Educating staff to manage threatening paranoid patients. *Amer. J. Psychiat.*, 136:333–335.

Donlon, P. T., Hopkin, J., & Tupin, J. P. (1979), Overview: Efficacy and safety of the rapid neuroleptization method with injectable haloperidol. *Amer. J. Psychiat.*, 136:273–278.

Eaton, M. E., Stetten, I. W., & Kitchen, A. D. (1971), The Missouri automated psychiatric history: Symptom frequencies, sex differences, use of weapons, and other findings. *Comprehen. Psychiat.*, 12:264–276.

Hackett, T. (1977), Management of the violent patient. Syllabus, Course in Emergency Psychiatry and Crisis Intervention. Massachusetts General Hospital and Harvard Medical School, Department of Continuing Education.

Kalogerakis, M. G. (1971), The assaultive psychiatric patient. *Psych. Quart.*, 45:372–381.

Lenefsky, B., de Palma, T., & Lorirers, D. (1978), Management of violent behaviors. *Persp. Psychiat. Care*, 16:212–217.

Leroy, P., & Hartocollis, P. (1976), Nursing aides and patient violence. *Amer. J. Psychiat.*, 133:429–431.

Lion, J. R. (1972), *Evaluation and Management of the Violent Patient*. Springfield, IL: Charles C. Thomas.

——— (1975), Conceptual issues in the use of drugs for the treatment of aggression in man. *J. Nerv. Ment. Dis.*, 160:76–81.

——— Bach-y-Rita, G., & Ervin, F. R. (1968), The self-referred violent patient. *J. Amer. Med. Assn.*, 205:91–93.

——— ——— ——— (1969), Violent patients in the emergency room. *Amer. J. Psychiat.*, 125:1706–1711.

——— Levenberg, L. B., & Strange, R. E. (1972), Restraining the violent patient. *J. Psychiat. Nurs. Ment. Health Serv.*, 10:9–11.

——— Pasternak, S. A. (1971), Countertransference reactions to violent patients. *Amer. J. Psychiat.*, 130:207–210.

MacDonald, J. M. (1971), The threat to kill. *Amer. J. Psychiat.*, 127:1473–1478.

Madden, D. J., Lion, J. R., & Penna, M. W. (1976), Assaults on psychiatrists by patients. *Amer. J. Psychiat.*, 133:422–425.

Mason, A. S., & Granacher, R. P. (1976), Basic principles of rapid neuroleptization. *Dis. Nerv. Syst.*, 12:547–551.

Rockwell, D. A. (1972), Can you spot potential violence in a patient? *Hosp. Physician*, 8:52–56.

Stewart, A. T. (1978), Handling the aggressive patient. *Persp. in Psychiat. Care*, 16:228–232.

Tauson, V. B. (1971), The psychiatrist and the violent patient. *Dis. Nerv. Syst.*, 32:764–768.

Whitman, R. M., Armao, B. B., & Dent, O. B. (1976), Assault on the therapist. *Amer. J. Psychiat.*, 133:426–429.

Commentary

Karen J. Evanczuk, M.S.N., Ph.D.

Dubin offers a practical and sound schema for dealing with the violent patient in the emergency room setting. Although addressed primarily to the psychiatric emergency service physician, his recommendations should be of great value to multidisciplinary staff and for a general emergency or outpatient setting as well.

In the introduction, the author appropriately urges a preventive approach to the management of violence. He outlines diagnostic groupings of patients having a high risk for violence. But, in addition to the need to be skilled in recognizing salient diagnostic and behavioral cues, there are other precautionary measures that can be implemented in emergency or outpatient settings. The following are important adjuncts to prevention that can help minimize violent occurrences and thereby decrease injury to patients and staff.

Special Concern File. Maintaining a file of patients who have a known history of violence, who have been armed with lethal weapons, or who have been previously assaultive to inpatient or outpatient staff, is a powerful tool for prevention. This file can be linked to computer systems. When conducting a computerized name search for patients arriving at our emergency department, the names of patients included in the special concern file are flagged, further information is obtained from the file, and proper precautions are taken (e.g., search for weapons, summoning of security personnel, etc.).

Electronic Door Lock. An electronic locking device on the emergency department exit door may be a useful adjunct to prevention. The unit receptionist can operate the device at the request of a clinician to prevent the elopement of a committable, dangerous patient (e.g., homicidal, suicidal) who may bolt from the service area during the evaluation process.

Searches. The employment of search measures for patients who are actively threatening, who have histories of assaultiveness, or who are known to have carried a weapon into the facility in the past is a useful precautionary measure. Patients who are paranoid may be hiding a weapon for use in protecting themselves. Knowing the state law regarding patient searches is essential in implementing this measure. Ultimately, the evaluation team may need to judge whether it is safe to interview the patient without the search, whether involuntary commitment should be considered, or whether the risk to staff and other patients is too great to proceed with the evaluation. In the latter case, the physician may elect to refuse to interview the patient.

The above is not an exhaustive list of measures. We could also consider the employment of alarm systems (i.e., "panic buttons") and the use of appropriate modes of dress by staff who deal with violent patients.

A final recommendation is the implementation of adequate training, not only for security personnel, but also for clinical staff and trainees. For only with ongoing training in the use of verbal, nonverbal, and physical control techniques will staff acquire the confidence and skill necessary to interact with the potentially violent patient.

Annotated Bibliography

Shevitz, S. (1978), Emergency management of the agitated patient. *Primary Care*, 5(4):625–634.

A brief overview of the problem of the agitated and/or assaultive patient in an emergency setting. Such behaviors are symptoms, not disorders unto themselves. Therefore, the management of such patients (including the use of pharmacologic restraints) clearly depends on the etiology of the behavior. The authors identify four major diagnostic categories that represent risk conditions: (1) functional psychoses; (2) organic brain syndromes (infection, trauma, dementia); (3) toxic psychoses; and (4) withdrawal from alcohol, barbiturates, and other central nervous system depressants.

Guirguis, E. F. (1978), Management of disturbed patients: An alternative to the use of mechanical restraints. *J. Clin. Psychiat.*, 39:295–303.

A brief outline of some of the causes of violence in clinical settings and step-by-step guidelines for the management of such behaviors. The guidelines include the effective use of medication and the actual physical handling of violent patients. Emphasizing staff education, as well as the importance of careful treatment planning, the author points out the dangers and abuses of mechanical restraints.

Richmond, J. S., & Ruparel, M. K. (1980), Management of violent patients in a psychiatry walk-in clinic. *J. Clin. Psychiat.*, 41(11):370–373.

Although not directed specifically to the emergency department, this paper discusses a systems approach for managing violent psychiatric outpatients. Multiple care giving and brief visits in an outpatient walk-in clinic setting can provide empathic care for those violent patients who become too threatened by the intimacy of individual therapy, and who often reject treatment. The authors use case vignettes to illustrate how the walk-in clinic treats violent patients with a variety of diagnoses, and prepares them for eventual acceptance of more traditional therapies.

Jacobs, D. (1983), Evaluation and management of the violent patient in emergency settings. *Psych. Clin. N. Amer.*, 6(2):259–269.

A brief discussion of a systematic approach to the violent emergency room patient.

Rofman, E. S., Askinawzi, C., & Fant, E. (1980), The prediction of dangerous behavior in emergency civil commitment. *Amer. J. Psychiat.*, 137(9):1061–1064.

Complementing chapter 11 by Monahan, the authors compared committed and noncommitted psychiatric patients with respect to the number of assaults noted during the first 45 days of hospitalization. The authors point out that most of the assaults occurred during the last 10 days of hospitalization. The committed group had a .41 probability and the control group a .08 probability of committing an assault. The occurrence of an actual act of battery before admission did not predict assault in the hospital to a greater degree than did a veral threat. The authors concluded that it was possible to make short-term predictions of assaultiveness in the hospital.

Burgess, A. W., & Holmstrom, L. L. (1974), The rape trauma syndrome. *Amer. J. Psychiat.*, 131(9):981–986.

A relevant and still timely paper. The reported study followed patients admitted over a one-year period to an emergency department with a presenting complaint of having been raped. The authors attempted to document the existence of a rape trauma syndrome and delineate its symptomatology as well as that of two variations, namely, compounded reaction and silent reaction. Specific therapeutic techniques seem to be required for each of these reactions.

Huber, G. A., Roth, L. H., Appelbaum, P. S., & Ore, T. M. (1982), Hospitalization,

Arrest, or Discharge: Important Legal and Clinical Issues in the Emergency Evaluation of Persons Believed Dangerous to Others. *Law Contemp. Prob.*, 45:99–123.

This thorough article, written by several faculty members of the University of Pittsburgh and invited commentators in this volume, examines the legal obstacles that hinder implementation of the suggestion that responsibility for control of dangerous persons with alleged mental illness be transferred to the criminal justice system. The issue is explored from the perspective of the psychiatric emergency room. The article shows that the present legal and ethical obligations of caregivers in the emergency setting all but preclude the possibility of shunting violent persons, once they have been evaluated, out of the system of psychiatric care.

Talbert, S., White, S. D., Bowen, J. D., Stephens, L. M., Mapstone, S. J., Spisso, K. R., & Edlich, R. F. (1980), Improving emergency department care of the sexual assault victim. *Ann. Emerg. Med.*, 9(6):293–297.

Complementing Burgess and Holmstrom (1974), this multiauthored and multidisciplinary paper provides an organized approach to the care of victims of sexual assault. The authors point out that such victims face the multiple threats of disease, unwanted pregnancy, psychological trauma, and physical injury. This is further complicated by an often exhaustive and sometimes embarrassing police investigation. The authors recommend that the care of victims, from arrival in the emergency room to rehabilitation, be coordinated by a nurse. This professional should be specially trained and serve as a liaison between the patient and other health professionals and the police team.

Jacobs, D., (1982–1983), Evaluation and care of suicidal behavior in emergency settings. *Internat.J. Psychiat. in Med.*, 12(4):295–310.

A relatively recent and comprehensive paper, in which the author comments first on the complicated matter of assessment of suicidal behavior. He points out the heterogeneity of suicidal patients across the full spectrum of psychiatric illnesses. He suggests that the focus of suicidal assessment should not be the suicide but the treatment and protection of the distressed person. Effective treatment would include recognition and management of the clinician's own feelings, delineating the suicidal crisis, contacting a significant other, calling a therapist, and dispensing medication if necessary.

13

Child Psychiatric Emergencies: A Research Note

M. E. Garralda

The need for prompt medical intervention in pediatric/psychiatric conditions such as drug overdoses is self-evident. That purely psychiatric disorders of children and adolescents require urgent treatment is less obvious. Children's psychiatric symptomatology is often linked to external events in their lives, and even relatively minor changes in the environment can substantially relieve acute childhood disturbance.

Although a number of nonpediatrically linked child psychiatric services provide emergency consultations (Ewing, 1978), the determinants of emergencies have not been extensively studied. Empirical studies have looked at the clinical characteristics in children that lead to urgent assessment. Increased anxiety, aggression, school refusal, and suicidal and bizarre behavior have figured prominently in previous partly uncontrolled reports (Burks and Hoekstra, 1964; Mattisson, Hawkins, and Seese 1967; Morrison and Smith, 1975; Shafi, Whittinghill, and Healy, 1979). Epidemiological and observational studies

This chapter was first published in *Journal of Child Psychology and Psychiatry* (1983), 24:261–267, and it is reprinted by permission.

have emphasized the importance of parental attitudes as determinants for referrals to child psychiatric clinics (Shepherd, Oppenheim, and Mitchell, 1966; Johnson and Lobitz, 1974). But for emergency presentations, the relationship between symptomatology in the children, on the one hand, and family and social features, on the other, remains little known.

The present report is a preliminary controlled investigation of child symptomatology, and family and social factors in emergency referrals to a child psychiatric clinic.

METHOD

Description of the Service

The study was carried out in the outpatient child and adolescent psychiatric department of a London psychiatric teaching hospital. As well as a routine service based on waiting list appointments, the department runs a walk-in emergency service during normal working hours. The various multidisciplinary teams that take up routine cases are on emergency call one day a week in rotation. Staff making the original emergency assessments continue to follow the cases themselves. Children requiring more technical medical intervention, for example, after overdoses, are usually seen in the neighboring pediatric unit of a general hospital and do not therefore feature in this report.

Selection of Cases

During the period of study from July 1977 to December 1978, emergency presentations constituted 8.2 percent of all the cases seen in the department. A considerable number of therapists were involved with emergencies, who presented to the hospital at any time during the day. This made it impracticable for the author to study all cases, and so 22 (40 percent) were selected for study. The 22 cases were representative of the global group of emergencies seen during that period for age, sex distribution, socioeconomic level, and predominant clinical features. Emergencies were defined as new or closed cases seen within three days of referral. Twenty controls, defined simply as nonemergency cases, were also selected. The only specific source of bias excluded from the control group was that of cases referred by other psychiatrists for a second opinion.

Measures and Analysis

Parents of the 42 cases were asked to complete a questionnaire on their first visit to the hospital. The first section of the questionnaire dealt with the child's presenting symptoms and any recent deterioration. The second section consisted of questions about current parental psychological and physical symptoms, features of marital and family dysfunction, and on any recent deterioration in these areas. The third section included details of extended family and social supports, and recent changes in their availability.

The case notes of all the patients were scrutinized and information collected on a variety of diagnostic, symptomatic, familial, social, and demographic variables.

The information was coded and the emergency group was compared with the controls on the items under study. Tests of statistical significance (χ^2; Wilcoxon rank sum two-sample test) were used when appropriate.

Some measure of reliability of the instruments used was established by comparing the scores obtained from case notes, with the scores available from questionnaires. This was done for items that had been systematically covered by both sources (duration of illness, referral symptoms, parental psychiatric and physical symptoms, marital discord, and social agency involvement). Agreement between the two sources was high, on the whole above the 80 percent level.

RESULTS

General data on the comparative study between emergencies and control are given in Table 13.1.

The age range was 5–15 years. In the emergency group the mean age was 12.3 years, with a standard deviation of 2.8; the corresponding figures for the controls were 11.3 and 2.8 (a nonsignificant difference on the Wilcoxon rank sum two-sample test).

The time between referral and assessment at the clinic was, on the whole, between one and three months for the controls. There were

Table 13.1
General Data

General data	Emergencies (*n* = 22)		Controls (*n* = 20)	
Age: 12 to 15 years	77%	(17)	50%	(10)
Females	54%	(12)	45%	(9)
Males	45%	(10)	55%	(11)
Referral agent				
General practitioners	68%	(15)	65%	(13)
Schools	18%	(4)	15%	(3)
Parents	9%	(2)	15%	(3)
Others	4%	(1)	5%	(1)
Waiting Period				
Less than 3 days	100%	(22)		—
1 to 3 months		—	65%	(13)
Socio-economic level				
I–II	20%	(4)	15%	(3)
III	54%	(12)	80%	(16)
IV–V	18%	(4)	5%	(1)
Not established	9%	(2)		—
Parents born in the U.K.	77%	(17)	75%	(15)
Local residents	63%	(14)	60%	(12)

hardly any differences between the two groups in terms of sex distribution, referral agent (usually the general practitioner), area of domicile, ratio of immigrant parents, or socioeconomic level.

Table 13.2 shows a number of significant differences in the symptomatology of the children. In the emergencies, the psychiatric diagnosis was more commonly mixed or emotional disorder, with fewer of the relatively uncommon conditions that present to a psychiatric clinic, such as simple developmental delays or a Gilles de la Tourette syndrome. In line with this finding, the presenting symptoms tended to be emotional or mixed behavioral/emotional. As expected from the previously quoted studies, all the symptoms listed in the table were more frequently in emergencies (anxiety, school refusal, wandering away from home and truancy, and aggression). However, only depression, and suicidal and psychotic symptoms reached statistical significance. Depression, with sadness, persistent crying, and general unhappiness, was present in over half the emergencies. Suicidal symptoms consisted of gestures or threats, with the exception of one child who had taken an overdose. Psychotic symptoms included either perceptual disorders or more rarely delusional ideation; they were reported in five emergencies. Although the nature of these symptoms suggested a psychotic disorder, only two of the subjects were given a final diagnosis of psychosis (schizophrenia in one case and acute psychotic reaction in another), the other three fell within the emotional/conduct disorder categories.

A shorter duration of illness of less than six months was relatively more common in emergencies, and at a statistically significant level more emergencies reported a deterioration in the child's condition over the previous weeks or months.

The family aspects of the comparison between the groups are listed in Table 13.3.

Table 13.2
Diagnosis and Symptomatology in the Children

Symptoms and Diagnosis	Emergencies ($n = 22$)		Controls ($n = 20$)	
Psychiatric diagnosis*				
Emotional disorder	36%	(8)	30%	(6)
Conduct disorder	18%	(4)	25%	(5)
Mixed conduct—Emotional	31%	(7)	5%	(1)
Psychosis	9%	(2)	—	
Other	4%	(1)	25%	(5)
Nil	—		15%	(3)
Presenting symptoms*				
Emotional	22%	(5)	5%	(1)
Behavioral	31%	(7)	25%	(5)
Mixed emotional–behavioral	18%	(4)	5%	(1)
Other	4%	(1)	45%	(9)
Not given in questionnaires	22%	(5)	20%	(4)
Symptoms				
Anxiety	45%	(10)	20%	(4)
Depression*	54%	(12)	20%	(4)
Suicidal*	31%	(7)	—	
School refusal	27%	(6)	15%	(3)
Wandering away	18%	(4)	5%	(1)
Aggression	45%	(10)	25%	(5)
Psychotic-type*	22%	(5)	—	
Duration				
Under 6 months	31%	(7)	10%	(2)
Over 3 years	22%	(5)	45%	(9)
Recent Deterioration*	54%	(12)	25%	(5)

*$p < 0.05$.

There was a slight trend for emergencies not to be living with two natural parents. There were also more problems in the mother–child relationship and a more recent increase in marital tension. Marginally more emergency parents rated themselves as irritable or anxious. Only two family items reached significance: a poor father–child relationship (50 percent of emergencies versus 5 percent of controls), and a parental self-rating of depression (63 percent of emergencies versus 25 percent of controls).

There were no significant differences in the use of extended family and social supports (Table 13.4). Social agency support, usually

Table 13.3
Family Aspects

Family aspects	Emergencies (n = 22)		Controls (n = 20)	
Living with two natural parents	59%	(13)	70%	(14)
Disturbed relationship with				
Mother	59%	(13)	30%	(6)
Father*	50%	(11)	5%	(1)
Marital tension	40%	(9)	30%	(6)
Recent deterioration	27%	(6)	5%	(1)
Family tension	31%	(7)	25%	(5)
Recent deterioration	13%	(3)	5%	(1)
Parental self-ratings of				
Irritability	50%	(11)	40%	(8)
Anxiety	50%	(11)	40%	(8)
Depression**	63%	(14)	25%	(5)
Aches and pains	13%	(3)	40%	(8)
Recent deterioration in parental symptoms	36%	(8)	15%	(3)

*$p < 0.05$; **$p < 0.01$.

Table 13.4
Social Supports

Social supports	Emergencies (n = 22)		Controls (n = 20)	
Social agencies involved	45%	(10)	25%	(5)
Frequent contact with extended family	63%	(14)	60%	(12)
Confidants	72%	(16)	70%	(14)
Having many friends	45%	(10)	55%	(11)

through local authority social workers, was more commonly used by emergencies (about half to a quarter of the controls), but contact with the extended family was similarly maintained by about two-thirds in each group. About half the parents reported having many friends and almost three-fourths said they had confidants, defined as somebody they could talk to if they were in difficulties or had any troubles.

Parental depression and a poor father–child relationship were studied in the 42 cases in relation to various symptomatic and social features to clarify the way in which those two factors could have contributed to emergency referrals. Depressed mood in parents was significantly linked to mixed or antisocial symptoms in the children on referral ($p = .02$) and with suicidal symptomatology; the latter was present in 31 percent of children of self-rated depressed parents and only 4 percent of the rest ($p = .05$).

In the group with disturbed father–child relationships, there were more natural parents living apart and more children living with their mother and a stepfather ($p = .005$). Interestingly, all the children living with stepfathers (4) had a poor relationship with them, and they all fell into the emergency group.

DISCUSSION

The sample in this study is small and the techniques somewhat crude. This calls for caution in interpreting the results. Unlike previous studies that have looked at aspects of family function and social environment (Brown and Rutter, 1966; Brown and Harris, 1978; Henderson, 1981), our measures were global and assessment of the social support system did not attempt detailed descriptions. The preliminary nature of the study needs to be emphasized in this connection. Because of the relative dearth of studies on the subject, we explored a number of issues in a general way, in order to identify areas deserving further and more sophisticated investigation.

Contrary to our original expectation that emergencies would reflect psychological problems in the child as much as tension in the family, significant differences between the emergency referrals and the control group were largely confined to the field of symptomatology in the children. In line with American findings (Morrison and Smith, 1975; Mattisson et al., 1967), emergencies reported emotional symptoms on referral, and depressive, suicidal, and psychotic symptomatology as part of the clinical picture, more often than controls. It can be concluded that early assessment and treatment of these children was well justified.

The excess of parents describing themselves as depressed in the group of emergency referrals is of interest, as is the association between depression in the parents and suicidal and antisocial behavior in the children. Parental depression could have induced suicidal threats in the children as a dramatic way of showing their desperation at the parents' state, and their naughtiness could be viewed as a means of shaking their parents out of their depression. Alternatively the depressed parental mood could have been a response to the alarming nature of the children's symptomatology, or have colored the parents' appraisal of the severity of the children's condition (Criest, Wells, and Forehand, 1979; Sandberg, Wieselberg, and Shaffer, 1980). Elucidation of the direction of this association and of the nature of the parental depression itself is called for and could have useful therapeutic implications.

The finding of an excess of disturbed relationships with the father among emergency referrals suggests that the current emphasis on the importance of fathers in the psychiatric treatment of their children is particularly relevant in those cases.

It does not appear from our results that social isolation was a factor that substantially influenced emergency referrals. These had, in fact, social agencies involvement more frequently than the controls, but this difference did not reach statistical significance, maybe due to the small number of cases studied. As with previous findings, a more sophisticated investigation of this is needed.

Lastly, we do not know what relevance our findings may have for work in other settings, such as psychiatric units attached to pediatric hospitals. The factors that lead families to seek urgent psychiatric help for their children rather than treatment in a casualty department for physical complaints or an overdose remain an interesting area for further study.

SUMMARY

In a controlled study, emergency referrals to a child psychiatric clinic showed increased depressive and suicidal symptomatology and more perceptual abnormalities. There was also more commonly a recent deterioration in the presenting condition. Parents rated themselves as depressed more frequently and there were more problems in the father–child relationship. There were no significant associations between emergency referrals and ratings of family dysfunction, availability of an extended family or contact with social agencies, but there was a trend toward increased use of the latter by the emergency group. The results highlight the need for early child-centered psychiatric intervention in a minority of conditions of children and adolescents.

REFERENCES

Brown, G. W., & Harris, T. O. (1978), *Social Origins of Depression*. London: Tavistock.

——— Rutter, M. (1966), The measurement of family activities and relationships: A methodological study. *Hum. Relat.*, 19:241–263.

Burks, H. L., & Hoekstra, M. (1964), Psychiatric emergencies in children. *Amer. J. Orthopsychiat.*, 34:134–137.

Criest, D., Wells, K. C., & Forehand, R. (1979), An examination of the predictors of maternal perceptions of maladjustment in clinic-referred children. *J. Abnorm. Psychol.*, 88:277–292.

Ewing, C. P. (1978), *Crisis Intervention as Psychotherapy*. New York: Oxford University Press.

Henderson, S. (1981), Social relationships, adversity and neurosis: An analysis of prospective observations. *Brit. J. Psychiat.*, 138:391–396.

Johnson, S. M., & Lobitz, G. K. (1973), The personal and marital adjustment of parents as related to observed child deviance and parenting behaviors. *J. Abnorm. Child Psychol.*, 2:193–207.

Mattison, A., Hawkins, J. W., & Seese, L. R. (1967), Child psychiatric emergencies: Clinical characteristics and follow-up results. *Arch. Gen. Psychiat.*, 17:584–592.

Morrison, G. C., & Smith, W. R. (1974), Child psychiatric emergencies: A comparison of two clinic settings and socio-economic groups. In: *Emergencies in Child Psychiatry: Emotional Crises of Children, Youth, and Their Families*, ed. G. C. Morrison. Springfield, IL: Charles C. Thomas.

Sandberg, S. T., Wieselberg, M., & Shaffer, D. (1980), Hyperkinetic and conduct problem children in a primary school population: Some epidemiological considerations. *J. Child Psychol. Psychiat.*, 21:303–311.

Shafi, M., Whittinghill, R., & Healy, M. H. (1979), The pediatric-psychiatric model for emergencies in child psychiatry: A study of 994 cases. *Amer. J. Psychiat.*, 136:1600–1602.

Shepherd, M., Oppenheim, A. N., & Mitchell, S. (1966), Childhood behaviour disorders and the child guidance clinic. *J. Child Psychol. Psychiat.*, 7:39–52.

Commentary

Joaquim Puig-Antich, M.D.

Chapter 13 represents a modest start to ascertaining the differences between emergency and nonemergency child psychiatric cases. In spite of relatively simple methods of measurement and the limited attention paid to their reliability and other psychometric properties, two findings emerge quite clearly: (1) that no significant differences appeared in familial functioning and social supports between the two groups and (2) that major differences in rates of certain of the child's presenting symptoms and behavior were found: depressive mood, suicidal threats, gestures, or acts, and "psychotic" symptoms were found to be significantly higher in the emergency group. One other finding, increased rate of parental depression by self-rating, is likely to be related to the fact that affective illness and suicidal behavior tend to aggregate in families.

These conclusions have to be tempered by the presence of several methodological shortcomings: (1) It is not clear what method was used to select the 22 percent of emergency cases and the 20 control cases studied out from all the cases seen at the hospital during the time period being considered. (2) The data were obtained either by self-administered questionnaire or from record review, none by semistructured clinical interview, and the assessment of reliability is short of what is desirable. (3) The sample sizes are rather small and many findings fall short of significance probably by lack of proper statistical power.

With these limitations in mind the findings clearly indicate that child symptomatology is the primary determinant of emergency presentations in child psychiatry and suggest that careful symptom assessment by interviewing the child and the parent is crucial if proper treatment is to be implemented. It also implies the futility, in such cases, of the widespread practice of looking at the child primarily as the expressor of a "system malfunction," it being the school, the family, or the peer group, before a systematic assessment of symptoms has been carried out. This does not seem to be considered by the author who focuses in the discussion, on the teleology of the depression in the children vis-à-vis the same diagnosis in the parent.

There is a puzzling statement in the chapter regarding restricting psychotic disorder diagnoses to only some of the children with hallucinations or delusions. One would expect that among the suicidal and depressed patients major depression psychotic subtype and/or mixed bipolar disorder would predominate. It is hard to reconcile a diagnosis of emotional or conduct disorders with the presence of hallucinations, unless these categories are defined so as to become meaningless.

In summary, the results of this preliminary study indicate that depression, psychotic symptoms, and suicidality predominate among child psychiatric emergencies, compared to other referred cases. Probably a variety of other symptoms like school refusal and aggression also predominate but the power was too low to detect them at a significant level.

Annotated Bibliography

Turgay, A. (1982), Psychiatric emergencies in children. *Psychiat. J. Univ. Ottawa*, 7:254–260.

This is one of the few published papers on psychiatric emergencies in children. The theoretical framework of pediatric–psychiatric crisis intervention is reviewed and a system of classification is proposed. In addition to looking at epidemiological features, some general family characteristics of child psychiatric emergencies are reviewed. The importance of a rapid and effective assessment is stressed as well as the importance of immediate therapeutic intervention.

Pfeffer, C. R. (1981), Suicidal behavior of children: A review with implications for research and practice. *Amer. J. Psychiat.*, 138:154–159.

The first of two papers by the same group, which examines the environmental and psychological factors associated with increasing suicidal behavior of 6- to 12-year-old children. Assessment of a child's suicidal potential using a developmental approach should focus on such issues as depression, family communication patterns, the child's concept about death, and the state of ego functioning. The need for more systematic investigations of suicidal behavior among children, more precise methods of interviewing including the utility of symptom inventories, recognition of at-risk signs and symptoms, and widespread public education about this life-threatening condition is emphasized.

——— Plutchnik, R., & Mizruchi, M. S. (1983), Suicidal and assaultive behavior in children: Classification, measurement, and interrelations. *Amer. J. Psychiat.*, 140:154–157.

A complementary and follow-up paper to Pfeffer (1981), investigating dangerous behaviors in 102 children aged 6 to 12 years seen in a municipal psychiatric facility. The authors identified four groups of suicidal and assaultive behaviors. Logistic regression analysis suggested that neurosis, intellectualization, and low levels of aggression predicted membership in the nonassaultive–nonsuicidal group; intense aggression, parental suicidal behavior, parental assaultive behavior, and compensation predicted membership in the assaultive–suicidal group; depression, a minimum of aggression, and adjustment disorder predicted membership in the suicidal-only group; and intense aggression and absence of depression predicted membership in the assaultive-only group.

14

Geriatric Psychiatry in the Emergency Department: Evaluation and Treatment of Geriatric and Nongeriatric Admissions

Howard M. Waxman, Ph.D., William Dubin, M.D., Melissa Klein, M.A., M.C.P., Kenneth J. Weiss, M.D., and Erwin A. Carner, Ed.D.

Hospital emergency departments offer one possible avenue of referral for the increasing numbers of older patients in need of acute psychiatric attention. As such, emergency departments are important settings in which to better understand the multiple problems of elderly patients with psychiatric symptoms and to begin to evaluate the care

This chapter was first published in the *Journal of the American Geriatric Society* (1984), 32:343–349, and it is reprinted by permission.

they receive (Waxman, Carner, and Dubin, 1982; Bassuk, Minden, and Apsler, 1983). Appropriate medical evaluation is particularly critical for elderly psychiatric patients, as many physical conditions can manifest with acute psychiatric symptoms. As a result, life-threatening physical disease can easily be misdiagnosed when the presenting symptoms are predominantly psychiatric. Many of these conditions are treatable or even reversible with appropriate intervention (Libow, 1973; Butler, 1980; Jarvik and Perl, 1981; Weingarten, Rosoff, Eisen, et al., 1982). However, failure to properly identify medical illness in these cases can result in the misapplication of therapeutic efforts, which may lead to increased morbidity and mortality and unnecessary nursing home placement. These considerations are especially important in an emergency department, where the difficulty of conducting a thorough evaluation adds to the risk of misdiagnosis.

In a previous study we compared the demographic and admission information abstracted from the medical records of 49 elderly and 49 middle-aged patients seen in an urban hospital's psychiatric emergency service (Waxman et al., 1982). We found enough significant differences in the characteristics of these two groups to suggest that increased attention be given to the special needs of elderly emergency department patients. Compared with middle-aged patients, the elderly patients lacked a history of psychiatric illness (33 percent of middle-aged patients lacked such a history, versus 66 percent of elderly patients) and were much more likely to have been accompanied to the emergency department by a relative rather than being self-referred. The elderly patients were less likely to have been diagnosed with a schizophrenic disorder and/or a substance abuse disorder and more likely to have been diagnosed as having an organic brain syndrome. In fact, a striking finding of this study was that almost 40 percent of the elderly patient sample was given a diagnosis of organic brain syndrome without any specified etiology. This finding concerned us, as it raised the possibility that the primary problems of these patients may have been medical rather than psychiatric in origin. Thus, it called into question the adequacy of an emergency department medical evaluation for patients who may have organic brain syndrome.

For these reasons, we continued our study of geropsychiatry in the emergency department by evaluating the workup and treatment given to elderly patients by the psychiatric service in an emergency department. We were interested to identify factors that may have influenced diagnostic and treatment decisions for groups of elderly patients with and without a diagnosis of organic brain syndrome. Of particular interest was which laboratory tests and procedures were performed on these patients, and the results. We therefore reviewed the results of the physical examinations, laboratory tests, and mental status examinations and compared these findings with (1) those from similar groups of middle-aged patients and (2) those from a group of elderly medical patients from the emergency department who were not seen by the psychiatry service.

MATERIALS AND METHODS

Thomas Jefferson University Hospital is located in downtown Philadelphia. The Psychiatric Emergency Service (PES), which is located within the hospital's emergency department, is staffed by psychiatric nurses, a staff psychiatrist, and a psychiatric resident. The PES treats approximately 4,000 patients per year, or about 10 percent of the 40,000 patients seen annually in the emergency department. Upon entry of a patient into the emergency department, a triage nurse determines whether the patient's primary problem is psychiatric or medical. A more complete description of the PES and of the characteristics of the patient population is available in our previous report (Waxman et al., 1982).

Most subjects for this study were selected retrospectively from all patients admitted to the PES during 1981. Patients were randomly selected from all admissions so as to have roughly equal numbers in each of four groups. One group consisted of elderly (over 65 years) PES patients who received a diagnosis of organic brain syndrome—Elderly/OBS ($n = 30$). Another group consisted of elderly PES patients who received another psychiatric diagnosis—Elderly/Psych ($n = 27$). Two corresponding middle-aged groups were selected—Middle-aged/OBS ($n = 28$) and Middle-aged/Psych ($n = 30$). In addition, a fifth group was created by randomly selecting charts of elderly patients who were seen in the emergency department during 1981 but who were not sent to the PES—Elderly/Medical ($n = 30$).

Two psychiatrists (WRD and KJW) reviewed the physical examination, laboratory testing, and mental status findings that were recorded on each chart. This material was supplemented by basic demographic and admission data obtained from the medical records. The admission data included such information as presenting complaints, psychiatric and medical history, social status, current medications, and admission priority. The admission priority code for all emergency department patients at Jefferson is a high-priority, medium-priority, low-priority rating system.

After evaluating each chart, the reviewing psychiatrists determined if, in their judgment, additional medical or psychiatric evaluation was needed beyond what the patient had received and if any medications in use by the patient could have been responsible for the psychiatric symptoms. Finally, the treatment plan was examined, including referral agencies and prescribed medications. Any missing or ambiguous information was coded as a missing variable. Chi-square and analysis of variance statistical techniques were employed for data analysis.

RESULTS

Demographic and Admission Data

The demographic and admission data for all five groups are presented in detail in Table 14.1. Differences between the groups included proportionately more men among the two organic brain syndrome groups than among the other two psychiatric groups ($\chi^2 = 4.28$; $p < 0.05$); more black and single patients among the four psychiatric groups than among the Elderly/Medical group (black patients: $\chi^2 = 4.06$; $p < 0.05$; single patients: $\chi^2 = 6.29$; $p < 0.05$); and more patients in the Elderly/Medical group assigned a higher priority rating for treatment than in the Elderly/OBS or Elderly/Psych groups ($\chi^2 = 5.6$; $p < 0.05$). Also, patients in the two elderly psychiatric groups were much less likely to have had a previous psychiatric hospitalization than were patients in the two middle-aged groups ($\chi^2 = 10.9$; $p < 0.001$).

From the medical records of all 115 patients seen by the PES, it was possible in 110 cases to determine that 89 patients (80.9 percent) were sent directly by the triage nurse to PES (direct referral), while the remaining 21 patients (19.1 percent) were evaluated first in the medical side of the emergency department and then referred to the PES (indirect referral). Sixteen (76.2 percent) of the 21 indirect-referral

Table 14.1
Demographic and Admission Characteristics of Elderly and Middle-Aged Emergency Department Patients

	Elderly/OBS (n = 30)	Elderly/Psych (n = 27)	Middle-Aged/OBS (n = 28)	Middle-Aged/Psych (n = 30)	Elderly/Medical (n = 30)
Sex					
Male	17	9	11	12	13
Female	13	18	17	17	17
Missing data	0	0	0	1	0
Race					
Black	13	9	11	13	5
White	17	18	16	16	24
Missing data	0	0	1	1	1
Mean age (years)	75.8	70.8	54.2	50.8	75.4
Marital status					
Married	6	4	5	9	11
Single	9	5	7	10	5
Divorced	0	3	2	2	1
Widowed	7	12	0	6	4
Missing data	8	3	14	3	9
Admission priority					
High	0	0	0	1	5
Medium	11	10	7	8	16
Low	9	8	8	10	3
Missing data	10	9	13	11	6
Brought in by					
Self	5	10	10	15	5
Relative	11	5	2	6	8
Other	14	12	16	9	17
Missing data	0	0	0	0	0
Previous psychiatric hospitalization					
No	20	11	4	9	
Yes	7	7	11	14	
Missing data	3	9	13	7	

patients were from the Elderly and Middle-aged/OBS groups. Significantly fewer direct-referral patients (42 out of 89, or 47.2 percent) came from these two groups ($\chi^2 = 4.6$; $p < 0.05$).

Presenting Complaints

The 10 most frequent presenting complaints of all psychiatric patients are listed in Table 14.2. Elderly/OBS and Middle-aged/OBS patients were more likely to present with "inappropriate behavior" ($\chi^2 = 5.7$; $p < 0.05$) and "confusion" ($\chi^2 = 10.8$; $p < 0.001$), and less likely to present as being "depressed" ($\chi^2 = 6.2$; $p < 0.05$) than were Elderly/Psych and Middle-aged/Psych patients. Middle-aged/OBS and Middle-aged/Psych patients were more likely to describe a "substance abuse" problem ($\chi^2 = 7.7$; $p < 0.01$) than were Elderly/OBS and Elderly/Psych patients.

Medical Evaluation

The six most common organ systems in which findings from the physical examination were documented included ear, nose, and throat (ENT), pulmonary (Pulm), cardiovascular (Chest), gastrointestinal (GI), neurologic (Neuro), and vital signs (V-Signs). The laboratory tests included a complete blood count (CBC), electrocardiogram (ECG), chest radiograph (Chest-X), rapid plasma reagin (RPR), and Sequential Multiple Autoanalyzer 6/60® (SMA-6/60, e.g., serum glucose, urea nitrogen, and electrolyte concentrations). Table 14.3 lists the number of patients in each group for whom each of 12 different tests was reported as having been conducted, as well as whether the findings were normal or abnormal. Elderly/Medical patients received the most extensive physical examinations of any group, with the greatest overall number of tests reported ($F = 17.1$; $p < 0.001$). The 58 Elderly and Middle-aged/OBS patients received more physical examinations and laboratory tests than the other psychiatric patients ($F = 4.7$; $p < 0.05$). However, 27 of these 58 patients (46.5 percent) had no reported pulmonary examination, 33 (56.8 percent) had no reported chest radiograph, 23 (39.6 percent) had no reported clinical chemistry (SMA-6/60) tests, and 40 (68.9 percent) had no ECG. A few patients in each group had evidence that a test was performed, but the results of the test were not recorded. (These cases are listed as missing data

Table 14.2
Presenting Complaints of Elderly and Middle-Aged Psychiatric Emergency Department Patients[a]

	Elderly/OBS (n = 30)	Elderly/Psych (n = 27)	Middle-Aged/OBS (n = 28)	Middle-Aged/Psych (n = 30)	Total (n = 115)
Inappropriate behavior	12	2	12	6	32
Substance abuse	3	0	11	8	22
Somatic complaints	4	3	7	7	21
Confused	10	1	7	2	20
Family problems	5	4	4	4	17
Irritable	7	2	2	5	16
Eating disorder	7	4	1	4	16
Sleep disorder	4	6	1	5	16
Depressed	0	2	1	11	14
Auditory hallucinations	2	1	6	2	11

[a] Up to four complaints were recorded for each patient

in Table 14.3.) Many Elderly/Psych patients (11 out of 27, or 40.7 percent) had no report of any of these tests being conducted.

There was a high incidence of abnormal laboratory findings when these tests were performed. For example, seven of the 13 (63.8 percent) Elderly/OBS patients for whom results of chest radiographs were reported had abnormal findings; seven of 19 (36.8 percent) had abnormal CBCs; four of 11 (36.4 percent) had abnormal ECGs; and three of 18 (16.7 percent) had abnormal results on the SMA-6/60. In all, 75.0 percent of those Elderly/OBS patients who had physical examinations and/or laboratory tests had at least one abnormal finding. Corresponding figures for the other groups were: Elderly/Psych, 75.0 percent; Middle-aged/OBS, 72.7 percent; Middle-aged/Psych, 50.0 percent; and Elderly/Medical, 96.7 percent. To determine if there were any differences in the extent of medical illness, a ratio of abnormal test results to total tests conducted was computed for every patient who received at least one of the tests, and these ratios were then converted to percentages. While the group of Elderly/Medical patients had the highest mean proportion of abnormal findings (50.2 percent) and the Middle-aged/Psych patients the least (30.5 percent), this analysis did not yield a statistically significant difference between the groups.

Psychiatric Evaluation

Psychiatric evaluation findings, where reported, included ratings on behavior, thought, mood, orientation, affect, appearance, judgment, suicidal ideation, memory, and speech. Some findings (e.g., thought, orientation) were more commonly reported than others and inconsistencies existed between the groups. The Elderly/OBS and Middle-aged/OBS patients were rated as being especially abnormal on the orientation and memory dimensions. Orientation findings were reported on 41 of the 58 OBS patients. Twenty-nine of these 41 patients (70.7 percent) were rated as abnormal, compared with only three of the other 27 psychiatric patients (11.1 percent) who had reported results ($\chi^2 = 20.9$; $p < 0.001$). Sixteen of the 20 OBS patients (80.0 percent) who were rated for memory were reported as abnormal, compared with only one of the 14 patients (7.1 percent) from the other psychiatric groups ($\chi^2 = 14.7$; $p < 0.001$). Mental status evaluation of the OBS patients found them to be significantly more impaired than the other psychiatric patients in thought ($\chi^2 = 5.3$; $p < 0.05$), appearance (χ^2

Table 14.3
Physical and Laboratory Test Results for Elderly and Middle-Aged Emergency Department Patients

	Elderly/OBS (n = 30)	Elderly/Psych (n = 27)	Middle-Aged/OBS (n = 29)	Middle-Aged/Psych (n = 30)	Elderly/Medical (n = 30)
ENT					
Normal	9	6	7	4	8
Abnormal	6	2	7	3	15
Missing data	3	3	2	3	0
Total tested	18	11	16	10	23
Total not tested	12	16	12	20	7
Pulm					
Normal	8	7	10	8	20
Abnormal	6	0	2	0	8
Missing data	3	4	2	3	0
Total tested	17	11	14	11	28
Total not tested	13	16	14	19	2
Chest					
Normal	7	3	10	7	10
Abnormal	8	4	2	1	17
Missing data	3	4	2	3	0
Total tested	18	11	14	11	27
Total not tested	12	16	14	19	3
GI					
Normal	9	6	9	5	16
Abnormal	5	1	3	0	10
Missing data	3	4	2	3	0
Total tested	17	11	14	8	26
Total not tested	13	16	14	22	4
Neuro					
Normal	9	5	7	3	9
Abnormal	5	0	2	2	4
Missing data	3	4	2	3	0
Total tested	17	9	11	8	13
Total not tested	13	18	17	22	17

Table 14.3 (cont.)

V-Signs					
Normal	12	7	14	11	12
Abnormal	6	8	7	7	17
Missing data	3	3	2	3	0
Total tested	21	18	23	21	29
Total not tested	9	9	5	9	1
CBC					
Normal	12	2	9	3	6
Abnormal	7	3	4	0	6
Missing data	3	4	3	3	5
Total tested	22	9	16	6	17
Total not tested	8	18	12	24	13
ECG					
Normal	7	0	4	1	7
Abnormal	4	3	0	0	8
Missing data	2	4	1	3	2
Total tested	13	7	5	4	17
Total not tested	17	20	23	26	13
Chest X					
Normal	6	1	3	1	1
Abnormal	7	1	4	1	4
Missing data	2	4	3	3	4
Total tested	15	6	10	5	9
Total not tested	15	21	18	25	21
RPR					
Normal	1	0	0	0	1
Abnormal	0	0	0	0	1
Missing data	2	4	3	3	0
Total tested	3	4	3	3	2
Total not tested	27	23	25	27	28
SMA-6/60®					
Normal	15	2	9	3	4
Abnormal	3	3	1	1	8
Missing data	3	0	4	4	5
Total tested	21	5	14	8	17
Total not tested	9	18	14	22	13

$= 5.4$; $p < 0.05$), judgment ($\chi^2 = 5.3$; $p < 0.05$), and speech ($\chi^2 = 4.3$; $p < 0.05$).

The physicians' review of the medical records revealed that over 30 percent of all patients were in need of further medical evaluation (Table 14.4). This assessment was based on such factors as the condition and presenting complaints of each patient and the number, type, and results of conducted tests. Additional evaluation was thought to be required for more Elderly/OBS patients than for any other group ($\chi^2 = 12.7$; $p < 0.005$). Corresponding reviews of the need for additional psychiatric workup (not reported in the table) also revealed significant differences between the groups, with the reviewing physicians also suggesting further evaluation was required for more Elderly/OBS patients than for any other group ($\chi^2 = 16.2$; $p < 0.001$).

Current Medications

Medications were noted as having been taken by at least 84 of the 115 psychiatric patients. For 5 patients, no medications were indicated, and for 26, there was no mention of whether medications were taken or not. According to the reviewing physicians, medications could have been implicated in the disorders of 47 of the 84 patients on medication, or 55.9 percent. This was more often the case for elderly patients than middle-aged patients, with 24 (70 percent) of the 35 elderly compared with 23 (45 percent) of the 49 middle-aged patients having possible drug-induced symptoms ($\chi^2 = 3.9$; $p < 0.05$).

Treatment and Disposition

All patients seen in the PES were treated for their psychiatric illness. Treatment involved supportive psychotherapy alone or with medication. Fifty-four (47 percent) of the 115 PES patients were prescribed medication in addition to supportive therapy following their evaluation; the remaining 61 (53 percent) received supportive therapy alone. There was no significant age or diagnostic difference as to whether medications were prescribed. Of those 54 patients who were prescribed medications, 26 (48.1 percent) were given antipsychotic medications. A much smaller number were either prescribed antianxiety (2 patients) or antidepressant medications (2 patients).

Following treatment, patients were either admitted to the hospi-

Table 14.4
Need for Further Medical Evaluation among Elderly and Middle-Aged Emergency Department Patients

	Elderly/OBS (n = 30)	Elderly/Psych (n = 27)	Middle-Aged/OBS (n = 28)	Middle-Aged/Psych (n = 30)	Elderly/Medical (n = 30)
Yes	16	7	9	3	8
No	14	17	19	26	20
Missing cases	—	3	—	1	2
Total	30	27	28	30	30

tal's inpatient psychiatric unit, referred for outpatient treatment, or discharged. This disposition status could be ascertained for 99 of the 115 PES patients: 48 or 48.5 percent were admitted to the hospital; 33 or 33.3 percent were treated and then referred to outpatient services, and 18 or 18.2 percent were treated and then discharged. Patients in the four age/diagnostic groups were equally likely to have been admitted, referred, or discharged.

DISCUSSION

A hospital's psychiatric emergency service (PES) provides immediate evaluation and treatment or referral of patients with acute behavioral disturbances. Previous studies have identified patients referred to psychiatric emergency services with unrecognized medical illnesses (Eilenberg and Whatmore, 1961; Eastwood, Mindham, and Tennant, 1970; Carlson, Nayar, and Suh, 1981; Dubin, Weiss, and Zeccardi, 1983). Of particular concern to us was the possibility that older patients who present with psychiatric symptoms to an emergency department are inappropriately being referred to the department's PES when they are in fact medically ill. In an earlier study we found that while only 5 percent of all PES patients in our hospital are elderly, almost 40 percent received a diagnosis of organic brain syndrome. In contrast, the prevalence of this diagnosis for all age groups is less than 2 percent (Waxman et al., 1982).

Our initial concern about the adequacy of the evaluation of older emergency department patients was justified by the findings of the present study. A large number of these patients failed to receive the in-depth medical evaluation necessary to detect potential medical causes for their psychiatric symptoms. Our physicians' assessment of the medical records underscored this concern by indicating a greater need for additional medical evaluation for all elderly patients but particularly the organic brain syndrome patients compared with middle-aged patients. Moreover, our review of the medical records documented many abnormal laboratory and physical findings that were suggestive of medical illness but were never followed up.

The presence of medical illness among elderly psychiatric patients is not a new finding, but our study does confirm and extend other reports that have shown a relationship between physical and mental health in older individuals (Bassuk et al., 1983; Brody and Kleban, 1983; Waxman, Carner, and Blum, 1983). It is distressing to note that there were actually as many signs of physiologic disorder among the Elderly/OBS patients whose records we examined as were found among the Elderly/Medical patients. While it is not possible in a retrospective research project to definitively demonstrate specific relationships between abnormal physical and laboratory findings and psychiatric symptoms in any patient, it is clear from this study that such potential relationships were not ruled out.

Another major concern is the referral of medically ill patients to the PES after they have been "medically cleared." This phenomenon has been previously noted in psychiatric emergency departments in studies of younger patients (Weissberg, 1979; Slaby, 1981). In the current study, these patients were the indirect-referral patients, individuals who were first seen by medicine and then referred to psychiatry but who had many physical findings and abnormal laboratory test results. The referral of a patient to psychiatry as "medically clear" after physical evaluation should imply that all necessary testing is complete and the results followed up. We question the value of having these patients declared "medically clear" and referred for what is presumed to be a functional psychiatric problem when this has not been done. Our reviewing physicians' indication of a need for additional medical workup and the large numbers of abnormal findings suggest that many patients were sent to the psychiatric service inappropriately or at least prematurely. This raises the question of what factors cause an emergency department to refer elderly patients who have symptoms of organic brain syndrome to a psychiatric service, while other patients are routed into the general medical emergency department.

When patients are brought into an emergency department, there may be a tendency to dichotomize them into medical or psychiatric categories on the basis of an initial impression. This initial decision may be based on a single piece of data, a single symptom, a single item of past history, or a previous diagnosis. The vagueness of elderly patients' complaints or their disturbed behavior may lead to the perception of a psychiatric problem by the triage nurse at the front desk or by the physician in the medical emergency department. Past experience with the difficult behavior of some elderly patients or, perhaps, some biases toward treating elderly patients, especially those perceived as having a psychiatric problem, may predispose an inappropriate referral to psychiatry. Aggression, belligerence, disorganized thought, hallucination, or delusion often mislead physicians into overlooking the medical illness that may underly these symptoms. The patients diagnosed with organic brain syndrome presented with a significantly greater degree of inappropriate behavior and confusion in our study. A perception of a behavioral problem with a concurrent failure to recognize the various manifestations of organic brain syndrome probably resulted in the inadequate evaluation. It would appear that ongoing educational efforts to familiarize emergency department staff with the multifaceted nature of organic brain syndrome is mandatory to enhance patient care.

While the generalizability of these findings has not yet been demonstrated, it is likely that other emergency departments in other hospitals also have difficulty in differentiating behavioral from physiological disorders in elderly patients. The large number of elderly psychiatric emergency service patients who have medical problems has been observed in at least one study in another hospital (Bassuk et al., 1983). However, to judge the full extent of the problem, it would be important to repeat the present study in other settings, including a nonteaching urban hospital and a community hospital, particularly one that might not have a psychiatric service in the emergency department.

We recommend that emergency departments provide a more thorough medical evaluation of elderly patients who have behavioral disturbances rather than providing early referral to psychiatry. Elderly medical patients could also benefit from mental-status examinations to detect symptoms of organic brain syndrome. The latter may also help to alleviate the well-recognized problem of psychiatric problems that are not treated and are assumed to represent chronic or irreversible disease. Such additional evaluation may prevent the high personal, financial, and social costs of unnecessary hospitalizations and nursing-home placements that may result from the failure to recognize and treat reversible physical and psychiatric disorders of older patients.

REFERENCES

Bassuk, E., Minden, S., & Apsler, R. (1983), Geriatric emergencies: Psychiatric or medical? *Amer. J. Psychiat.*, 140:539–542.

Brody, E., & Kleban, M. (1983), Day-to-day mental and physical health symptoms of older people: A report on health logs. *Gerontol.*, 23:75–85.

Butler, R. (1980), Senility reconsidered: Treatment possibilities for mental impairment in the elderly. *J. Amer. Med. Assn.*, 244–259.

Carlson, R., Nayar, N., & Suh, M. (1981), Physical disorders among psychiatric patients. *Can. J. Psychiat.*, 26:65–67.

Dubin, W., Weiss, K., & Zeccardi, J. (1983), Organic brain syndrome: The psychiatric imposter. *J. Amer. Med. Assn.*, 249:60–62.

Eastwood, M., Mindham, R., & Tennant, T. (1970), The physical status of psychiatric emergencies. *Brit. J. Psychiat.*, 116:545–550.

Eilenberg, M., & Whatmore, P. (1961), Physical disease and psychiatric emergencies. *Comprehen. Psychiat.*, 2:358–363.

Jarvik, L., & Perl, M. (1981), Overview of physiologic dysfunctions related to psychiatric problems in the elderly. In: *Neuropsychiatric Manifestations of Physical Disease in the Elderly*, eds. A. Levenson & R. Hall. New York: Raven Press.

Libow, L. (1973), Pseudo-senility, acute and reversible organic brain syndromes. *J. Amer. Geriat. Soc.*, 32:112–120.

Slaby, A. (1981), Emergency psychiatry: An update. *Hosp. Commun. Psychiat.*, 32:687–698.

Waxman, H.M., Carner, E., & Dubin, W. (1982), Geriatric psychiatry in the emergency department: Characteristics of geriatric and nongeriatric admissions. *J. Amer. Geriat. Soc.*, 30:427–432.

——— ——— Blum A. (1983), Depressive symptoms and health service utilization among the community elderly. *J. Amer. Geriat. Soc.* 31:417–420.

Weingarten, C., Rosoff L., Eisen, S. et al., (1982), Medical care in a geriatric psychiatry unit. *J. Amer. Geriat. Soc.*, 30:738–743.

Weissberg, M. (1979), Emergency room medical clearance: An educational problem. *Amer. J. Psychiat.*, 136:787–790.

Commentary

Robert S. Marin, M.D.

Chapter 14 is really two reports in one. As the introduction describes, it is the second of two studies carried out by the authors to evaluate the care received by geriatric patients in an emergency room. The first report offered a demographic profile of a similar subject population, whereas the present one addresses the content of the medical evaluation received by these patients. Together the two provide a window into the areas of overlap between the principles and practice of geropsychiatry and emergency psychiatry. By addressing both the social and medical dimensions of elderly psychiatric patients, the two studies encompass one of the central principles of competent geriatric care, namely that it must be comprehensive, and more specifically, multidisciplinary. This is, of course, a guiding principle in any health service field and in the management of any psychiatric emergency, but with elderly patients in whom serious medical and social liability is so much more likely, failure to attend to it intensively is likely to lead to important treatment errors.

The authors suggest that psychiatric patients are often "cleared" prematurely by physicians in the medical emergency services so that psychiatrists who then see them have to carry out medical evaluations that should have been completed before referral. It is implicit that agist attitudes among professionals and a higher prevalence of medical problems compound this problem for elderly patients. In fairness, the issue is not so much when the evaluation is done, but how it is done, by whom, and why. Premature referral may not reflect deficiencies in clinical judgment regarding the adequacy of a medical evaluation, for example, for dementia. Rather, it may occur because of administrative and quasi-political disagreements regarding which specialty services oversee the medical evaluations of what kinds of patients. Resolution of such problems is as much a prerequisite for good care as are sound clinical knowledge and good clinical judgment; unfortunately, it may be more difficult to realize.

Chapter 14, of course, addresses only a few aspects of emergency geropsychiatric care. More interesting than the observation of increased cognitive symptoms among patients with organic mental disorders would be data on the number of organic behavioral syndromes that present *without* cognitive disturbance. These are undoubtedly at greater risk for being overlooked. The interested reader also might wish to consider the application to the emergency room setting of such geropsychiatric principles as the relationship of late life loss (e.g., job loss, illness, death, change in residence) to psychiatric presentation; the role and integration of the family into the emergency room setting; the organization of crisis intervention for the older patient; and the establishment of linkages to community resources.

Annotated Bibliography

Waxman, H. M., Carner, E. A., Dubin, W., & Klein, M. (1984), Geriatric psychiatry in the emergency department: Characteristics of geriatric and non-geriatric admissions. *J. Amer. Geri. Soc.*, 30:427–432.

This paper is part I of a study, of which chapter 14 is part II. In this one, 49 elderly and 49 middle-aged patients seen in an urban hospital psychiatric emergency service are compared regarding demographic and admission information, psychiatric treatment history, presenting complaints, symptoms, diagnoses, and final disposition status. The findings raise important issues concerning the unique psychosocial needs of elderly patients.

Herst, L. D. (1983), Emergency psychiatry in the elderly. *Psychiat. Clin. N. Amer.*, 6:271–280.

This paper stresses the need to take extra time to assess the mental status of geriatric patients in emergency settings. Special presentations of geriatric depression, the consequences of various sensory deprivations, and the impact of complex medical problems and of changes in the environment are some of the factors that must be considered in any such evaluation.

Wells, C. E. (1978), Geriatric organic psychoses. *Psychiat. Annals*, 8:466–478.

A comprehensive review article that addresses the process of differential diagnosis in geriatric organic psychoses. Three questions serve as the framework for this "meaty" article: Do the patient's symptoms and signs result from (1) functional or from organic brain disease? (2) focal or diffuse cerebral disease? (3) delirium or dementia?

Bassuk, E. L., Minden, S., & Apsler, R. (1983), Geriatric emergencies: Psychiatric or medical? *Amer. J. Psychiat.*, 140:539–542.

A rather brief, but substantial, paper completing those by Waxman et al. (1984, chapter 14) which looks at how the elderly use the emergency room. The authors compared emergency patients age 65 and older with younger patients in terms of demographics, clinical factors, patterns of emergency room use, and clinician response. Like younger patients the elderly had scanty social supports, but unlike the younger patients, came for care repeatedly with somatic complaints. As noted by other studies, the elderly had coexisting medical and psychiatric illnesses, and yet they were generally treated by one service. The need for a holistic, psychobiologic approach to the care of the elderly emergency patient is emphasized.

15

Chronic Crisis Patients: A Discrete Clinical Group

Ellen Bassuk, M.D., and
Samuel Gerson, Ph.D.

Psychiatric emergency services positioned at the interfaces between the community and the hospital and between inpatient and outpatient facilities sensitively mirror changes in the ideology and provision of mental health services. With the dramatic reduction in the population of state hospital inpatient units, ambulatory services have gradually assumed greater responsibility for the care of the chronically ill patient (Talbott, 1978). This shift in the locus of care has been a major factor in the phenomenal expansion of psychiatric emergency services during the last two decades and will undoubtedly contribute to increasing demands on these services in the next decade (Bassuk and Gerson, 1979). To meet the challenge of providing acute management for the broad spectrum of psychiatric patients effectively, it is becoming increasingly important to delineate subgroups of patients who share common characteristics and for whom specific treatment approaches can be developed.

This chapter was first published in the *American Journal of Psychiatry* (1980), 137:1513–1517, and it is reprinted by permission.

One such group of patients are those who, despite persistent efforts to engage them in ongoing treatment, keep returning to the emergency ward. Difficulties in providing continuity of care and preventing these patients, known as repeaters, from becoming part of the emergency ward revolving door is a major problem facing the clinician in this setting.

Previous studies of repeaters (Ungerleider, 1960; Miller, 1968; Raphling and Lion, 1970; Bauer and Balter, 1971; Schwartz, Weiss, and Miner, 1972) have reported that 7–17.9 percent return to the emergency ward within six months of the initial visit. Although one study (Miller, 1968) reported no demographic differences between repeaters and nonrepeaters, another (Bauer and Balter, 1971) concluded that more than 90 percent of repeaters were women and 56 percent were divorced, widowed, or separated. In the latter study, repeaters were described as having a slightly different symptom profile characterized by a higher level of suicidal ideation, depression, psychomotor retardation, and anorexia.

In a study of repeaters to a 24- to 48-hour holding facility (Schwartz et al., 1972), the authors found that 13.1 percent were seen two to seven times. An interesting observation was that multiple visits were related to a single episode of illness and generally occurred within days of each other. Most of these patients were women with chronic personality disorders, frequently accompanied by alcoholism and drug dependence. In contrast, most of the nonrepeaters were given the diagnosis of transient situational disorders.

To our knowledge, the only report in the literature discussing the clinical issues in the management of the repeater group is an anecdotal description of 15 patients who each made 7–30 visits to the emergency ward within one year (Raphling and Lion, 1970). During at least one admission most were labeled as borderline, although five were also diagnosed as having chronic schizophrenia. This group returned repeatedly during recurrent crises with urgent demands for immediate relief of their distress related in a provocative, often help-rejecting style. Their manner of relating may significantly contribute to their difficulties in becoming engaged in a stable psychotherapeutic relationship and, therefore, to their frequent use of emergency services.

A rational treatment approach to the clinical management of these difficult patients demands an elaboration of their common distinguishing characteristics. Patients comprising this group represent a sizable proportion of most emergency ward populations and consume an even greater percentage of personnel time. To improve patient care and the efficient use of resources, we designed a study to clarify our understanding of the repeater group and the reactions they elicit in their caretakers.

METHOD

This study was conducted at the Beth Israel Hospital in Boston, Massachusetts, a private general hospital affiliated with a medical school. The psychiatric emergency service, located in the emergency unit, provides 24-hour care 7 days a week and is primarily staffed by first-year psychiatric residents and first-year psychology interns. Approximately 1,400 psychiatric patients are seen each year. The overall pattern of utilization is similar to that reported in the many descriptive studies in the literature of similar urban settings.

The total sample consisted of 307 patients treated by 18 therapists. Of these, the 50 patients (16.3 percent) who were seen in the psychiatric emergency service more than once during the previous 12 months were defined as repeaters. The choice of one year as the time frame for defining repeaters was based on the clinical assumption that most repeaters return for subsequent treatment within that period.

At the conclusion of the assessment and disposition of each patient, data on a variety of demographic and clinical variables were gathered. The tests used included the Brief Psychiatric Rating Scale (BPRS) (Overall and Gorham, 1962), which measures the patient's clinical characteristics, and the Global Assessment Scale (GAS) (Endicott, Spitzer, Fleiss, et al., 1976), which measures the overall severity of the patient's functional impairment. In addition, the therapist's affective response to the patient was measured on a self-report scale consisting of nine items, each scored on a seven-point scale, rating rapport with, interest in, and emotional reactions to the patient. A total score of 63 is possible on this scale; scores of 23 or lower represent an intense negative response, and scores of 50 or higher represent a strong positive response to the patient (Gerson, 1979).

To delineate patient characteristics associated with frequent use of psychiatric emergency services, the repeater group of patients was compared with the nonrepeaters on the following six dimensions; demographics, psychiatric treatment history, social supports, clinical symptomatology, therapist's affective response, and disposition.

RESULTS

Demographically, the 50 repeaters and 257 nonrepeaters differed significantly only on the age variable; there was a significantly greater likelihood of being a repeater if the patient was between 31 and 50 years of age ($\chi^2 = 24.91, p < .001$). Although there was a tendency for more women and housewives to be repeaters, the results were not significant. Race, marital status, and socioeconomic class did not differentiate the two groups.

The current and past psychiatric treatment of the repeaters significantly differed from that of the rest of the emergency ward patients (see Table 15.1). More of the repeaters were involved in ongoing psychotherapy, and more of them also had received previous inpatient treatment. Of the patients who had been previously hospitalized, the repeater group had a significantly greater number of inpatient episodes.

The network of social supports available to repeaters was signif-

Table 15.1
Psychiatric History of Patients with Repeated Visits and Patients with Single Visits to a Psychiatric Emergency Service

Variable	Percentage of repeaters	Percentage of nonrepeaters
Past inpatient treatment (N = 307)[a]		
Yes	86	36.2
No	14	63.8
Number of previous hospitalizations (N = 136)[b]		
1–2	30.2	74.2
3–5	23.3	18.3
6 or more	46.5	7.5
Current and past psychotherapy (N = 307)[c]		
Never in therapy	18.0	50.6
Currently in therapy	60.0	29.2
Not currently but previously in therapy	22.0	20.2

[a] $x^2 = 40.10$, df = 1, P<.001
[b] $x^2 = 32.31$, df = 2, P<.001
[c] $x^2 = 21.50$, df = 2, P<.001

icantly more sparse than that available to nonrepeaters; 46 percent of the repeaters, but only 26.4 percent of the nonrepeaters, said they had one or no supports ($\chi^2 = 15.36, p < .001$). The scanty social supports of the repeaters was also evidenced in the finding that the great majority of repeaters (84 percent) arrived on the emergency ward unaccompanied by friend or family, compared with only 38.5 percent of the nonrepeaters ($p < .001$).

The major clinical difference between the two groups of patients was in their response to the emergency ward therapists. The repeaters were rated as significantly more hostile, suspicious, and uncooperative than the nonrepeaters (see Table 15.2). The groups did not differ significantly on ratings reflecting the clinical symptoms of acute psychoses, affective disorders, or anxiety reactions. Overall ratings of psychopathology (total BPRS score) and functional impairment (GAS score) were significantly higher for the repeater patients.

Approximately one-half of the repeaters were considered to have character disorders and one-half psychoses, compared with approximately one-third of the nonrepeaters for each of these categories.

Measurements of the therapist–patient interaction revealed that the repeaters as a group tended to elicit a generally negative affective response from their emergency ward therapists. Thirty-two percent of the repeater group but only 4.3 percent of the nonrepeaters were found to be intensely disliked (therapists' scores of 12–23); only 8 percent of the repeaters, compared with 31.5 percent of the nonrepeaters, were found to engage in a highly positively toned interaction with the therapist (scores of 50–62) ($\chi^2 = 45.05, p < .001$).

Fifty-two percent of the repeaters and 33.9 percent of the nonrepeaters were referred for hospitalization ($\chi^2 = 16.78, p < .01$).

DISCUSSION

The data indicate that the repeaters represent a discrete clinical group characterized by a common symptom profile, a similar treatment history, and a typical manner of interacting with therapists. These three dimensions are interrelated, continuously reinforcing each other, and resulting in a self-defeating style of seeking help and then rejecting it. The repeater group can be defined as chronic crisis patients; they share similar symptomatic and historical characteristics with a group

Table 15.2
Clinical Characteristics of 307 Patients Seen on a Psychiatric Emergency Service

Variable	t^a
BPRS symptom	
Somatic concern	2.57[b]
Anxiety	−1.16
Emotional withdrawal	−1.08
Conceptual disorganization	1.71
Guilt feelings	−6.42[c]
Tension	− .87
Mannerisms and posturing	1.83
Grandiosity	1.16
Depressive mood	−1.22
Hostility	4.53[c]
Suspiciousness	2.57[b]
Hallucinatory behavior	1.89
Motor retardation	−2.04[d]
Uncooperativeness	4.29[c]
Unusual thought content	2.10[d]
Blunted affect	1.30
Total BPRS score	2.14[d]
Global Assessment Scale (GAS) score	6.10[c]
Degree of Suicidal threat	.46
Degree of Homicidal threat	.28

[a] Positive t values indicate that the symptom was more prevalent in repeaters.
[b] $p < .01$
[c] $p < .001$
[d] $p < .05$

of borderline patients described in a recent study conducted on an emergency ward (Perry and Klerman, 1980). A cross-sectional analysis of their behavior illustrates the patterns that generate and maintain their status as repeaters.

Beginning with the symptom profile, these patients relate to caretakers in a generally negativistic manner and have been described as "entitled demanders" and "manipulative help rejecters" (Groves, 1978). Often they come to the emergency ward with the unrealistic expectation of immediate gratification of their wishes and instant relief of their discomfort. Their neediness is accentuated by their inability to effectively communicate reality-based wishes and their ambivalence about involvement in a potentially close relationship. They transmit intense anger and communicate in a provocative style. As our findings indicate, the therapist responds to this symptom profile with feelings of anger and dislike and has difficulty establishing a relationship.

The lack of rapport and the therapist's intense negative affect may contribute to the greater likelihood of hospitalizing such patients. The finding that repeaters and nonrepeaters did not differ significantly in the degree of acute psychotic, suicidal, homicidal, anxious, or depressive symptomatology suggests that other factors were involved in planning the disposition of the patient. The tendency to hospitalize repeaters more frequently than nonrepeaters may therefore be more of a reflection of the difficulty in establishing meaningful contact with the former group than of the clinically based need for inpatient care.

Further support for the decision to hospitalize may come from the striking paucity of the repeaters' social network. Clinical experience and historical data suggest that the manner in which these patients communicate their needs often leaves other persons emotionally exhausted and depleted, not unlike the feelings that the emergency ward therapist experiences in attempting to manage this group. Over a period of time this is likely to result in a gradual recession of potential resources, a factor that has been shown to be a major determinant in dispositional decision making (Gerson and Bassuk, 1980).

The psychiatric history of the repeater patient appears to be another nonclinical factor that affects decision making. For example, the finding that repeaters were diagnosed as psychotic more frequently than were nonrepeaters, even though the two groups did not generally differ in clinical ratings of psychotic symptomatology, may illustrate the influence of the patient's history. With regard to disposition, therapists may be overly influenced by the impressively large number of previous hospitalizations and may regard this as the treatment of choice. The resulting hospitalization only seems to perpetuate the cycle of rejection of help. A similar process may also occur in an outpatient treatment context.

To bypass this pattern the therapist should view the engagement and containment of these patients in any setting as a protracted process characterized by frequent flights from the helper. This disengagement is an expectable part of the behavior of some patients when involved in treatment. It partially reflects their incapacity to negotiate a comfortable distance without feeling isolated or a reasonable closeness without feeling engulfed. They are unable to tolerate the limits of a relationship and defend against it by seeking an alternative source of support, again repeating the cycle.

For the purpose of discussing an approach to the more effective emergency ward management of repeaters, they can be divided into two subgroups: those currently involved in a treatment program and those without therapeutic support. As the data indicate, many repeaters who visit the emergency ward are seeing an outside therapist and often have concerns and complaints about their treatment. This commonly is a manifestation of a transference bind and should be viewed as an inevitable part of the process of psychotherapy. Often when the patient cannot tolerate ambivalent feelings about the therapist, he or she may use the defense mechanism of splitting (Kernberg, 1966). The patient may view the therapist as the bad, devalued object and the emergency ward clinician as the good, overidealized object or vice versa. The emergency ward clinician should recognize this defensive operation and attempt to delineate the precipitant of the visit, focus on the therapeutic relationship, reality test some of the patient's distortions about the therapist, and encourage the patient to return and discuss his or her feelings with the therapist. In addition, and after discussion with the patient, the emergency ward clinician should notify the therapist of the patient's visit and develop an integrated approach to his or her management (Skodol, Kass, and Charles, 1979).

Treatment of the repeater who does not have a therapist is more difficult. As previously described, these patients may be repeatedly hospitalized because they lack a support network, tend to reject help, and have a history of psychiatric treatment. However, the same principles of management should be applied to this subgroup. Most importantly, an attempt should be made to engage these patients in ongoing treatment. For those few repeaters who have not been previously hospitalized or been in psychotherapy, strenuous efforts should be made to engage them in treatment. This may sometimes necessitate a short-term inpatient stay to complete a diagnostic assessment and initiate treatment. Such an inpatient stay should be weighed against the possibility of a severe regression, which often marks the clinical course of these patients.

Most repeaters have made abortive attempts to become involved in psychotherapy or in various treatment programs. As Raphling and Lion (1970) have suggested, these patients should be managed on the emergency ward and their repeated visits should be viewed as opportunities to engage them in a therapeutic relationship. Consistent with the principles of aftercare, some of these patients will ultimately form a transference to the emergency ward that will help to contain them effectively at an optimal level of functioning (Safirstein, 1967). This approach might dilute the intensity of the transference, but it may sacrifice the possibility of working through aspects of the patient's problems with closeness in relationships. To manage patients in this setting successfully and to avoid further splitting, it is essential to have frequent and consistent communication with each member of the emergency ward staff who comes into contact with the patient. Most often the patient's previous behavior and history can offer clear indications for the most appropriate therapeutic stance.

What is most difficult in the management of these patients, however, is not the development of a dispositional approach, but rather the management of the therapist's feelings in response to the repeaters' provocative style. Because these patients are often intensely hostile, manipulative, uncooperative, and devaluing, the therapist experiences anxiety, helplessness, and even hate (Perry and Klerman, 1980). To manage these feelings, the therapist must repeatedly remind himself or herself that the patient's style repeats aspects of the troubled early mother–child relationship. It is, in part, a learned response and has become a model for later relationships despite its distortions. An understanding of this will help the therapist remain empathetic in the face of the patient's provocativeness. The therapist should make every attempt to bypass the struggle while acknowledging to himself or herself the intensity and discomfort of these feelings. Often it is necessary to set limits on the patient's inappropriate behavior while simultaneously providing support and reassurance and clarifying aspects of the patient's help-rejecting stance.

CONCLUSIONS

Although the general hospital is gradually assuming some of the functions of the state hospital, it has not yet developed a comprehensive range of intermediate services such as partial hospitalization, halfway houses, and community residences. In addition, in many cases formal affiliation agreements that directly guide the flow of patients through the complex mental health system have not been defined. It is our clinical impression, supported by discussions with other emergency ward directors, that repeaters use multiple points of entry simultaneously, thereby establishing many opportunities for splitting and for sabotaging the existing therapeutic relationship or preventing one from developing. Communication through a committee of regional directors of emergency ward services can often help in the management of this difficult group of patients.

Identifying one facility as the major caretaker and notifying it of the patient's use of other settings will further improve the patient's care. Community mental health centers with many integrated and diverse treatment components might be more appropriate settings for the management of the repeater group because they offer a wider range of treatment alternatives within a centralized setting. However, if the patient has access to multiple psychiatric facilities within the geographic region, broader communication among these services must be established. The most important principle in the care of these patients is that a single treatment facility, such as the emergency ward, be identified as the primary therapist and be responsible for planning a consistent treatment approach. This offers the patient the greatest possibility of containment, engagement in a treatment process, and eventual resolution of his or her problems.

REFERENCES

Bassuk, E., & Gerson, S. (1979), Into the breach: Emergency psychiatry in the general hospital. *Gen. Hosp. Psychiat.*, 1:31–45.

Bauer, S., & Balter, L. (1971), Emergency psychiatric patients in a municipal hospital. *Psychiat. Quart.*, 45:382–393.

Endicott, J., Spitzer, R., Fleiss, J., et al. (1976), The global assessment scale. *Arch. Gen. Psychiat.*, 33:766–771.

Gerson, S. (1979), Determinants of psychiatric emergency room disposition. *Diss. Abs. Internat.*, 39(11):552-B.

——— Bassuk, E. (1980), Psychiatric emergencies: An overview. *Amer. J. Psychiat.*, 137:1–11.

Groves, J. (1978), Taking care of the hateful patient. *N. Eng. J. Med.*, 298:883–887.

Kernberg, O. (1966), Structural derivatives of object relationships. *Internat. J. Psycho-Anal.*, 47:236–253.

Miller, W. (1968), A psychiatric emergency service and some treatment concepts. *Amer. J. Psychiat.*, 124:924–933.

Overall, J., & Gorham, D. (1962), The brief psychiatric rating scale. *Psychol. Rep.*, 10:799–812.

Perry, J., & Klerman, G. (1980), Clinical features of the borderline personality disorder. *Amer. J. Psychiat.*, 137:164–173.

Raphling, D.L., & Lion, J. (1970). Patients with repeated admission to a psychiatric emergency service. *Commun. Ment. Health J.*, 6:313–318.

Safirstein, S. (1967). Institutional transference. *Psychiat. Quart.*, 41:557–566.

Schwartz, D., Weiss, A.T., & Miner, J. (1972). Community psychiatry and emergency service. *Amer. J. Psychiat.*, 129:710–715.

Skodol, A., Kass, F., & Charles, E. (1979). Crisis in psychotherapy: Principles of emergency consultation and intervention. *Amer. J. Orthopsychiatry*, 49:585–597.

Talbott, J.A. (1978). *The Chronic Mental Patient*. Washington, DC: American Psychiatric Press.

Ungerleider, J.T. (1960). The psychiatric emergency: Analysis of six months experience of a university hospital's consultation service. *Arch. Gen. Psychiat.*, 3:593–601.

Commentary

Cleon Cornes, M.D.

Bassuk and Gerson have addressed an extremely important and difficult problem in our current mental health system. Emergency rooms in psychiatric hospitals and in general medical hospitals have been increasingly burdened by repeated visits of chronic mental patients. Their study was done in a setting where psychiatric services are readily available to emergency room personnel. Unfortunately, that is often not the case, and the responsibility of dealing with large numbers of psychiatrically ill patients in general medical settings has led to much anger being directed toward these patients, as well as psychiatrists and other mental health professionals. We need to develop more effective ways of understanding and treating chronic patients, and chapter 15 provides a useful step in that direction.

The authors review earlier studies that described frequent visits during an episode of illness. In my experience that is particularly true of patients with schizophrenia or affective disorder, who will begin calling or visiting an emergency room during the prodromal phase of an acute episode. Other observers have noted that "repeaters" often lack social supports, have long-standing personality disorders, and abuse drugs and alcohol. These patients have repeated crises, come to the emergency room demanding immediate relief of their distress, relate in a "provocative help-rejecting manner," and utilize large amounts of staff time and energy. Their styles of relating may contribute to their difficulty engaging in stable therapeutic relationships and thus to their repeated use of emergency services.

The chapter describes a discrete clinical group of patients (16.3 percent) with repeated visits to the emergency room. They were more likely to be between the ages of 31 and 50; to be involved in ongoing psychotherapy, and have a history of repeated inpatient treatment; to have fewer social supports and arrive in the emergency room alone; to be more hostile, suspicious, uncooperative, and have high ratings of psychopathology and functional impairment; to receive a diagnosis of psychosis or character disorder; to elicit negative responses from the staff; and to be admitted to the hospital. In my opinion, the authors have accurately described and adequately differentiated this group of chronic patients from other patients seeking emergency care less frequently. They describe some similarity between this group and borderline patients, and suggest that they are more frequently admitted because of their problems in establishing meaningful contact, poor social networks, and history of previous hospitalizations. I agree that the important dynamic issues seem to be their difficulty negotiating a comfortable distance without feeling isolated or a reasonable closeness without feeling engulfed. Doctors Bassuk and Gerson make several useful suggestions about treatment, such as avoiding splitting and enhancing communication with everyone involved in their care. I emphasize the need to help therapists deal with their anger through consultation and case conferences. At the Western Psychiatric Institute and Clinic we have also developed comprehensive treatment plans for each patient, which need to be updated frequently and kept in the emergency room.

16

Death and Dying

Kevin M. O'Keeffe, M.D.

INTRODUCTION

In 1949, Evelyn Waugh deftly skewered the American attitude toward death in his novel, *The Loved One*. In a more documentary fashion, Jessica Mitford showed how only the funeral industry had seemingly kept its finger on the "pulse" of the contemporary mode of dealing, and not dealing, with death in *The American Way of Death* (1964).

It was, however, Elizabeth Kübler-Ross, M.D., with the commencement of her research in 1965 and the publication of her work, *On Death and Dying*, in 1969, who rescued the medical profession from the embarrassing position of even lagging behind society in its attention to what should be a key physician role. Following media attention and heightened public interest in the ensuing years, we have been deluged by material concerning death.

Nevertheless, there is little written on death in the emergency department. Most articles are based on inpatient or chronic outpatient care (Kübler-Ross, 1974; Steinfels, 1975). Ironically, there is probably no portion of the health care system that sees more death or with more intensity than emergency services.

This chapter was first published in the *Journal of the American College of Emergency Physicians* (1979), 8:275–279, and it is reprinted by permission.

Because of our experiences in the emergency department of a large city–county hospital, we have developed some guidelines for dealing with death. House staff in the emergency department were generally uneasy and uninterested in dealing with this problem. Nor is death and dying a subject that lends itself to classic research methodology. My subsequent experience in a private community emergency department has not been significantly different from that in the city–county hospital setting.

SPECIAL CHARACTERISTICS

The general characteristics of death and dying as experienced by patient, family, and health personnel are covered in the literature (Kübler-Ross, 1969, 1974). The emergency department milieu is not well explored. The facets of that setting that alter this experience include the nature of the event and its pressures on victim and family, the intensity surrounding care needed, largely felt by providers, and the setting itself, which makes sensitive interaction between parties difficult.

First, unlike inpatient and/or chronic care, death in the emergency department usually involves a sudden medical event, such as a myocardial infarction, or a violent injury. Neither the patient, if sentient, nor his loved ones, have time for evolution through the stages of accepting death (Kübler-Ross, 1969). For every death observed in the aged with chronic illness, there are many more unanticipated deaths that often seem unjust. The emotions surrounding traumatic deaths in young and vital patients are often compounded in intensity because they result from careless accidents, self-destruction, or criminal violence. Probably only someone who has personally experienced it can fully understand the powerful emotional and psychological forces that the grief-stricken must deal with. Their lack of an opportunity for a last goodbye makes death even more unacceptable. In the case where someone is spared in the same accident in which a spouse or other close person died, there are additional emotions relating to the acceptance of the accident itself and the risk of developing postaccident neurosis (O'Connor, 1970; Mattson, 1975).

The physician carries a real burden as well. The emergency physician has no prior rapport with the victim, or the family, and no basis for them to trust his competence, which can put the physician in a defensive posture. Particularly in public hospitals, the physician and family interact across social and cultural barriers with that associated hostility. Most emergency physicians have not had training to assist in developing rapid rapport. Often there is little that the physician can tell the family regarding the circumstances leading to the death. Even with the highest clinical competence, death, or pending death, has resulted, and the family's current state will give the physician little feeling of reward for his labors.

The typical emergency department is an appalling place for the sensitive handling of death and dying, perhaps due to the perceived need for cold efficiency for acute care but also the continuing neglect of human values in emergency department design and operation. No more hurried, impersonal, and seemingly random setting exists, particularly when observed by those not deadened by prolonged exposure. There is often no suitable area in which the family can wait out a resuscitation of their loved one. Other patients and visitors are generally preoccupied with themselves and display no sensitivity. Unfortunately, an equal insensitivity can be often displayed by ambulance attendants, police, or the clerks, and their early contact with patients and visitors can affect later relationship with the physician. Privacy is almost nonexistent, and even resuscitated patients have reported inappropriate comments during their care (*Reader's Digest,* April 1979).

The family is isolated from their loved one in these last minutes with little or no effect on what is being, or should be, done. Rather than being impressed with an efficient but cold technical response to the emergency, they are distracted by it, and often resentful.

One final subtle factor, not appreciated during the emotional turmoil, is the matter of expense. A few minutes of even a futile resuscitation can prove extremely expensive. When the bill later arrives, the sensitivity with which families' concerns were dealt, rather than competency alone, will affect their reaction.

DYING IN THE EMERGENCY DEPARTMENT

In the emergency department, death is encountered more often than the process of dying. Still, our society has made it difficult to die at home, a reversal of the time at the turn of the century when most people died at home (Sampson, 1977). Even patients who have died in their own homes, or nursing homes, are often sped posthaste and postmortem to the emergency department. It is the rare family who will accept a terminally ill patient dying at home. Also, often it is the family physician who persuades the family to take the patient to the hospital, even in opposition to the wishes of patient and family.

However, should a terminally ill patient present without any acute threat to life, but because of family concern regarding pain, anorexia, constipation, or weakness, the emergency physician should not reflexively hospitalize the patient. He should be carefully evaluated and his condition discussed with the patient and family. Consulting the patient's medical record, and preferably, the patient's physician, can help to arrive at a careful decision. If hospitalization is not felt necessary by agreement of all parties, unnecessary expense and, more importantly, medical interference with the dying process, are avoided.

Symptomatic relief and care of reversible conditions, such as dehydration and mild heart failure, can be initiated and, above all, the patient and family reassured and supported in their ability to manage the patient at home. Arrangement for visiting nurse follow-up is of great assistance. The family should be told of support available from their regular physician when deciding on home care, and given the important "lifeline" of being able to call or return to the emergency department as necessary. They should be given instruction or what can be done for the patient, and what progression might be expected—without being unrealistically predictive.

There is no justification for a rigid approach. Unfortunately, many times one can see the patient's recognition that the family could not cope and thus, a reluctant agreement to admission. Since it is difficult to reverse the social factors that make death at home difficult, perhaps "hospices" for dying patients, as in England, will provide a reasonable alternative (Saunders, 1977).

If terminally ill patients must be admitted, it should not be routine that they go to an intensive care unit. If acutely moribund, it is, however, preferable that they be hospitalized because the emergency department is an unsuitable place for dying.

Many patients are effectively dead but are kept alive by advanced life suport, which raises the question of organ donation. Despite much publicity, there seems to be little use of the process outlined by the National Uniform Anatomic Gift Act and supported by legislation in all 50 states. Similarly, there are few "living wills" encountered with written documentation that the patient does not want extreme measures in life support.

In general, all patients who present in arrest should have reasonable resuscitation attempts with modification of the duration of efforts and the extent of measures employed as appropriate to known etiology, patient's age, and adequacy of prehospital care. The emergency physician need not wrestle, to any extent, with the problems of worth or eventual success of resuscitation. At my former institution, the incidence of long-term coma following resuscitation was much rarer than feared (Yarnell, 1976). In my experience, resuscitation successes generally result in secondary arrest in the first few hours in the hospital, where an easier decision regarding further resuscitation can be made.

The policy of universal attempts at resuscitation in the emergency department relates to the basic concept of the emergency care mission and, hence, emergency staff morale. We have repeatedly heard complaints by ambulance personnel of their dismay and reluctance to bring "codes" where aggressive resuscitation is not done.

As to using organs from patients "halted in dying" by technology, this has been well covered by Rosenberg (Rosenberg, Krome, and McDonald, 1975) and Gennich (1977). We only stress that, while such cases are initially encountered in the emergency department, the final disposition must be based on written guidelines developed by the medical staff of the hospital. Other than the adequate maintenance of vital organs, disposition should be by the appropriate inpatient service.

PRONOUNCEMENT OF DEATH

The legal definition of death is in flux. Emerging specifications require prolonged observation and sophisticated procedures such as brain flow studies and electroencephalograms (Black, 1975, 1978). The evolving uncertainty tends to make some emergency physicians unduly cautious. The question of brain death is best left to inpatient physicians. While there is confusion about the present statutory definition of death, to the best of my knowledge, there has been no overturning of the traditional precedent in common law that a patient is dead when a licensed physician says so. Thus, the physician need not be overcautious in pronouncing a patient dead on the basis of long used guidelines (i.e., the appearance of cardiac death with lack of spontaneous and/or effective cardiac action). Pupillary dilation may not be a uniformly useful guide but actual observation of cessation of retinal artery flow can help.

There are, however, entities that are exclusions to such criteria as that of the Harvard Committee, namely severe central nervous system sedative overdose or hypothermia below 32 C (89.6 F) (Harvard Medical School, 1968). As noted elsewhere, hypothermia (as opposed to postmortem cooling of the body) can subtly mimic death. A more thorough analysis for vital activity by electrocardiogram or Doppler is called for (O'Keeffe, 1977). In effect, the emergency physician may be comfortable in making pronouncements of cardiac death, but should leave the determination of brain death to inpatient services.

CERTIFICATION AND AUTOPSY

Emergency physicians are commonly called on to complete the death certificate. Too often, the only history is that of a nonspecific cardiorespiratory arrest. If the emergency physician feels he has no realistic basis for assigning cause of death beyond that entity (which is in many jurisdictions not acceptable as an initial cause of death), he is not obligated to do so. The responsibility for completion of the death certificate then lies with the coroner, hospital pathologist, or patient's physician.

The majority of emergency department deaths fulfill the usual criteria of state or local law to be classified as "coroner's cases." Using the California code (Section 10250, Health and Safety Code, State of California) as a reference, the following situations constitute a coroner's case (some states or counties use the district attorney or a medical examiner in lieu of a coroner system): any death (1) in which the patient was not seen by an attending physician in less than the prior 10 days; (2) which resulted at any point in time following mechanical, environmental, or thermal trauma; (3) with any suspicion of homicide, suicide, abortion (even therapeutic), or accidental poisoning; (4) involving possible occupational hazard or communicable disease; and (5) in which the attending physician is unwilling to state the cause.

There are other situations when the emergency physician should consult with his county coroner. A request for postmortem approval by the family should not precede release of the body by the coroner to avoid the appearance of coercion. Incomplete postmortems are of little use or validity and should not be done unless requested by court order. Most coroners will do an "academic" postmortem if requested. Certainly, a desire for a postmortem examination beyond legal necessity should follow only from genuine concern regarding possible cause of death or complications of care, rather than a need for good institutional statistics. Until a postmortem examination is decided against, all "tubes" should be left in place and any postresuscitation practice sites marked (and preferably avoided in cases that might prove legally entangled). Most major faiths found in Western culture generally permit a postmortem examination to be done, within certain limits.

ANNOUNCEMENT AND BEREAVEMENT

The most significant, and certainly most difficult, element of death and dying has been left for last—namely the informing of family and friends and the beginning of the initial grief process. I prefer to break this up into four essential phases—alerting, notifying, facilitating, and following through. The first three involve the emergency department with arrangements for the fourth preferably made by the staff.

If at all possible, during a lengthy resuscitation attempt, a nurse, or preferably a physician, should briefly inform the family as to the status of the patient. Ideally, there should be a comfortable and private room for the family.

The family is, therefore, aware that all measures are being employed and begins preparations for possible grieving. One must walk a realistic line between being a "crepe hanger" so that one "can't lose" no matter what the outcome, or a "sunshine boy" (Siegler, 1975). It is best to give a brief plan of what is being and will be done, and the hoped-for results, and state that the family will be kept closely apprised of the situation. One can usually sense the family's tense anticipation of death at this time, as well as their initial grief response if the arrest will be called.

If the resuscitation is successful, inform the family of the initially favorable outcome, what efforts will be continued, and who will be caring for the patient. Without giving a precise prognosis, stress the uncertainty of the first few days postarrest. Percentages do not apply to individual patients.

If the arrest is called, the responsible physician should inform the family himself. We feel that the closest person to the deceased should be informed directly, although others employ the "no bad news by a stranger" philosophy and use a less affected relative or friend to relay the news.

More important than what the physician says is how he receives and responds to the family's feelings. A brief phrase of sincere regret that efforts were unsuccessful and an offer of sympathy is usually sufficient at first. Too often an uncomfortable vacuum is filled with statements about "everything possible being done," and "there being no pain," which may not even be heard by those numbed and preoccupied with their grief.

Grief must be accepted as a normal and necessary process. Nothing has refuted this as classically noted by Lindemann (1944). The physician can, more by tone and posture, and possibly touch, rather than by verbal content, help this necessary grief process.

This can be done without losing impartiality and observation of the impact on the family. We are often concerned in our society about the disastrous impact of bad news on the bereaved. In fact, there are anecdotal reports of sudden death of spouses or others in the first few days after a loved one's death (Engel, 1971). There is an increased mortality among widowers following death of a spouse (Young, Benjamin, and Wallis, 1963). Despite these obvious risks, there is no evidence that these deaths are preventable by avoiding the bad news. Family members are often overly concerned about a spouse's "heart or nerves" more because of their own reluctance to deal with that person's grief than any objective likelihood of emotional shock causing harm. If a survivor has bona fide organic cardiovascular disease, there may be some reason to alter the manner of announcement.

Nevertheless, using this rare occurrence to justify a reluctance to open up the grieving process is undoubtedly collectively much more harmful. Large scale experience (DeVaul and Zisook, 1976) has shown that, if grieving is not experienced, there is a high likelihood of somatic equivalents, including headaches, job and social withdrawal, and the actual onset of organic illness, such as ulcerative colitis and rheumatoid arthritis.

Since the emergency physician will not follow the grieving person through the whole process, he can only help its onset and observe the initial reaction. He should observe the personal response as well as be aware of how different cultures usually express grief. As a generality, persons of Latin, Mediterranean, and African cultures are usually much more expressive than those from northern cultures. However, adequate delineation of these variations is not possible and individual exceptions are common.

The most common initial response is denial of death, particularly if unanticipated. One might also see initial anger at abandonment or guilt at being thought of as responsible for the death.

As with all psychological distress, one must help the person put his feelings in perspective. Don't have them deny sorrow, anger, guilt, or disbelief, or attempt to explain away these feelings. View them as realistic and normal for the grieving person.

Sometimes denial can be extreme. In one episode, two workers in their thirties were killed in a freak cave-in accident. The bereaved spouse of one was already present when the second wife arrived. She completely blocked the reality of her husband's death, going from the belief that he was only hurt, to that he wasn't even there. She even expressed compassion for his co-worker's spouse while not accepting that sympathy from her. Her strong need to deny was not attacked but was not allowed to exist as being consented to either. A relative verified the death to her. Finally, she agreed to view the body (as is generally advisable, she was told of the presence of the endotracheal and other tubes, as well as any visible disfigurements). She immediately rushed away, denying that it was her husband, saying that "she had to go home and prepare his dinner." Rather than further pressuring her, other family members were advised of the situation. We enlisted a home mental health worker to stay with her until impact did occur, with instructions to bring her back to the emergency department if denial persisted or hyperreaction occurred.

A clear example of sublimation of a grief reaction was given by a young Mexican-American who was the only man among the bereaved sisters, daughters, and cousins of his deceased mother. He was initially calm, acting as moderator to the overt and markedly emotional responses of the women. Nevertheless, less than 10 minutes later, he was brought back with a full-blown hyperventilation syndrome. He stated, "Everyone else was crying and I wanted to cry too, but I felt I should be strong."

The emergency physician is often wounded by a seeming lack of appreciation for his efforts by the family because he is unaware of the normal detached state of a grieving person. He may, in fact, become the focus of anger because of the family's annoyance with their own doctor, ambulance service, county hospital, impolite clerk, etc. This is not uncommon and is another defense mechanism, a displacement of their anger toward the lost one and/or of guilt. The physician should not respond defensively to such an attitude.

Requests are often made for sedatives for the grief-stricken. I feel that this generally blocks the necessary grief process and recommend only the minimal use of a hypnotic for the first few nights. It is better to rely on family, cultural, and, if present, religious support. While the person most directly involved is not going to remember much of what the physician says, I try to educate quickly someone who seems fairly responsible that grief is "OK" and, in fact, necessary, and that the family must accept, not block, genuine feelings.

Ideally, there should be some mechanism available for grief follow-through to aid "good" grief and detect pathologic grief. The family physician will rarely do so and may fall back on using tranquilizers. Psychiatrists, or general mental health clinics, are not needed for the routine grief process. The extended family and a strong cultural and religious tradition seem to carry the best prognosis for a favorable outcome. It is unfortunate that the readily available information and follow-up services for Sudden Infant Death Syndrome episodes are not matched for other death and dying episodes (Friedman, 1974).

The physician can initiate the healthy process of grief by manifesting apparent personal acceptance of that fact. The physician's willingness to risk the opening up of grief, the direct confrontation in stating that death has occurred, and the acceptance of normal reactions by the family, all encourage a normal and healthy period of bereavement. Clichés of sympathy as a verbal defense against the family's feelings and the physician's own sense of inadequacy should be avoided.

Generally, most grieving persons are helped by viewing the body and this option should be offered. Both the body, and the grief-stricken, should be prepared for this viewing. It is best not to have the head covered. The physician can invite the family to be more intimate by placing a hand on the body. This generally helps the families act on any desire to touch and even kiss the body without embarrassment.

Whatever the physician's personal religious views on death, he should offer the assistance of a chaplain. These ministers of comfort are often the only help available.

Distracting details of consent, billing, and arrangements for the body should be kept to a minimum so that the family can give full attention to their emotional needs. If a postmortem examination other than by the coroner is advised, the need and method of this procedure should be realistically appraised. There should be no coercion by playing on guilt, or expectation of unrealistic bencfits of what might be discovered.

In summary, after death of a patient, the emergency physician must now consider his responsibility to the grief-stricken. In his preoccupation with the cure, the physician must never forget his ability to care.

REFERENCES

Black, P. (1975), Criteria of brain death. *Postgrad. Med.*, 57:69–74.

——— (1978), Medical progress: Brain death. *N. Eng. J. Med.*, 299:338–344.

DeVaul, R. A., & Zisook, S. (1976), Unresolved grief. *Postgrad. Med.*, 59:267–271.

Engel, G. (1971), Sudden and rapid death during psychological stress. *Ann. Intern. Med.*, 74:771.

Friedman, S. (1974), Psychological aspects of sudden death in infants and children. *Pediat. Clin. N. Amer.*, 2:103–111.

Gennich, J. M. (1977), The emergency physician and organ donation. *J. Amer. Coll. Emerg. Physicians*, 6:21–25.

Harvard Medical School, Faculty of (1968), Report of the ad hoc committee of the Harvard Medical School to examine the definition of brain death. *J. Amer. Med. Assn.*, 205:337

Kübler-Ross, E. (1969), *On Death and Dying*. New York: Macmillan.

——— (1974), Questions and answers on death and dying. *Collier*, p. 177.

Lindemann, E. (1944), The symptomatology and management of acute grief. *Amer. J. Psychiat.*, 101:141–148.

Mattson, E. (1975), Psychological aspects of severe physical injury and its treatment. *J. Trauma*, 15:217–234.

Mitford, J. (1964), *The American Way of Death*. New York: Fawcett.

O'Connor, G. (1970), Psychiatric changes in the acutely injured. *Postgrad. Med.*

O'Keeffe, K. M. (1977), Accidental hypothermia. A review of 62 cases. *J. Amer. Coll. Emerg. Physicians*, 6:491–496.

Rosenberg, J. C., Krome, R. L., & McDonald, F. D. (1975), Identifying and managing the potential transplant donor in the emergency department. *J. Amer. Coll. Emerg. Physicians*, 4:328–331.

Sampson, W. (1977), On dying at home. *Emerg. Med.*, 137–139.

Saunders, C. (1977), On living with dying. *Man & Med.*, 227–252.

Siegler, M. (1975), Pascal's wager and the hanging of crepe. *N. Eng. J. Med.*, 17:853–857.

Steinfels, P. (1975), *Death Inside Out*, ed. R. Veatch. Scranton, PA: Harper & Row.

Waugh, E. (1949), *The Loved One*. New York: Grosset.

Yarnell, P. (1976), Neurologic outcome of prolonged coma in survivors of out-of-hospital cardiac arrests. *Stroke*, 3(7):279–282.

Young, M., Benjamin, B., & Wallis, C. (1963), The mortality of widowers. *Lancet*, 2:454–456.

Commentary

Lynn H. Hackett, M.D.

Ernest Becker (1973) has written that "of all things that move man, one of the principal ones is his terror of death." Indeed, death is the most absolute of all events confronting the physician. Although the causes of the cessation of a life are legion, once the terminal event occurs we are left with the inescapable fact that a member of our species has ceased to be. Acculturation and our own temperaments dictate how we respond. For the emergency room staff, who deal with death as a regular event, the routine, mechanized aspects of evaluation and resuscitation impel analysis, discussion, and ideally careful, considered training so that the human response might be as skillful and as therapeutic as possible. That the latter is not the general case is well known. I expect those of us who practice medicine recall receiving little or no formal instruction in coping with death, either on the wards or in the emergency room. The event occurred, the patient was pronounced, and we went to the telephone or to the waiting room to inform the family. For a new physician this is a deeply felt and terrifying experience.

Chapter 16 may be viewed as a first attempt to address the problem of death in the emergency room, and its implications for the bereaved family and the professionals who face death as a part of everyday life. As Dr. O'Keeffe points out, the process of dying, that is, the stages both the dying person and his or her family pass through, is well covered in the literature. Grief and bereavement, both normal and pathological, are discussed in the classic article by Lindemann (1944), a work that still serves as the standard reference on this subject. But sudden, traumatic, and violent death and the response to it on the part of both professional and family systems have been neglected in medical writing. In contrast, Elizabeth Kübler-Ross (1969) discusses the objectification of the dying person who is rushed by ambulance to the emergency room, suggesting that the mechanized approach to the patient, while having the explicit intent of efficient resuscitation, may also serve as a distancing device for the medical staff face-to-face with death. Recognition and explication of this phenomenon could provide a useful heightening of self-awareness on the part of the emergency room personnel. This is especially critical for the new nurse or doctor, who, by simply following the modeling provided by his or her mentors without an enlightened understanding of the process observed, might likely perpetuate the problematic behaviors the author appears to criticize.

Dr. O'Keeffe notes such circumstances as the intensity of the response when the dying person arrives in the emergency room, the fact that the rapid progression of events allows the family no passage through the generally accepted phases of confrontation with death, and even that the physical environment of most emergency rooms provides no protected place for the family to wait out the frightening procedures of resuscitation. Dr. O'Keeffe shifts course, then, to supply information on what might be termed the logistics of death. The reader is provided with discussions on such topics as admission of the terminally ill, organ donation, resuscitation, pronouncement of death, the completion of the death certificate, and the delicate issue of autopsy. Certainly, this material is useful, but this is already taught traditionally in hospital and emergency settings, and some of the details vary from state to state. The author later returns to the effect of the death on the bereaved, describing the procedure of informing the family of the bad outcome, the manifestations of the initial grief reaction, and methods to facilitate the emergence of normal grieving.

Clearly, Dr. O'Keeffe has accurately sensed that the issues of dying in the emergency room and the attendant process are important ones, demanding reasoned attention. His thesis should serve as a stimulus to further investigation into a neglected area of medical care.

References

Becker, E. (1973), *The Denial of Death*. New York: The Free Press.

Kübler-Ross, E. (1969), *On Death and Dying,* New York: Macmillan.

Lindemann, E. (1944), The symptomatology and management of acute grief. *Amer. J. Psychiat.*, 101:141–148.

Annotated Bibliography

Perlmutter, R. A. (1983), Family involvement in psychiatric emergencies. *Hosp. & Commun. Psychiat.*, 34 3:255–257.

A short but important study that assessed the impression that many of the cases seen in a psychiatric emergency room reflect family problems in psychopathology. The results of the study show a discrepancy between the number of patients who were actually referred for family treatment and the larger number of patients who, it appeared, should have benefited from this therapeutic modality. The author concludes that there is a high need for training in family intervention skills, underscored by the findings of this study.

Pittman, F. S., III, (1973), Managing acute psychiatric emergencies: Defining the family crisis. *Sem. in Psychiat.*, 5/2:219–227.

It is proposed that a central element in managing an acute breakdown of the family is defining the family systems crisis. The author outlines seven phases in family crisis therapy, offers a classification of crisis-producing stressors, and discusses ways of resolving the crisis.

Goodstein, R. K., & Page, A. W. (1981), Battered wife syndrome: Overview of dynamics and treatment. *Amer. J. Psychiat.*, 138/8:1036–1044.

In this important paper the authors review some key factors associated with the battered wife syndrome, including definitions, incidence, characteristics of wives, injury profiles, setting of the violence, psychodynamics, role of alcohol, family backgrounds, characteristics of husbands, coping responses of wives, seeking help, social support systems, recognition of the battering syndrome, prevention and treatment, and group therapy. The authors point out that although force has long been used as a resource in family interactions, we have just started to understand some of its precipitants, and treatment options.

Purdie, F. R. J., Honigman, B., & Rosen, P. (1981), The chronic emergency department patient. *Ann. Emerg. Med.*, 10/6:298–301.

Another article about the chronic emergency room patient. The tremendous waste of resources is pointed out. Examining a population of 16 frequent or chronic emergency room visitors, the authors indicate that these visitors were predominantly single, had an average age of 48, the vast majority were suffering from a chronic psychiatric condition, often were dependent on government support, and lived alone. Ambulance transport was used for 84 percent of the visits but in only 6 percent was hospital admission required. The authors point out that this group is at high risk for medical and traumatic illness, and offer suggestions for disposition.

Robbins, E., Stern, M., Robbins, L., & Margolin, L. (1980), Unwelcome patients: Where can they find asylum? *Hosp. & Commun. Psychiat.*, 29:44–46.

An article about 23 specific patients of Bellevue Hospital in New York who were constantly seeking admission but did not cooperate with treatment. They appeared to respond to stress with rage, often augmented by substance abuse. They were mainly male and lacked vocational and social skills. The authors suggest the development of therapeutic units in which such patients would be sheltered, protected from their impulses, and taught and encouraged to become self-sufficient.

Lansley, D. G. (1978), Three models of family therapy: Prevention, crisis treatment or rehabilitation. *J. Clin. Psychiat.*, 39:792–796.

While not focusing exclusively on emergency room issues, this paper has pertinence to therapeutic efforts in this setting. It describes three models of intervention at a family level: prevention, crisis intervention, and rehabilitation. The second model, crisis intervention, suggests that early identification and prompt intervention may avoid the development of more serious decompensation.

III

MANAGEMENT AND DISPOSITION ISSUES

Having reviewed specific forms of behavioral emergency, the third part of the book will examine broad therapeutic and organization of care issues. Certain psychotherapies and somatotherapies particularly relevant to the emergency setting are considered first. The decision to hospitalize, probably the most crucial one made in the emergency department is considered next. Chapters 20 and 21 deal with organization of care; that is, the contributions of the psychiatric professional in a general hospital emergency department and the planning of care delivery systems.

Specific questions considered include the following: How should crisis theory concepts be implemented in an emergency setting? What steps are required for a sound use of psychotropic drugs and what is the role of such specific drugs as neuroleptics and sedatives? What are the aspects of the clinical condition most pertinent to hospitalization decisions, and what is the contribution of comprehensive diagnostic formulations in this process? What are the medical, social, and emotional factors involved in the work of a psychiatric consultant in a general emergency department? How can patterns of patients' needs and service use be employed in the strategic planning of emergency care?

17

Crisis-Intervention: Theory and Practice

Larry L. Smith, D.S.W.

According to Howard J. Parad (1971, p. 196) crisis intervention is "a process for actively influencing the psychosocial functioning of individuals during a period of disequilibrium." Most experts (Aguilera, Messick, and Farrell, 1970; Morley, 1970; Parad, 1971; Rapoport, 1970) consider Erich Lindemann (1944, 1956) to be the father of crisis-intervention theory and practice. Parad (1971) believes Lindemann's classic study (1944) of the bereaved disaster victims of the Coconut Grove nightclub fire in 1943 set the stage for the study and development of crisis theory and practice. Even so, others (Bloom, 1963; Lukton, 1974; Mackey, 1968; Pasewark and Albers, 1972; Smith, 1975, 1976) believe crisis intervention is not yet a well-defined theory or treatment model. Darbonne (1968) reports that the crisis-intervention model is still unclear and cannot at this time be considered a proven method of social intervention. Smith's (1975) review of the literature on crisis intervention, found that other authors share Darbonne's criticism. This chapter will review the current status of crisis-intervention theory and practice. The first part of the review will concentrate on crisis-inter-

This chapter was first published in *Community Mental Health Review* (1977), 2:4–13, and it is reprinted by permission.

vention theory. This will be followed by a review of crisis-intervention practice across the following areas: (1) childhood and adolescent crises; (2) mental health problems; (3) marital and family conflicts; (4) emergency hospitalization; and (5) suicide prevention. Other practice areas, of course, have been written about, although the author will limit his discussion to these five areas.

CRISIS-INTERVENTION THEORY

What Is a Crisis?

In describing the characteristics of acute grief, Lindemann (1944) established the basic framework for defining the symptomatology of a crisis reaction. Lindemann concludes that most people experiencing the crisis of acute grief or bereavement usually have five related reactions: (1) somatic distress, (2) preoccupation with the image of the deceased, (3) guilt, (4) hostile reactions, and (5) loss of patterns of conduct. Lindemann also found that the stages and duration of a bereavement reaction seem to depend on the success with which a person does his "grief work." This grief work includes achieving emancipation from the deceased, readjustment to the environment in which the deceased is missing, and the formation of new relationships.

Gerald Caplan (1964) was the first theorist to associate the concept of homeostasis with crisis intervention. According to Caplan, the human organism constantly endeavors to maintain a homeostatic balance with the outside environment. When this delicate balance is threatened by either physiological or psychological forces, the human organism engages in problem-solving activities designed to restore this delicate balance. In a crisis situation, however, the individual is faced with a problem that appears to have no immediate solution, hence the idea that a crisis is an upset of a steady state.

Rapoport (1962a) defines a crisis as an upset of a steady state where an individual finds himself in a hazardous situation. After rephrasing some of Caplan's (1964) ideas on homeostasis, Rapoport adds that in a state of crisis the normal problem-solving mechanisms of the individual are not adequate to achieve a balanced state, which throws the individual into disequilibrium. Rapoport believes that three related factors usually produce a state of crisis: (1) a hazardous event, (2) a threat to life goals, and (3) an inability to respond with adequate coping mechanisms. Parad (1966) adds to this definition by saying that a crisis is an upset in a steady state characterized by (1) a specific and identifiable stressful event, (2) the perception of that event as meaningful and threatening, (3) the response to the event, and (4) the coping tasks involved in successful adaptation.

Sifneos (Golan, 1969) identifies four components of an emotional crisis: (1) the hazardous event, (2) the vulnerable state, (3) the precipitating factor, and (4) the state of active crisis. This conceptual framework of a crisis is interesting because Sifneos makes a distinction between the hazardous event and the precipitating factor. According to his framework, the hazardous event leads to the crisis while the precipitating factor is that final event or circumstance that makes the hazardous event unbearable and results in the crisis. Sifneos's interactive concept of hazardous event and precipitating factor offers an explanation of why some people have a higher tolerance to certain crisis situations only to succumb finally when a less serious event occurs.

Schulberg and Sheldon (1968) have devised a conceptual framework that attempts to predict how an individual, family, group, community, or even nation might react to a future crisis situation. Their conceptual framework incorporates three factors: (1) the probability that a hazardous event will occur, (2) the probability that an individual will be exposed to this event, and (3) the vulnerability of the individual to the event.

Bloom (1963) wanted to determine if highly skilled clinicians could agree on what circumstances constitute a crisis. After administering case histories to crisis theorists and clinicians at the Harvard School of Public Health, he found that the judgment of what constitutes a crisis is made significantly more often when there is a known precipitating event. Other theorists (Bonstedt, 1970; Brandon, 1970; LaSor and Strickler, 1970; Cohen and Walder, 1971; Rusk, 1971) have also identified the importance of a precipitating event in determining what is a crisis.

In adding to this list of definitions, the author (Smith, 1975, 1976) believes a crisis exists when an individual is faced with any problem he perceives as serious that has no immediate solution. Many times the problem seems hopeless because the individual cannot resolve the crisis with his customary problem-solving skills. Despite the seriousness of the crisis, however, most theorists (Caplan, 1960; Caplan, Mason, and Kaplan, 1965; Parad and Caplan, 1960; Parad, 1965a,b; Rapoport, 1962a, 1967) stress that it can be a period of important personality growth and development. This is an important concept to remember and one that Erikson (1950, 1956) discusses in his theory of human development.

Stages of a Crisis Reaction

Caplan (1964) considers a crisis to be a time-limited period of disequilibrium that usually lasts 5 to 8 weeks and follows four characteristic stages. The first stage is the initial rise in tension that results from the crisis-provoking event. When this tension begins to mount, the individual will usually try to resolve the crisis by using familiar patterns of problem-solving behavior. The second stage of crisis is characterized by increased tension because the individual has not yet resolved the crisis. If emergency problem-solving skills fail to alleviate the tension, the individual enters the third stage of crisis. Now the tension becomes so great that the individual may experience acute depression or try to strike back at whatever appears to be causing the crisis. In the fourth stage of crisis, one of two outcomes may occur. If tension continues to increase, the individual may have a major emotional breakdown (Brown and Birley, 1968). Another individual may resolve the crisis by using maladaptive forms of behavior that reduce tension but also impair his future social functioning.

Rapoport (1962a, 1967, 1970) identifies three phases of a crisis reaction: (1) initial or beginning, (2) middle, and (3) end. During the initial phase, there is a rise in tension because of the stressful precipitating event that the individual attempts to alleviate with habitual problem-solving mechanisms. If these habitual problem-solving mechanisms fail, the individual moves into the middle phase of the crisis. Now emergency problem-solving mechanisms such as denial, flight into health, and so on, are applied to the crisis. These emergency mechanisms result in one of three conclusions: (1) problem solved, (2) problem redefined, or (3) problem denied. All crisis reactions have an end phase when some type of equilibrium is restored. This equilibrium, however, can be equal, lower, or higher than the precrisis level of functioning.

Hill (1949, 1958), apparently working independently from Lindemann and Caplan, developed his own stages of a crisis reaction involving individuals and families. According to Hill (1949), the course of an individual's or family's reactions to a crisis follows a roller-coaster pattern. First, upon meeting a crisis, the individual is numbed by the blow. Then, as the full impact of the situation forces the individual to face the reality of the crisis, there follows a downward slump in behavior wherein the individual often becomes confused, disoriented, and helpless. After this brief period of disorganization, the individual attempts to recover from the crisis by using emergency coping skills.

Sachs (1968) has taken these concepts and, using Hill's earlier illustration, developed the diagram of a crisis reaction shown in Figure 17.1

This illustration shows that a crisis first leads to a period of disorganization. Yet, based on how the individual copes with the crisis, the eventual outcome may find the individual in an even better state of functioning. Which outcome state finally occurs, of course, is often the result of the kind of help a person receives from others during the crisis. Most crisis theorists (Aguilera et al., 1970; Brandon, 1970; Caplan, 1964; Forer, 1963; Lindemann, 1944; Parad, 1966; Rapoport, 1970) state that effectively used techniques of crisis intervention are designed to return the individual to at least his precrisis level of functioning, and hopefully even improve it.

Different Types of Crises

Although Lindemann presents only a brief description of the different types of crises, Caplan discusses them in depth using Erikson's (1950, 1956) model of developmental and accidental crises. Caplan (1964) has defined developmental crises as transitional periods in personality development characterized by cognitive and affective upset. Common examples of these types of crises are birth, infancy, childhood, ado-

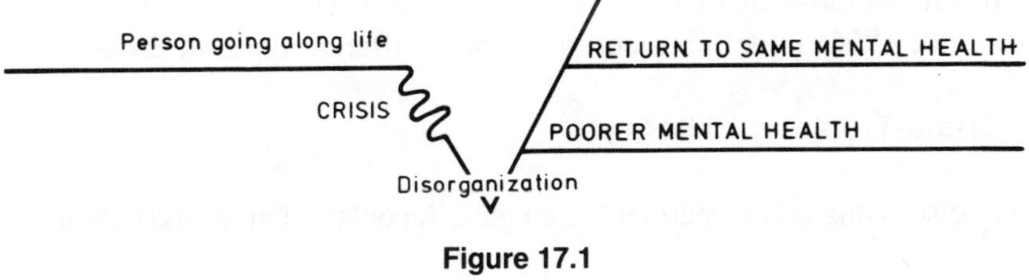

Figure 17.1

lescence, adulthood, and old age. Accidental crises are described as periods of psychological and behavioral upset that are precipitated by life hazards involving significant losses such as illness and death. Caplan also emphasizes that developmental and accidental crises are transitional periods that present the individual with both an opportunity for personality growth as well as emotional and mental deterioration.

Unlike the other major crisis theorists, Jacobsen (1965a,b, 1970; Jacobsen, Strickler, and Morley, 1968) does not classify different crises according to Erikson's framework of developmental and accidental crises. Instead, Jacobsen et al. (1968) state that any classification of crises must include references to the social, intrapsychic, and somatic factors involved or the biopsychosocial field. The social factor of crisis refers to any role changes or other alterations in interpersonal behavior. The intrapsychic factors of crisis emphasize the changes in a previously existing equilibrium within the psychic apparatus that involve unconscious as well as conscious processes. In discussing the somatic classification of crisis, Jacobsen refers to pathogenic grief that may result in chronic psychosomatic illnesses.

Hill (1949, 1958) has developed a conceptual framework to describe different types of family crises. According to Hill (1958), family crises are either intrafamily or extrafamily in nature, and fall under the following categories: (1) dismemberment only, (2) assession only, (3) demoralization only, (4) demoralization plus dismemberment or assession. The category "dismemberment only" would include such crises as the death of a child, spouse, or parent while the category of "assession only" includes crisis situations like an unwanted pregnancy, some adoptions, or an aged relative's coming to live with a family. Crises that cause demoralization include nonsupport, infidelity, alcoholism, and drug abuse, while divorce and suicide can have a demoralizing and dismembering effect on the family.

In defining the characteristics of different types of crises, most of the other writers (Malamud, 1927; Kaplan, 1962; Klemme, 1970; Rogers, 1970) added little to the knowledge base of crisis intervention. In fact, almost all of them point to the pioneering work of Erikson (1950, 1956) in defining and describing different types of crises.

Crisis-Treatment Theory

In discussing crisis treatment strategies, Jacobsen et al. (1968) identify two separate approaches, the generic and the specific, and then discuss the treatment techniques of each model. The central thesis of the generic approach to crisis treatment is that for each crisis, such as bereavement, prematurity, divorce, etc., there are certain identifiable patterns that require specific psychological tasks if the crisis is to be resolved successfully. In Lindemann's (1944, p. 147) study on bereavement, he states that the following tasks have to be accomplished by the grieving client:

1. Accept the pain of bereavement.
2. Review his relationship with the deceased and become acquainted with the alterations in his own modes of emotional reaction.
3. Express sorrow and a sense of loss.
4. Find an acceptable formulation of his future relationship to the deceased.
5. Verbalize his feelings of guilt and find persons around him whom he can use as "primers" for the acquisition of new patterns of conduct.

In implementing the treatment strategies of the generic approach, emphasis is placed on accomplishing these specific psychological tasks with each client regardless of his individual differences. The accomplishment of these tasks, however, requires that the client and worker engage in mutually directed problem-solving activity. In addition, any evaluation or assessment of crisis treatment must be based on how well these psychological tasks were accomplished by the client.

The specific or individual approach to crisis treatment differs from the generic model in its emphasis on the clinician's professional assessment of the individual in crisis. This individual concern for the client is reflected in Parad's (1971) three initial questions: (1) What is troubling the client? (2) Why does he come for help now? (3) What can I do to help? Specifically, the therapist needs to assess why the client's normally effective patterns of coping are no longer sufficient and what can be done to enhance his coping abilities. This requires extensive knowledge and experience in assessing the psychological and psychosocial pressures that are interacting with the client. The author believes this is an inherent weakness of the individual approach to crisis treatment because many workers will not have this clinical expertise.

Paul (1966, pp. 142–143) asserts that in crisis therapy the worker must accomplish four tasks:

1. Identify (to yourself) the precipitating event.
2. Discern (for yourself) the defensive maneuvers employed against the responses to the precipitating stress event.
3. Acquaint the client with the main (most powerful) defenses he is using against recognizing and feeling the responses.
4. Acquaint him with the precipitating event and the responses to it he is warding off.

This step-by-step guide to crisis intervention does not clarify how the crisis is finally resolved, however. It seems wise to add a fifth task: Identify with the client the psychological tasks associated with resolving the crisis and work with him in completing these tasks. This approach tends to follow Jacobsen et al.'s (1968) concept of generic crisis intervention, because the worker follows the same treatment plan with all clients.

In summarizing the important features of crisis treatment, Aguilera et al. (1970, p. 16) emphasize the following points that she and Morley (1970) developed:

1. It is essential that the therapist view the work that he is doing not as a "second-best" approach but as the treatment of choice with persons in crisis.
2. Accurate assessment of the presenting problem, not a diagnostic evaluation, is essential to an effective intervention.
3. Both the therapist and the client should keep in mind throughout the contacts that the treatment is sharply time-limited and persistently direct their energies toward the resolution of the presenting problem.
4. Dealing with material not directly related to the crisis has no place in an intervention of this kind.
5. The therapist must be willing to take an active and sometimes directive role in the intervention. The relatively slow-paced approach of more traditional treatments is inappropriate in this type of therapy.

6. Maximum flexibility of approach is encouraged. Such diverse techniques as serving as a resource person or information giver, taking an active role in establishing liaison with other helping resources, and so forth, are often appropriate in particular situations.
7. The goal toward which the treatment is striving is explicit. His energy is directed entirely toward returning the individual to at least his precrisis level of functioning.

CRISIS INTERVENTION PRACTICE

Children and Adolescents

In discussing crisis intervention with children, most of the writers (Epstein, 1965; Baldwin, 1968; Lang and Oppenheimer, 1968; Keith-Lucas, 1969; Sze, 1970; Stein, 1970; Blaufarb and Levine, 1972; Galdston and Hughes, 1972; Ewalt, 1973; LaVietes, 1974) focus either on child-guidance clinics or child hospitalization services. Crisis practice with adolescents (Deeths, 1970; Armsby, 1971; Bonier and Koplovsky, 1971; Denison, 1971; Hart, 1971; Riscalla, 1971) seems to deal primarily with adolescent clinics and correctional facilities for youth in trouble with the law.

One of the first articles written about children and crisis practice is Rosenfeld and Caplan's (1954) study of Jewish immigrant children entering Israel during the late 1940s and early 1950s. They discuss the efforts of the Lasker Mental Hygiene Center of Hadassah in meeting the emotional and physical needs of 16,000 unaccompanied immigrant children from the ages of 6 to 17. Periodically, about 10 to 15 percent of these children were referred to the Lasker Center because of "neurotic symptoms." It was at this stage that the crisis consultants were involved in the treatment of the children.

Epstein (1965) discusses the Child and Family Services Center in Chicago which offers substitute or supplementary child care through the use of homemakers. This service was initiated and directed by a crisis consultant who helped the agency staff begin appropriate crisis procedures to assist a troubled child. Cain and Fast (1966) explain that disturbed children are usually referred to their centers by parents who are also experiencing a crisis. They discuss in depth the disturbed child who is referred by the surviving parent after the other parent has committed suicide. Lang and Oppenheimer (1968) and Morrisey (1964) discuss the reactions and crisis treatment of children who are suffering from a fatal illness. Both studies refer to the crisis of childhood leukemia.

Shifting to adolescent crisis practice, Garrell (1969), Armsby (1971), Bonier and Koplovsky (1971), and Denison (1971) describe direct services offered by community centers in meeting the needs of adolescents in crisis. Armsby (1971) describes the Adolescent Unit at the Hawaii State Hospital that treats emotionally disturbed adolescents between the ages of 12 and 19. Bonier and Koplovsky (1971) discuss a crisis treatment plan given to 28 adolescents at the McLean Hospital Outpatient Clinic.

In other articles, Deeths (1970), Riscalla (1970), Villeponteaux (1970), and Hart (1971) describe the crisis treatment of adolescent offenders. Deeths (1970) discusses a crisis-treatment service that uses psychodrama with male drug users at a correctional facility in Stockton, California. Villeponteaux's (1970) article deals with the Horizon House, a 3-year pilot project in Charleston, South Carolina, sponsored by the Junior League, that helps adolescents on probation for serious offenses.

By conducting follow-up interviews, Armsby (1971) assessed some of the long-term effects of crisis treatment. Of the 106 families treated by the crisis team at the Hawaii State Hospital, 74 (70 percent) were still together as family units 6 months later. In addition, the mean score of family functioning for all treated families had significantly improved based on the 20-item Periodic Evaluation Community Record Form.

In discussing the use of specific crisis techniques, Strickler and Allgeyer (1967), Morley and Brown (1969), and Allgeyer (1970) discuss the crisis group and its use at the Benjamin Rush Center. The crisis group is designed to meet the needs of persons ordinarily underrepresented in mental health facilities; that is, families with incomes of less than $4,000, blacks, Mexican-Americans, and blue-collar workers.

Marital and Family Conflicts

The literature on crisis intervention with families centers around four subject areas. First, there are a number of writers (Duckworth, 1967; Langsley et al., 1968; Langsley and Kaplan, 1968; Argles and Mackenzie, 1970) who discuss the practice of crisis intervention in family counseling centers. Other writers (Koos, 1948; Caplan, 1960; Dyer, 1963; Caplan et al., 1965, Rosenberg, 1975, Wiseman, 1975) describe family crisis intervention with specific problems such as premature births, parenthood, and divorce. A third group of crisis-intervention theorists (Lindemann, 1956; Parad and Caplan, 1960; Klein and Lindemann, 1961) present generic conceptual frameworks for studying and helping families in crisis. A final series of writers (Richman and Davidoff, 1971; Eisler and Hersen, 1973) presents two specific approaches to crisis intervention with families: behavioral therapy and interaction testing.

Probably the best description of crisis intervention with families is presented by Langsley and Kaplan (1968), Kaplan (1968), and Langsley et al. (1969). Their articles discuss in detail family crisis intervention at the Family Treatment Unit of the Colorado Psychiatric Hospital. The Family Treatment Unit was established to test whether family crisis therapy could provide an effective alternative to emergency psychiatric hospitalization by meeting with the prospective patient and his family before hospitalization. After the study was completed, Langsley et al. (1969) found that 29 percent of the patients receiving more traditional forms of psychiatric treatment were readmitted within 6 months, while only 13 percent of the family-crisis-treatment patients were hospitalized during the same period. Langsley's study also found that family crisis treatment cost one-sixth or less than the cost of traditional hospital treatment. In fact, the mean patient cost for family crisis therapy was $200, compared to $1,300 for more traditional emergency psychiatric services.

Mental Health Problems

The articles reviewed on crisis practice in community mental health centers focus on three main areas. First, a number of writers (Polak, 1967; Gebbie, 1968; Morley and Brown, 1969; Hiatt and Spurlock, 1970; Clarke, 1971) describe certain crisis-oriented clinics such as the Benjamin Rush Center in Los Angeles or the nationwide services by the Travelers Aid Society. The focus of another group of writers (Allgeyer, 1970; Sutherland and Scherl, 1970; Brown, 1971; Fox and

Scherl, 1972) is on more specific techniques that mental health centers can use in working with the crisis reactions that often accompany rape or drug abuse. The final groups of writers (Gottschalk et al., 1967; Brown, 1969; Birnbaum, 1973; Schild et al., 1974; Strickler and Bonnefil, 1974) discuss related aspects of crisis practice in mental health programs.

According to Jacobsen (1965a), Strickler (1965), and Paul (1966), the Benjamin Rush Center is a community-based, walk-in center for individuals and families suffering from various intensities of psychological stress. The center's 24-hour walk-in service is available to anyone over 17½ years of age who lives in the encatchment area. Treatment, in the words of Jacobsen (1965a, p. 210), "focuses on the immediate problem or crisis, rather than on long-standing pathology or on well established character patterns." The crisis services are brief, usually lasting no longer than six 1-hour visits spread over 6 weeks or more.

Clarke (1971) discusses the emergency services of a mental health department in a London borough. Serving an catchment area of about 210,000 people, this mental health department also maintains a 24-hour emergency service. Unlike the Benjamin Rush Center, emergency callers at the London clinic are first contacted by phone after their initial phone inquiry. When the mental health officer returns their call, he decides at that time whether or not to deal with the situation as a crisis. In comparison, Hiatt and Spurlock's (1970) discussion of Travelers Aid presents some valuable treatment concepts for people caught in "crisis-flight."

Polak (1967) discusses the crisis of emergency psychiatric care at the Fort Logan Mental Health Center. As part of the emergency-care procedures, each patient when referred for admission is requested to come with at least one family member to the next admission-assessment meeting. In this way, the crisis team believes they are better able to evaluate the seriousness of the crisis. Polak also reports that 90 percent of a sample of 104 male patients requesting admission at the Fort Logan Mental Health Center had a presenting crisis that precipitated the admission request. In 60 percent of these crisis situations, the crisis focused on the family's unwillingness or inability to tolerate the client's behavior any longer.

Argles and Mackenzie (1970) present a model of family crisis therapy for multiproblem families who have not been helped by more traditional forms of social welfare services. In their series of articles, Caplan (1960), Rapoport (1962b), and Caplan et al. (1965) discuss the family crisis experienced by a premature birth and treatment techniques that can help a family resolve this crisis effectively. These writers stress the completion of certain psychological or behavioral tasks in dealing successfully with the crisis of prematurity. Other writers (LeMasters, 1957; Dyer, 1963; Signell, 1969) deal with the resolution of family crises such as parenthood or unwed motherhood. Signell (1969) explains how the family-crisis worker can consult with other "professional caregivers" such as school counselors, religious leaders, etc., in gaining additional community resources and support for the unwed mother.

Parad and Caplan (1960) present practice models for helping families in crisis that stress three main areas: (1) family-life-style, (2) intermediate problem-solving mechanisms, and (3) need-response patterns. Klein and Lindemann (1961, p. 289) discuss a model for family crisis therapy that promotes a community approach so "knowledge of neighborhood patterns, community resources, and current community concerns that may have relevance to the specific predicament is added to the planning of the clinical team."

Emergency Hospitalization

The theorists who have written about crisis practice in hospital settings analyze a variety of crisis situations. A number of writers (Kritzer and Pittman, 1968; Munoz, Tuason, and Dick, 1970; Langsley, Mackotha, and Flomenhaft, 1971; Decker and Stubblebine, 1972) discuss the crisis of emergency psychiatric hospitalization. Aguilera (1971), Eisendrath, (1969), and Oppenheimer (1967) describe crisis intervention with the patient who is hospitalized with a fatal illness such as cancer or leukemia. Other writers (Burnside, 1970; Oberleder, 1970; Florell, 1971; Foreman and Zerwehk, 1971) describe additional hospital crises experienced by geriatric and orthopedic patients. Finally, Birley and Brown (1970) and Kirshner and Kaplan (1970) describe how sudden life crises can precede the onset of acute schizophrenia or ataxia.

In Decker and Stubblebine's (1972) publication, they discuss the crisis treatment of 225 young adults at San Francisco General Hospital who voluntarily or involuntarily sought emergency hospitalization. With few exceptions, these young adults were treated on an outpatient basis by an interdisciplinary crisis team. Kritzer and Pittman (1968) describe how overnight care in a general hospital emergency room was used to avert more serious crisis reactions and help the crisis team at the Colorado Psychiatric Hospital extend crisis intervention to troubled individuals. Raphling and Lion (1970) discuss the emergency crisis clinic at Massachusetts General Hospital where all walk-in patients are treated on a 24-hour basis.

Eisendrath (1969) explores the role of grief and fear in dying kidney-transplant patients. He reports that those patients who died were distinguished either by a sense of being abandoned during their illness by significant others or by anxiety approaching panic about their ultimate fate. Oberleder (1970) discusses a crisis treatment program at the Bronx State Hospital in New York City where 12 geriatric patients received crisis therapy. These 12 patients were randomly selected from the 1,000-bed mental hospital complex where one-third of all patients were geriatric cases. Burnside (1970) also presents guidelines for hospital staffs to follow in crisis intervention with aged hospital patients.

Oppenheimer (1967) presents one of the clearest conceptualizations of crisis practice in hospital settings. In his article, he discusses crisis intervention with the hospitalized cancer patient and his family. Oppenheimer (1967, p. 45) asserts that:

> The techniques for intervention and change in this crisis situation, as in other crises, are focused on (1) helping the patient or family develop conscious awareness of their problem, (2) assessing quickly and accurately the total situation for the patient and family, and (3) enabling the patient and family to make a new use of their existing ego-adaptive techniques or to develop new and more effective mechanisms.

Suicide Prevention

In recent years, a great deal of information has been written about suicide prevention and emergency telephone services. The majority of publications fall into four areas. The first group of articles focuses on writers (Heilig and Klugman, 1965; Berliner, 1970; Farberow, 1970; Litman, 1970; Pretzel, 1970; Tabacknick and Klugman, 1970) who discuss the services offered by the Los Angeles Suicide Prevention Center. The second group (Waltzer and Hankoff, 1965; Brockopp, 1970a,b,c,d; Juechter, 1971; Mikawa, 1971; Musgrave, 1971, Torop and Torop, 1972) describes other suicide prevention and telephone hot-line services operating throughout the United States. The third group (Murphy et al., 1969; Lester, 1970a,b,c,d,e, 1971a,b,c; Sokolow et al., 1971; Speer, 1971) deals with such topics as how to evaluate a suicide-prevention center, who calls a suicide center, and how workers on the telephone can assist a person suffering from a bad drug trip. The final set of writers (McGee, 1965; Noyes, 1970) discuss the worldwide problem of suicide and how community mental health programs can meet the increasing need for services through crisis intervention.

Farberow (1970) discusses the growth and development of the Los Angeles Suicide Prevention Center. According to Farberow, 99 percent of their first contacts with clients is by telephone, with only 10 clients out of a monthly caseload of 500 seen for any length of time. In order to respond to a yearly caseload of over 6,000 callers, the center now has 30 offices, 12 phone lines, and a staff of nearly 100 professionals and volunteers. Most of the service demands are met by nonprofessional volunteers under the supervision and consultation of the professional staff. Services are available for anyone who calls for help, 24 hours a day.

Musgrave (1971) describes the telephone hotline service provided by the Los Angeles Children's Hospital. This hotline telephone service gives assistance to adolescents overwhelmed by their problems. By dialing Hotline, Musgrave (1971, p. 757) explains "a caller may have a 'tuned in, turned on' adult to listen to him; he may receive information about free clinics, drug counseling, or draft counseling; he may get the address of a crash pad." According to Musgrave, there are approximately 90 hotline services throughout the nation.

Mikawa (1971) explains how the University of Nevada in Reno developed a suicide-prevention and crisis call center to counter the high rate of suicide in the area. To deal with the threat of suicide and other crises, a crisis center staffed primarily by volunteers and open 24 hours a day was begun. Today the center has 34 nonprofessional volunteers along with nine professional consultants.

Yasser (1970) discusses how to work with the drug crisis problem of a bad trip. He believes the telephone therapist must engage the client in calm discussion, emphasizing that the experiences the patient is having stem from the drug and will end when the effect of the drug wears off. Consequently, the telephone worker maintains telephone contact until the caller begins to feel better.

UNRESOLVED ISSUES AND PROBLEMS

Conceptualizing the Crisis Model

Despite the contributions that have been referred to in this chapter, crisis theorists and practitioners are still struggling with some difficult problems. According to Rapoport (1970, p. 307), the "most glaring problem is that there is little systematic practice that consciously uses the crisis model." In other words, most crisis practitioners are not using accepted principles of crisis intervention in treatment. Unfortunately, after completing an extensive review of the literature, the author also found this to be true. Most crisis theorists present sketchy conceptualizations of practice that even the most skilled clinician would have difficulty in following. As theorists continue to refine crisis treatment, it will be much easier to follow a systematic body of crisis practice based on accepted principles of crisis intervention.

Parad (1971, pp. 201–202) believes the problem is much broader than specifying crisis treatment and lists the following knowledge areas where exploratory research is desperately needed.

1. Criteria for intervention.
2. The client's perception of the precipitating stressful event.
3. Whether and why the worker and client think there is a crisis and how serious it is.
4. The goals of treatment in specific rather than global terms.
5. The client's and the worker's perceptions of the time dimension.
6. Types of treatment techniques used.
7. How the worker and the client perceive outcome both at the time of termination and at prearranged time intervals following intervention.

In examining this list, it is apparent that most of Parad's research suggestions are an attempt to clarify what characterizes crisis treatment. In fact, there seems to be no real difference between Rapoport's research suggestions and those of Parad other than the fact that Parad attempts to identify specific treatment areas that remain unclear. Both theorists are saying that crisis treatment remains unclear and will probably remain so until more research is conducted. Yet before crisis treatment can be explored, theorists and practitioners must first take the time to conceptualize what constitutes crisis practice. In order to do this, they will have to identify and describe systematically the various aspects and stages of crisis treatment.

Recommendations and Suggestions

If the knowledge base and effectiveness of crisis intervention are to be enhanced, this author (Smith, 1975, pp. 231–233) believes crisis theorists, practitioners, and the agencies they represent should consider the following recommendations and suggestions.

1. Crisis theorists and practitioners must develop models of crisis intervention that focus on the process of treatment from the initial contact with the client or family through termination of services.
2. Instead of developing treatment models for specific crisis situations, theorists and practitioners should focus their efforts on a more general model of crisis intervention that can be applied to most practice settings.
3. Agencies offering crisis intervention services should seriously consider implementing the following list of administrative policies suggested by Parad (1971, p. 201):
    a. The elimination of waiting lists.
    b. The avoidance of complex intake screening so treatment will be simultaneous with diagnosis.
    c. The development of an open-door policy for those who may require further services when faced with a new crisis.
    d. The use of a built-in policy of preplanned follow-up interviews to provide feedback about the effectiveness of services.
4. Crisis intervention agencies should maintain up-to-date library facilities that contain research, reviews, and pertinent articles and publications on crisis theory and practice.
5. These same agencies should provide practitioners with treatment source books that discuss as many different crisis reactions as possible and the psychological tasks and problem-

solving activities that are suggested in helping individuals and families successfully resolve these crises.

6. National, state, and local mental health programs and facilities should consider adopting more extensive crisis-intervention programs that can markedly increase services while reducing the cost and duration of treatment.

Conclusion

This review of crisis-intervention theory and practice has demonstrated that although crisis intervention is a popular model of social intervention the model is still conceptually unclear to many critics. This seems to have occurred because most crisis theorists have not operationalized crisis theory into clear treatment plans. As theorists and practitioners conceptualize their models more completely, researchers will be able to conduct better studies and crisis knowledge should increase dramatically. As the model is refined, crisis intervention will more readily be acknowledged as the treatment of choice for individuals and families suffering from a crisis.

REFERENCES

Aguilera, D. C. (1970), Sociocultural factors: Barriers to therapeutic intervention. *J. Psychiat. Nurs. & Ment. Health Serv.*, 8(5):14–18.

——— (1971), Crisis: Moment of truth. *J. Psychiat. Nurs. & Ment. Health Serv.*, 9(3):23–25.

——— Messick, J. M., & Farrell, M. S. (1970), *Theory and Methodology*. St. Louis: C. V. Mosby.

Allgeyer, J. M. (1970), The crisis group—Its unique usefulness to the disadvantaged. *Internat. J. Group Psychother.*, 10(2):235–240.

Argles, P., & Mackenzie, M. (1970), Crisis intervention with a multi-problem family: A case study. *J. Child Psychol. & Psychiat. & Allied Discip.*, 11(3):187–195.

Armsby, R. E. (1971), The adolescent crisis team: An experiment in community crisis intervention. *Proceedings of the Convention of the American Psychological Association*, 6(2):735–736.

Baldwin, K. A. (1968), Crisis-focused casework in a child guidance clinic. *Soc. Casework*, 49(1):28–34.

Berliner, B. S. (1970), Nursing a patient in crisis. *Amer. J. Nurs.*, 70(10):2154–2157.

Birnbaum, F., et al. (1973), Crisis intervention after a natural disaster. *Soc. Casework*, 54(9):545–551.

Birley, J. L., & Brown, G. W. (1970), Crises and life changes preceding the onset or relapse of acute schizophrenia: Clinical aspects. *Brit. J. Psychiat.*, 116:327–333.

Blaufarb, H., & Levine, J. (1972), Crisis intervention in an earthquake. *Soc. Work,* 17(4):16–19.

Bloom, B. C. (1963), Definitional aspects of the crisis concept. *J. Consult. Psychol.*, 27(6):498–502.

Bonier, R. J., & Koplovsky, A. (1971), Borderline adolescent in crisis intervention. *Proceedings of the Convention of the American Psychological Association,* 6(1):437–438.

Bonstedt, T. (1970), Crisis intervention or early access brief therapy? *Dis. Nerv. Syst.*, 31(11):783–787.

Brandon, S. (1970), Crisis theory and possibilities of therapeutic intervention. *Brit. J. Psychiat.*, 117(541):627–633.

Brockopp, G. W. (1970a), Crisis theory and suicide prevention. *Crisis Interven.*, 2(2) Suppl.:38–41.

——— (1970b), A note on the telephone handling of the obscene caller. *Crisis Interven.*, 2(4):96–98.

——— (1970c), The telephone call: Conversation or therapy. *Crisis Interven.*, 2(3):73–75.

——— (1970d), Training the volunteer telephone therapist. *Crisis Interven.*, 2(3):65–72.

Brown, C. W., & Birley, J. L. (1968), Crises and life changes and the onset of schizophrenia. *J. Health & Soc. Behav.*, 9(3):203–214.

Brown, F. G. (1969), The zone concept in psychiatric care. *Amer. J. Nurs.*, 69(9):1923–1926.

Brown, T. E. (1971), Career counseling as a form of pastoral care. *Pastoral Psychol.*, 22(212):15–20.

Burnside, I. M. (1970), Crisis intervention with geriatric hospitalized patients. *J. Psychiat. Nurs. & Ment. Health Serv.*, 8(2):17–20.

Cain, A. C., & Fast, I. (1966), Children's disturbed reactions to parent suicide. *Amer. J. Orthopsychiat.*, 36(5):873–880.

Caplan, G. (1960), Patterns of parental response to the crisis of premature birth: A preliminary approach to modifying the mental health outcome. *Psychiatry,* 23(4):365–374.

——— (1964), *Principles of Preventive Psychiatry.* New York: Basic Books.

——— Mason, E., & Kaplan, D. (1964), Four studies of crisis in parents of prematures. *Commun. Ment. Health J.*, 1(2):149–161.

Clarke, J. (1971), An analysis of crisis management by mental welfare officers. *Brit. J. Soc. Work,* 1(1):27–37.

Cohen, S. I., & Walder, L. O. (1971), An experimental analog derived from crisis theory. *Amer. J. Orthopsychiat.*, 41(5):811–819.

Darbonne, A. (1968), Crisis: A review of theory, practice, and research. *Internat. J. Psychiat.*, 6(5):371–377.

Decker, J. B., & Stubblebine, J. M. (1972), Crisis intervention and prevention of psychiatric disability: A follow-up study. *Amer. J. Psychiat.*, 129(6): 725–729.

Deeths, A. (1970), Psychodrama crisis intervention with delinquent male drug users. *Group Psychother. & Psychodrama,* 23(1–2):41–44.

Denison, J. M. (1971), An unusual social experiment to help youth in crisis. *Can. Med. Assn. J.*, 104(1):15–19.

Duckworth, G. L. (1967), A project in crisis intervention. *Soc. Casework,* 48(4):227–231.

Dyer, E. D. (1963), Parenthood as crises: A re-study. *Marr. & Fam. Living,* 25(2):196–201.

Eisendrath, R. M. (1969), The role of grief and fear in the death of kidney transplant patients. *Amer. J. Psychiat.*, 126(3):381–387.

Eisler, R. M., & Hersen, M. (1973), Behavioral techniques in family-oriented crisis intervention. *Arch. Gen. Psychiat.*, 28(1):111–116.

Epstein, L. (1965), Casework process in crisis abatement. *Child Welf.*, 44(10):551–555, 562.

Erikson, E. H. (1950), *Childhood and Society*. New York: W. W. Norton.

——— (1956), Growth and crisis of the health personality. In: *Personality in Nature, Society and Culture,* eds. C. Kluckhohn & H. Murray. New York: Alfred Knopf.

Ewalt, P. L. (1973), The crisis-treatment approach in a child guidance clinic. *Soc. Casework,* 54(7):406–411.

Farberow, N. L. (1970), Ten years of suicide prevention—Past and future. *Bull. Suicidol.*, 6(Spring):6–11.

Florell, J. L. (1971), Crisis intervention in orthopedic surgery. *Diss. Abs. Internat.*, 32(6-B):3633.

Foreman, N. J., & Zerwekh, J. V. (1971), Drug crisis intervention. *Amer. J. Nurs.*, 71(9):1736–1739.

Forer, B. (1963), The therapeutic value of crises. *Psycholog. Rep.*, 13(1):275–281.

Fox, S. S., & Scherl, D. J. (1972), Crisis intervention with victims of rape. *Soc. Work,* 17(1):37–42.

Galdston, R., & Hughes, M. C. (1972), Pediatric hospitalization at crisis intervention. *Amer. J. Psychiat.*, 129(6):721–725.

Garrell, D. C. (1969), A hotline telephone service for young people in crisis. *Children,* 16(5):177–180.

Gebbie, K. M. (1968), Treatment drop-outs and the role of the crisis therapist. *J. Psychiat. Nurs. & Ment. Health Serv.*, 6(6):328–333.

Golan, K. (1969), When is a client in crisis? *Soc. Casework,* 50(7):389–394.

Gottschalk, L. A., et al. (1967), Prediction and evaluation of outcome in an emergency brief psychotherapy clinic. *J. Nerv. & Ment. Dis.*, 144(2):77–96.

Hart, T. F. (1971), The changing function of the London Girls' Remand Home: Crisis intervention and classification. *Internat. J. Offender Ther.*, 15(1):35–47.

Heilig, S. M., & Klugman, D. J. (1965), The social worker in a suicide prevention center. In: *Crisis Intervention: Selected Readings,* ed. H. J. Parad. New York: Family Service Association of America.

Hiatt, C. C., & Spurlock, R. E. (1970), Geographical flight and & its relation to crisis theory. *Amer. J. Orthopsychiat.*, 40(1):53–57.

Hill, R. (1949), *Families Under Stress*. New York: Harper & Brothers.

——— (1958), Generic features of families under stress. *Soc. Casework,* 39(2–3):139–149.

Jacobsen, G. F. (1965a), Crisis theory and treatment strategy: Some socio-cultural and psychodynamic considerations. *J. Nerv. & Ment. Dis.*, 141(2):209–217.

——— (1965b), Some psychoanalytic considerations regarding crisis therapy. *Psychoanal. Rev.*, 141(2):25–31.

——— (1970), Crisis intervention from the viewpoint of the mental health professional. *Pastoral Psychol.*, 21(203):21–28.

——— Strickler, M., & Morley, W. (1968), Generic and individual approaches to crisis intervention. *Amer. J. Pub. Health*, 58(1):338–343.

Juechter, J. K. (1971), Guidelines for suicide prevention in New York State colleges. *Diss. Abs. Internat.*, 32(5-A):2307.

Kaplan, D. M. (1962), A concept of acute situational disorder. *Soc. Work*, 7(2):15–23.

——— (1968), Observations on crisis theory and practice. *Soc. Casework*, 49(3):151–155.

Keith-Lucas, A. (1969), Structures in traditional agencies for crisis intervention. *Child Welf.*, 48(7):420–422.

Kirshner, L. A., & Kaplan, N. (1970), Conversion as a manifestation of crisis in the life situation: A report of seven cases of ataxia and paralysis of the lower extremities. *Comprehen. Psychiat.*, 11(3):260–266.

Klein, D. C., & Lindemann, E. (1961), Preventive intervention in individual and family crisis situations. In: *Prevention of Mental Disorders in Children: Initial Exploration*, ed, G. Caplan. New York: Basic Books.

Klemme, H. L. (1970), Mid-life crisis. *Menn. Perspect.*, 1(2):2–6.

Koos, E. L. (1948), *Class Differences in Family Reactions to Crisis*. New York: Duvall & Hill.

Kritzer, H., & Pittman, R. S. (1968), Overnight psychiatric care in a general hospital emergency room. *Hosp. & Commun. Psychiat.*, 19(10):303–306.

Lang, P. A., & Oppenheimer, J. R. (1968), The influence of social work when parents are faced with the fatal illness of a child. *Soc. Casework*, 49(3):161–166.

Langsley, D., et al. (1968), Family crisis therapy—Results and implications. *Fam. Proc.*, 7(2):145–158.

——— et al. (1969), Follow-up evaluation of family crisis therapy. *Amer. J. Orthopsychiat.*, 39(5):753–759.

Langsley, D. G., & Kaplan, D. M. (1968), *The Treatment of Families in Crisis*. New York: Grune & Stratton.

——— Mackotha, P., & Flomenhaft, K. (1971), Avoiding mental hospital admission. A follow-up study. *Amer. J. Psychiat.*, 127(10):1391–1394.

LaSor, B., & Strickler, M. (1970), The concept of loss in crisis intervention. *Ment. Hyg.*, 54(2):301–305.

LaVietes, R. L. (1974), Crisis intervention for ghetto children: Contraindications and alternative considerations. *Amer. J. Orthopsychiat.*, 44(5):720–727.

LeMasters, E. E. (1957), Parenthood as crisis. *Marr. & Fam. Living*, 19(4); 352–355.

Lester, D. (1970a), Recruitment of a counselor. *Crisis Interven.*, 2(2) Suppl.:34–37.

——— (1970b), Steps toward the evaluation of a suicide prevention center: I. *Crisis Interven.* 2(2) Suppl.:42–45.

——— (1970c), Steps toward the evaluation of a suicide prevention center: II. *Crisis Interven.* 2(1) Suppl.:12–18.

——— (1970d), Steps toward the evaluation of a suicide prevention center: III. *Crisis Interven.*, 2(1) Suppl.:19–21.

——— (1970e), Steps toward the evaluation of a suicide prevention center. IV. *Crisis Interven.*, 2(4):10–22.

——— (1971a), Attitudes toward death held by staff of a suicide prevention center. *Psycholog. Rep.*, 28(2):650.

——— (1971b), The evaluation of suicide prevention centers. *Internat. Behav. Scient.*, 3:40–47.

——— (1971c), Geographical location of callers to a suicide prevention center. Note on the evaluation of suicide prevention programs. *Psycholog. Rep.*, 28(2):421–422.

Lindemann, E. (1944), Symptomatology and management of acute grief. *Amer. J. Psychiat.*, 101(Sept.):141–148.

——— (1956), The meaning of crisis in individual and family living. *Teachers Coll. Rec.*, 57(5):310–315.

Litman, R. E. (1970), Suicide prevention center patients: A follow-up study. *Bull. Suicidol.*, 6(Spring):12–17.

Lukton, R. L. (1974), Crisis theory: Review and critique. *Soc. Serv. Rev.*, 48(3):384–402.

Mackey, R. A. (1968), Crisis theory. Its development and relevance to casework practice. *Fam. Coord.*, 17(3):165–173.

Malamud, W. (1927), Adaptation and growth. *Ment. Hyg.*, 11:584–598.

McGee, R. K. (1965), The suicide prevention center as a model for community mental health programs. *Commun. Ment. Health J.*, 1(2):162–170.

Mikawa, J. K. (1971), A university affiliated suicide prevention center. *Crisis Interven.*, 3(1):3–7.

Morley, W. E. (1970), Theory of crisis intervention. *Pastoral Psychol.*, 21(203):14–20.

——— Brown, V. (1969), The crisis-intervention group. A natural mating or a marriage of convenience? *Psychother.*, 6(1):30–36.

Morrissey, J. R. (1964), Death anxiety in children with a fatal illness. *Amer. J. Psychother.*, 27(4):606–615.

Munoz, R. A., Tuason, V. B., & Dick, E. (1970), Psychiatric emergency room service patterns. *Comprehen. Psychiat.*, 11(2):185–189.

Murphy, G. E., et al. (1969), Who calls the suicide prevention center: A study of 55 persons calling on their own behalf. *Amer. J. Psyhiat.*, 126(3):314–324.

Musgrave, L. C. (1971), Hot line takes the heat off. *Amer. J. Nurs.*, 71(4):756–759.

Noyes, R. (1970), Shall we prevent suicide? *Comprehen. Psychiat.*, 11(4):361–370.

Oberleder, M. (1970), Crisis therapy in mental breakdown of the aging. *Gerontol.*, 10(2):111–114.

Oppenheimer, J. R. (1967), Use of crisis intervention in casework with the cancer patient and his family. *Soc. Work*, 12(1):44–52.

Parad, H. J., ed. (1965a), *Crisis Intervention: Selected Readings*. New York: *Family Service Association of America*.

——— (1965b), Preventive casework: Problems and implications. In: *Crisis Intervention: Selected Readings*, ed. H. J. Parad. New York: Family Service Association of America.

——— (1966), The use of time-limited crisis intervention in community mental health programming. *Soc. Ser. Rev.*, 40(3):275–282.

——— (1971), Crisis Intervention. In: *Encyclopedia of Social Work,* 16th ed., Vol. 1, ed. R. Morris. New York: National Association of Social Workers.

——— Caplan, G. A. (1960), Framework for studying families in crisis. *Soc. Work,* 5(3):3–15.

Pasewark, R. A., & Albers, D. A. (1972), Crisis intervention: Theory in search of a program. *Soc. Work,* 17(2):70–77.

Paul, L. (1966), Crisis intervention. *Ment. Hyg.,* 50(1):141–145.

Polak, P. (1967), The crisis of admission. *Social Psychiat.,* 2(4):150–157.

Pretzel, P. W. (1970), The volunteer clinical worker at the suicide prevention center. *Bull. Suicidol.,* 6(Spring):19–34.

Raphling, D. L., & Lion, J. (1970), Patients with repeated admissions to a psychiatric emergency service. *Commun. Ment. Health J.,* 6(4):313–318.

Rapoport, L. (1962a), The state of crisis: Some theoretical considerations. *Soc. Ser. Rev.,* 36(2):211–217.

——— (1962b), Working with families in crisis: An exploration in preventive intervention. *Soc. Work,* 7(3):48–56.

——— (1967), Crisis-oriented short-term casework. *Soc. Ser. Rev.,* 41(1):31–43.

——— (1970), Crisis intervention as a mode of brief treatment. In: *Theories of Social Casework,* eds. R. W. Roberts & R. H. Nee. Chicago, IL: University of Chicago Press.

Richman, J., & Davidoff, I. F. (1971), Interaction testing and counseling as a form of crisis intervention during marital therapy. *Proceedings of the Convention of the American Psychological Association,* 6(1):439–440.

Riscalla, L. M. (1970), Crisis therapy with adolescents. *Internat. J. Offender Ther.,* 141:40–43.

Rogers, C. G. (1970), The use of alienation in crisis work. *J. Psychiat. Nurs. & Ment. Health Ser.,* 8(6):7–11.

Rosenberg, B. N. (1975), Planned short-term treatment in developmental crises. *Soc. Casework,* 56(4):195–204.

Rosenfeld, J. M., & Caplan, G. (1954), Techniques of staff consultation in an immigrant children's organization. *Amer. J. Orthopsychiat.,* 24(1):41–62.

Rusk, T. N. (1971), Opportunity and technique in crisis psychiatry. *Comprehen. Psychiat.,* 12(3):239–263.

Sachs, V. K. (1968), Crisis intervention. *Publilc Welf.,* 26(2):112–117.

Schild, J. S., et al. (1974), The influence of crisis intervention upon agency practice. *J. Jewish Commun. Serv.,* 50(4):332–339.

Schulberg, H. C., & Sheldon, A. (1968), The probability of crisis and strategies for preventive intervention. *Arch. Gen. Psychiat.,* 18(5):553–558.

Signell, K. A. (1969), The crisis of unwed motherhood: A consultation approach. *Commun. Ment. Health J.,* 5(4):304–313.

Smith, L. L. (1975), *Crisis Intervention Theory and Practice: A Source Book.* Washington, DC: University Press of America.

——— (1976), A general model of crisis intervention. *Clin. Soc. Work J.,* 4(3):162–171.

Sokolow, L., et al. (1971), The effect of distribution of information about crisis intervention services on number of calls to a suicide prevention center. *Crisis Interven.*, 3(4):91–92.

Speer, D. C. (1971), Rate of caller re-use of a telephone crisis service. *Crisis Interven.*, 3(4):86.

Stein, M. (1970), The function of ambiguity in child crises. *J. Amer. Acad. Child Psychiat.*, 9(3):462–476.

Strickler, M. (1965), Applying crisis theory in a community clinic. *Soc. Casework*, 46(3):150–154.

——— Allgeyer, J. (1967), The crisis group: A new application of crisis theory. *Soc. Work*, 12(3):18–32.

——— Bonnefil, M. (1974), Crisis intervention and social casework: Similarities and differences in problem-solving. *Clin. Soc. Work J.*, 2(11):36–44.

Sutherland, S., & Scherl, D. J. (1970), Patterns of response among victims of rape. *Amer. J. Orthopsychiat.*, 40(3):503–511.

Sze, W. C. (1970), A study of the effect of social variables on psychiatric emergency situations among children. *Diss. Abs. Internat.*, 31(1-A):475.

Tabacknick, N., & Klugman, D. (1970), Anonymous suicidal telephone calls. A research critique. *Psychiat.*, 33(4):526–532.

Torop, P., & Torop, K. (1972), Hotlines and youth culture values. *Amer. J. Psychiat.*, 129(6):730–733.

Villeponteaux, L. (1970), Crisis intervention in day school for delinquents. *Crime & Delinquency*, 16(3):317–323.

Waltzer, H., & Hankoff, L. D. (1965), One year's experience with a suicide prevention telephone service. *Commun. Ment. Health J.*, 1(4):309–315.

Wiseman, R. S. (1975), Crisis theory and the process of divorce. *Soc. Casework*, 56(4):205–212.

Yasser, A. N. (1970), Treating the bad trip by telephone. *Crisis Interven.*, 2(1) Suppl.:25–26.

Commentary

Stanley D. Imber, Ph.D.

Chapter 17 is a succinct, comprehensive review of the field. Although the better part of a decade has passed since its publication and the reference list might bear updating, it is noteworthy that the substance of Smith's paper holds firm today. In part this is a reflection of somewhat limited progress in the field, but it is also due to the fact that the thinking of such pioneers as Erich Lindemann and Gerald Caplan forms a central base for Smith's review, and their contributions still comprise the core material in crisis theory and practice.

The chapter has the special value of the broad and pragmatic perspective of a competent social worker. Probably more than any other professional discipline, social work provides the combined depth of conceptual background, direct clinical skills, and integration of community resources required for an understanding and effective practice of crisis intervention. Although the review provided here is a general one that goes beyond psychiatric crises per se, the nature of crisis is such that inevitably there are profound psychological and psychiatric implications regardless of the presenting problem. Nearly all references in the chapter are drawn from mental health sources.

The most useful section of the chapter is the last one where the author provides a thoughtful summary and recommendations. Particularly important is his admonition that "crisis theorists present sketchy conceptualizations of practice that . . . clinicians have difficulty following." Partly in response to this deficiency he notes a number of concrete suggestions that clinicians will find helpful, such as the avoidance of complex intake screening in order that treatment may proceed promptly, the need for follow-up interviews, and the advice that crisis agencies have readily accessible for practitioners treatment source books that deal with a variety of problem-solving activities. In connection with the latter, it may be added that in the time since the review was written, short-term psychotherapy methods have received a great deal of attention and refinement (Sifneos, 1979; Rush, 1982; Anchin and Kiesler, 1982; Budman and Stone, 1983) and several have been put in manual form (Mann, 1973; Horowitz, Marmar, Krupnick, Wilner, Kaltreider, and Wallerstein, 1984; Klerman, Weissman, Rounsaville, and Chevron, 1984; Luborsky, 1984; Strupp and Binder, 1984), facilitating training in those techniques. A number of them may be adapted for continuing or supplementary treatment with crisis patients and should be particularly advantageous in the prevention or moderation of future crisis episodes.

Finally, Smith's call for more and better research remains timely. The need here is not necessarily for large-scale sophisticated designs, but surely it will advance this critical area of patient care if there were something like a series of planned, systematic outcome studies of crisis intervention, including follow-ups, with some measure of controls.

References

Anchin, J. C., & Kiesler, D. J., eds. (1982), *Handbook of Interpersonal Psychotherapy*. New York: Pergamon Press.

Budman, S., & Stone, J. (1983), Advances in brief psychotherapy: A review of recent literature. *Hosp. & Commun. Psychiat.*, 34:939–946.

Horowitz, M., Marmar, C., Krupnick, J., Wilner, N., Kaltreider, N., & Wallerstein, R. (1984), *Personality Styles and Brief Psychotherapy*. New York: Basic Books.

Klerman, G., Weissman, M., Rounsaville, B., & Chevron, E. S. (1984), *Interpersonal Psychotherapy of Depression*. New York: Basic Books.

Luborsky, L. (1984), *Principles of Psychoanalytic Psychotherapy: A Manual for Supportive–Expressive Treatment*. New York: Basic Books.

Mann, J. (1973), *Time-limited Psychotherapy*. Cambridge, MA: Harvard University Press.

Rush, A. J., ed. (1982), *Short-term Psychotherapies for Depression*. New York: Guilford Press.

Sifneos, P. (1979), *Short-term Dynamic Psychotherapy*. New York: Plenum.

Strupp, H. H., & Binder, J. L. (1984). *Psychotherapy in a New Key: A Guide to Time-limited Dynamic Psychotherapy*. New York: Basic Books.

Annotated Bibliography

Peebles, M. J. (1983), Handling psychiatric urgency, or keeping one's diagnostic wits in a crisis. *Bull. Menn. Clin.*, 47:453–471.

In this paper the author discusses the challenge posed to the most seasoned clinician by psychiatric urgencies. Using a case example, she offers suggestions for the therapist to master urgency's state of heightened arousal and regressive pull. According to Peebles, ''If psychiatric diagnosticians, consultants and treaters are able to appreciate the 'doing' power inherent in the capacity to absorb and contain affect, to label, to 'pause' productively, and then to reflect and integrate, they will be more likely to 'do' based on reasoned sensitivity and efficient planning rather than because of a compelling need to 'do' for 'doing's' sake alone.''

Flegenheimer, W. V. (1978), The patient–therapist relationship in crisis intervention. *J. Clin. Psychiat.*, 39:348–350.

Using three case examples, the author illustrates how the crisis situation, because it engenders feelings of helplessness, promotes regression in the patient. It makes the patient susceptible to the rapid formation of an intense positive relationship between himself and the therapist. This requires constant monitoring on the part of the therapist lest dependency and regression be furthered. Techniques for avoiding such problems are discussed.

West, D. A., Litwok, E., Oberlander, K., & Martin, D. A. (1980), Emergency psychiatric home visiting: Report of four years experience. *J. Clin. Psychiat.*, 41:113–118.

The advantages of a multidisciplinary emergency psychiatric home visiting team are presented here. The team made 624 home visits to 443 patients in a four-year period. For patients who were psychotic, violent, or threatening violence, the team was successful at facilitating emergency care and defusing crisis situations. The team was less successful at preventing hospitalization. However, facilitation of hospitalization often became a more important function than its preempting. Few visits were for suicidal behavior. No team member was ever harmed in the course of a visit. The team also became the major psychiatric care provider to chronic patients and family utilizers of the service.

Darbonne, A. (1976), Crisis: A review of theory, practice. *Psychother.: Theory, Res. & Pract.*, 4:49–56.

A paper that challenges mental health specialists to convert impressions into hypotheses and clinical reports into experimental research. It reviews relevant studies from the forties to the sixties in three categories: situational aspects, interpersonal family and group aspects, and individual and psychodynamic aspects of crisis.

18

Psychopharmacology in Psychiatric Emergencies

Irl Extein, M.D.

Although the revolution in psychopharmacology of the past 25 years has yielded specific and sometimes definitive treatments for the major psychiatric syndromes, the time delay of usually several weeks from the start of treatment to full therapeutic effect limits the goals and expectations of emergency psychiatric treatment. The objectives of a psychopharmacologically knowledgeable physician in the emergency setting include careful medical and psychiatric evaluation; optimal management of agitation, violence, or psychosis; and referral to adequate treatment facilities. At times, specific pharmacological treatment can be started in an emergency setting. Fulfillment of these objectives requires, in addition to attention to the psychological needs of the patient and family, knowledge of psychiatric diagnosis that is oriented to delineating medication-responsive syndromes, and an understanding of the pharmacology of psychotropic medications. This chapter will emphasize the prompt and effective pharmacological treatment of patients who are out of control and agitated, violent, or psychotic. Optimal treatment of these patients depends on knowledge of

This chapter was first published in the *International Journal of Psychiatry in Medicine* (1980–1981), 10:189–204, and it is reprinted by permission.

a few basic principles of the pharmacology of antipsychotic and sedative-hypnotic drugs. The focus will be on the clinical effects and pharmacokinetics of haloperidol (Haldol), chlorpromazine (Thorazine), and diazepam (Valium), three of the medications most commonly used and most useful in psychiatric emergencies.

PHARMACOTHERAPY OF THE MAJOR PSYCHIATRIC SYNDROMES

The past 25 years has ushered in a new era in psychopharmacology. Medications are in common use that have specific efficacy in the major psychiatric syndromes, including schizophrenic psychosis, acute schizophreniform psychosis, mania, major depressions, and some severe anxiety states (Klein and Davis, 1968; Byck, 1975; Drugs for Psychiatric Disorders, 1976; Baldessarini, 1977). The major psychotropic medications—antipsychotics, antidepressants, and lithium—have specific indications in these syndromes, and can dramatically eliminate the syndromes and decrease the likelihood of their recurrence. The revolution in psychopharmacology of the past 25 years has been the development of these medications that allow specific and sometimes definitive treatment, rather than nonspecific treatment with partial alleviation of symptoms.

Table 18.1 lists the major adult psychiatric syndromes, the drugs of choice for each syndrome, and the number of days of treatment required before a therapeutic response can be expected. Antipsychotic medications (also called neuroleptics or major tranquilizers) have been demonstrated in a number of large-scale collaborative placebo-controlled double-blind studies to be effective in the treatment of schizophrenic psychosis. The antipsychotic effects are most readily observed in acute and florid cases of psychotic excitement with considerable anxiety and agitation. The target symptoms that respond consistently to antipsychotic drugs include combativeness, tension, hyperactivity, hostility, negativism, hallucinations, acute delusions, insomnia, poor self-care, and anorexia. Though many of the more florid symptoms can improve within the first few hours of aggressive treatment, maximal improvement in thought disorder and poor socialization can take up to six weeks or more on medication. Acute schizophreniform psychosis refers to schizophreniclike psychosis in an individual without the deterioration of chronic schizophrenia. This is sometimes called reactive or good prognosis schizophrenia and is treated in essentially the same manner with antipsychotic medications. Maintenance of antipsychotic medications exerts a prophylactic effect in reducing the likelihood of recurrent psychotic episodes.

A large number of controlled studies demonstrate the efficacy of lithium carbonate in acute mania, with improvement rates typically 70–80 percent in 10 to 14 days. Antipsychotic medications are often used in these first few days to control hyperactivity, insomnia, and aggression, and are then tapered as the lithium begins to work. Lithium also has prophylactic utility in preventing recurrent attacks of mania as well as depression in bipolar affective disorder. The term ''bipolar affective disorder'' has replaced the term manic-depressive illness,'' and refers to patients with a history of at least one major episode of depression and one episode of mania. Lithium can also be effective in the manias of patients with schizoaffective disorders.

Antidepressant medication, including the tricyclics and monoamine oxidase inhibitors (MAOI), has been shown in double-blind placebo-controlled trials to be effective in up to 80 percent of major depressions. It should be emphasized that the main usefulness of antidepressant medications is in major depressions, with persistent symptoms and endogenous features, rather than minor depressive syn-

Table 18.1
Specific Pharmacotherapy of Major Psychiatric Syndromes

	Medication of Choice	Days to Therapeutic Effect
Schizophrenic psychosis	Antipsychotic	1–42
Acute schizophreniform psychosis	Antipsychotic	1–42
Mania	Lithium	10–14
Major depression		
Unipolar	Tricyclic, MAOI	21–28
Bipolar	Tricyclic, MAOI, Lithium	21–28
Psychotic depression	Tricyclic plus antipsychotic (ECT)	21–28
Panic attacks in phobic-anxiety syndromes	Tricyclic, MAOI	3–14

dromes, often called reactive or neurotic depressions. Though tricyclics can begin to improve sleep almost immediately, tricyclics and MAOI take up to 3 or 4 weeks to exert their full therapeutic effect. Antidepressants can be effective in the depressions of schizoaffective disorders as well. Patients with bipolar depressions have been shown to have an antidepressant response to lithium, the time course of which is similar to that of the tricyclics or MAOI. Psychotic depressions, marked by delusions or hallucinations, often require treatment with a combination of antipsychotic and antidepressant medications or electroconvulsive therapy (ECT), still the most effective treatment known for major depressions.

Antidepressant medications can be quite specific and effective treatment for certain severe anxiety syndromes. These syndromes are referred to by such terms as *agoraphobia* and the *phobic-anxiety-depersonalization syndrome*. The panic attacks of patients with these syndromes can improve markedly after treatment for 3 to 14 days or more with tricyclics (Klein, 1964) or MAOIs. Although clinical drug trials have demonstrated sedative-hypnotic medications to have antianxiety effects greater than those of placebo, these effects are nonspecific and partial. The main usefulness of these agents is in the short-term treatment of relatively transient forms of anxiety (Baldessarini, 1977).

The above review of the pharmacological treatment of major psychiatric syndromes serves as a reminder of the variety of seriously ill patients who can be seen in emergency situations and can be reasonably expected to improve with adequate pharmacological treatment. Of crucial significance to the physician responsible for the treatment of psychiatric emergencies is the fact that the pharmacological treatment of the major psychiatric syndromes requires much more time than is available in the emergency setting, usually at least three or four weeks for optimal therapeutic benefits. The goals and expectations of the physician in an emergency setting must reflect this time constraint.

The first objective, that of diagnosis, though not the focus of this chapter, cannot be overemphasized. The diagnosis of medical illnesses that can present as psychiatric emergencies is very important. In diagnosing psychiatric illness, pharmcologically knowledgeable clinicians may be more familiar than others with the use of diagnostic categories that define specific medication-responsive syndromes. The third edition of *The Diagnostic and Statistical Manual* of the American

Psychiatric Association (DSM-III) has been adapted from Research Diagnostic Criteria (RDC), which were developed in part to define reliably major affective and schizophrenic disorders with characteristic responses to medications (Spitzer, Endicott, and Robins, 1975).

There is often a conflict between an optimal assessment of the patient's signs and symptoms in the unadulterated state, and the need to medicate the patient for his own safety and that of others. A "wait and see" approach can have advantages. For example, if the differential diagnosis of an acute psychotic episode includes an acute organic brain syndrome (OBS) secondary to drug ingestion or medical illness, delaying the use of psychotropic medication can help in making the diagnosis and indicate the correct treatment. If the psychosis resolves in a relatively short time, this might support the diagnosis of a drug-induced psychosis. If a medical illness is identified, the treatment of which resolves the psychosis, then the etiology and treatment of the psychosis have been established. Another situation in which a wait and see approach can have advantages is in the establishment of medication response. For example, if a psychotic patient displays elements of mania as well as schizophrenic psychosis, it might be better to delay antipsychotic medications and see if the syndrome resolves in 10 to 14 days on lithium alone. If an acutely anxious patient can be helped to calm down by interpersonal intervention alone, without medication, then this can be the first step toward the patient's learning to understand and control his own behavior. On the other hand, prompt use of medication can facilitate diagnosis and treatment by enabling the patient to give an adequate history and participate in his own treatment. The clinician must use his best judgment in each individual case to resolve these dilemmas.

There are a number of psychiatric emergencies wherein the decision to treat with psychotropic medications is dependent on diagnostic tests that themselves involve the use of medications. The response to an injection of anti-Parkinsonian agents benztropine (Cogentin) 1–2 mg intramuscularly (IM) or intravenously, or diphenhydramine (Benadryl) 25–50 mg IM or intravenously, can establish the diagnosis of akathisia versus exacerbation of schizophrenic symptoms, or akinesia versus catatonia. The response to a test dose of sedative-hypnotic drug, such as secobarbital (Seconal) or diazepam, can help establish the diagnosis of an alcohol or sedative-hypnotic withdrawal state versus other agitated states. The amytal interview has been used for a number of purposes, such as making the diagnosis of organic illness versus conversion reaction.

ANTIPSYCHOTIC AND SEDATIVE-HYPNOTIC MEDICATIONS IN PSYCHIATRIC EMERGENCIES

The main role of psychopharmacology in psychiatric emergencies is in the management of patients who are out of control. This includes severely agitated or violent patients, some of whom are psychotic. The keystone to the treatment of these patients is the IM injection of antipsychotic medications, such as haloperidol, which will be discussed in detail. Efforts to establish personal contact, explain the situation, and provide reassurance and a supportive environment for such patients, are usually an important addition to, not a replacement for, the injection of antipsychotic medication. Intramuscular administration of antipsychotic medication provides a safe and humane way to abort situations that are potentially dangerous to patient and staff and to facilitate diagnosis and treatment (Klein and Davis, 1968; Byck, 1975; Drugs for Psychiatric Disorders, 1976; Baldessarini, 1977; Donlon, Hopkin, and Tupin, 1979). The nonpharmacological treatments of the severely agitated or violent patient are not particularly effective, humane, or easy to use. They include physical restraints, wet sheet packs, use of seclusion rooms, and police custody.

The symptoms of a severely agitated or violent patient represent a final common pathway for a variety of psychiatric and medical illnesses. Loss of control with severe agitation or violence can occur in almost any psychiatric diagnostic group, but occurs most commonly in paranoid schizophrenic psychosis, acute schizophreniform psychosis, mania and hypomania, psychotic depressions, borderline syndromes, antisocial character disorders, dyscontrol syndromes, acute organic brain syndromes from many medical illnesses, and alcohol and drug intoxication, and withdrawal states. In these latter cases, assessment and specific treatment of the medical illness or drug withdrawal state can be tried if the situation allows. If not, then the agitation and violence need to be treated symptomatically, like the same symptoms from other causes, and more definitive diagnosis and treatment must be deferred.

Sedative-hypnotic medications such as diazepam can be useful in milder cases of anxiety and agitation. These are often transient situational reactions or exacerbations of neurotic or characterological disorders. Simply talking to the patient and family in an understanding way can be quite helpful in these cases. Diazepam is usually needed only in those cases in which interpersonal intervention has been tried unsuccessfully.

Table 18.2 compares the clinical effects of acute administration of diazepam as a representative sedative-hypnotic and haloperidol and chlorpromazine as representative antipsychotic medications. This table demonstrates some of the advantages of diazepam for the treatment of anxiety and agitation of mild to moderate degree, and some of the advantages of haloperidol and chlorpromazine in the treatment of severe agitation, violence, or psychosis. All three medications are available in preparations for oral (PO) administration or IM injection. Diazepam is approved for intravenous injection. Dosage varies according to clinical needs. All three are sedating drugs, though in dosages that calm an agitated patient and exert control over violent behavior, haloperidol is less sedating. All three have anxiolytic effects. Diazepam can be experienced as a mild "high" or cause a "spacy" feeling. Antipsychotic medications can cause a heavy and unpleasant feeling, particularly in nonpsychotic patients. Both haloperidol and chlorpromazine have specific antipsychotic effects independent of their sedating effects, a property not shared by diazepam.

A difference between haloperidol and chlorpromazine, and di-

Table 18.2
Comparison of Haloperidol, Chlorpromazine, and Diazepam in Psychiatric Emergencies

	Haloperidol (Haldol)	Chlorpromazine (Thorazine)	Diazepam (Valium)
Route of administration	IM, PO	IM, PO	IV, IM, PO
Dosage	1–10 mg	10–200 mg	2–20 mg
Sedation	Mild/moderate	Moderate/severe	Moderate/severe
Antipsychotic activity	Yes	Yes	No
Behavioral disinhibition	No	No	Sometimes
Major side effect	Dystonia	Orthostatic hypotension	Ataxia
Complications from regular use	Tardive dyskinesia	Tardive dyskinesia	Abuse, addiction

azepam that can be crucial in emergency situations is the tendency of the latter to cause behavioral disinhibition (DiMascio, Shader, and Giller, 1968). This refers to the paradoxical loss of control and rage reactions that sometimes follow sedative-hypnotic drug use. The differing tendency to produce disinhibition might best be understood in terms of the different mechanisms of action of antipsychotic and sedative-hypnotic drugs. The former selectively block dopaminergic neuronal transmission, which is involved in the subcortical arousal mechanisms, leaving cortical function relatively intact. The sedative-hypnotics suppress neuronal activity in a less discriminating manner, to which their ability to cause general anesthesia in high doses attests. Thus, sedative-hypnotics like diazepam can suppress the cortical functions that are needed to inhibit aggressive impulses and control behavior. This can exacerbate rather than help agitated, violent, or psychotic patients, whose own cortical control mechanisms are failing. Patients with loss of control secondary to obvious loss of cortical function, such as pathological alcohol intoxication or acute OBS, are particularly prone to behavioral disinhibition from sedative-hypnotics. Related to disinhibition is the tendency of sedative-hypnotics to cause confusion, particularly in the elderly. Antipsychotic drugs can produce calm in doses that do not produce disinhibition or confusion. This ability makes them invaluable in psychiatric emergencies in psychotic and nonpsychotic patients.

There are many antipsychotic medications, all sharing the ability to block dopamine receptors in the brain. They differ in potency but not efficacy. That is, all known antipsychotic medications are equally effective antipsychotic agents but require different doses to exert their antipsychotic effects. Table 18.3 includes antipsychotic medications commonly used in this country, with the dosage of each that is equivalent to 100 mg of chlorpromazine. Chlorpromazine was the first of the antipsychotic medications and has become a standard against which other agents are measured. The medications listed in Table 18.3 include drugs in five distinct chemical classes: phenothiazine (chlorpromazine, thioridazine, perphenazine, fluphenazine, and trifluoperazine); butyrophenones (haloperidol); indolones (molindone); thioxanthenes (thiothixene); and dibenzazepines (loxapine).

The antipsychotic medications can be broadly grouped into three groups based on potency and side effects. The least potent agents—chlorpromazine and thioridazine—are the most likely to cause

Table 18.3
Side Effects and Equivalent Dosages of Selected Antipsychotic Medications

Extrapyramidal effects (dystonia, akathisia, Parkinsonian rigidity and akinesia)	◄	———	———	► Sedation Orthostatic Hypotension Anticholinergic Effects	
Fluphenazine (Prolixin)	2.5 mg	Perphenazine (Trilafon)	10 mg	Chlorpromazine (Thorazine)	100 mg
Trifluoperazine (Stellazine)	5 mg			Thioridazine (Mellaril)	100 mg
Haloperidol (Haldol)	2.5 mg	Molindone (Moban)	10–20 mg		
Thiothixene (Navane)	5 mg	Loxapine (Loxitane)	15 mg		

sedation and orthostatic hypotension, and have the most intense anticholinergic effects. These are the least likely to produce extrapyramidal side effects. The most potent agents—fluphenazine, trifluoperazine, haloperidol, and thiothixene—are the most likely to produce extrapyramidal side effects including dystonias, akathisias, and Parkinsonian rigidity and akinesia. They are the least likely to produce sedation, orthostatic hypotension, and anticholinergic effects. Perphenazine, molindone, and loxapine are intermediate in potency and production of side effects. Any of these agents that are available for parenteral use could be used in psychiatric emergencies. It is advisable for the physician to become familiar with at least two of the antipsychotic medications, one from the least potent group and one from the most potent group. Chlorpromazine and haloperidol are the drugs from each of these groups with which the most experience has been accumulated, and will be the two antipsychotic medications on which this chapter will focus. The choice of antipsychotic medication is usually based on response of patient in the past, the range of side effects felt to be most easily tolerated, and the experience of the physician.

The sedative-hypnotic medications include the barbiturates and structural relatives of the barbiturates, propanediols such as meprobamate (Milltown), and the newer benzodiazepines such as diazepam, chlordiazepoxide (Librium), and flurazepam (Dalmane). These are sometimes referred to as minor tranquilizers or antianxiety drugs, but since the sedating dose is often not much greater than the anxiolytic dose, the older term sedative-hypnotic drug is preferable. Differences between one drug of this class and another as antianxiety agents or hypnotics for short-term use have not been well documented, but the benzodiazepines are clearly the safest. Many authorities now advise against prescribing the nonbenzodiazepine barbituratelike sedative-hypnotics for any reason except the treatment of epilepsy. Tolerance to them develops quickly, overdosage is often lethal, withdrawal symptoms can be severe, and interactions occur with many other drugs (Drugs for Psychiatric Disorders, 1976). For this reason, only the benzodiazepines will be discussed here. Diazepam is the most commonly used of this class, is available for parenteral use, and hence is a medication with which a clinician treating psychiatric emergencies should become familiar.

The potential side effects must be carefully considered in choosing the appropriate medication for a psychiatric emergency. Diazepam is probably the safest of all psychotropic drugs with regard to medical complications. It has an extremely high therapeutic index (ratio of lethal dose to effective dose), though some caution should be exerted in patients with underlying respiratory illness or who have ingested other respiratory depressant drugs, such as alcohol. The main side effects from use of diazepam in an emergency situation are sedation or ataxia, which are transient.

Haloperidol and chlorpromazine are likewise generally safe medications with very high therapeutic indices, though with potentially more distressing side effects than diazepam. Chlorpromazine, representative of the less potent antipsychotic, tends to produce orthostatic hypotension and anticholinergic side effects including dry mouth, blurred vision, exacerbation of glaucoma, tachycardia, constipation, and urinary retention. Orthostatic hypotension is particularly likely to occur after injection of high doses of chlorpromazine, and can cause syncope. This is a side effect to be avoided if the clinician intends for the patient to return home in the standing position after the emergency has been treated. Haloperidol might be a better choice than chlorpromazine in a patient with cardiovascular disease. Haloperidol, representative of the more potent antipsychotics, tends to produce extrapyramidal side effects. Dystonias are the extrapyramidal side effects that can occur in the first minutes or hours after initial treatment. Acute dystonias are moderate to severe contractions of the branchiomeric musculature of the neck, mouth, and tongue. Dystonias can be painful and very frightening to an agitated or psychotic patient. Oculogyric crisis is an extrapyramidal side effect that can also be quite distressing. Some physicians make a practice of administering 1 mg of benztropine along with the first dosage of haloperidol as prophylaxis against extrapyramidal side effects. Others wait to see if these side effects occur before treating them. There is no great disadvantage to using benztropine prophylactically in the emergency situation, though one would not want to continue an unnecessary medication on a long-term basis. Antipsychotics can cause impotence and disturbance of ejaculation. Some antipsychotic medications can lower seizure thresholds. More potent drugs, such as haloperidol, are thought to be the safest in patients with seizure disorders. The physician should always inquire about a history of allergic reactions to particular antipsychotic medications.

The possibility that a young woman might be pregnant must be considered (Drugs for Psychiatric Disorders, 1976; Baldessarini, 1977). There is some recent evidence that the benzodiazepines may be teratogenic, inasmuch as cleft lip and palate have been associated with their use in the first trimester of pregnancy. Benzodiazepines and other sedative-hypnotics should almost always be avoided if possible during pregnancy and lactation. The safety of antipsychotic agents in pregnancy and lactation has not yet been established. These agents pass the blood-placenta barrier as well as the blood-brain barrier, and are to some extent secreted in human milk. There is no evidence that they are responsible for an increased incidence of fetal malformation. The current consensus is that these agents should be avoided if possible during pregnancy and lactation. However, this might be weighted against clinical needs and possible risk to the fetus of not treating a pregnant woman in a psychiatric emergency.

Because use of a medication in an emergency situation can begin a lifetime pattern of treatment, one must consider the serious complications of long-term use. Tardive dyskinesia, for which there is no effective treatment, is a not uncommon complication of long-term treatment with antipsychotic medication. Sedative-hypnotic medications, including diazepam, are subject to abuse. Unlike antipsychotic medications, they are in some patients euphoric agents that cause a pleasant "high" that can lead to recreational use. Diazepam can become addicting with development of tolerance, physical dependence, and compulsive drug-seeking behavior.

Pharmacokinetic Principles

The physician treating a psychiatric emergency can maximize the effectiveness of antipsychotic and sedative-hypnotic medications by keeping basic pharmacokinetic principles in mind. Table 18.4 summarizes information on the pharmacokinetics of diazepam (Hillestad, Hansen, Melson, et al., 1974), chlorpromazine (Hollister, Curry, Derr, 1970), and haloperidol (Cressman, Bianchine, Slitnick, et al., 1974; Forsman and Ohman, 1976). The pharmacokinetics of other antipsychotics seem to be similar to those of chlorpromazine and haloperidol, which have been most extensively studied. The information in Table 18.4 can help inform decisions about dose, route of administration, and repeat administration. Haloperidol and chlorpromazine are absorbed more completely, with less variability, and more quickly after IM than oral administration. Peak plasma levels for haloperidol are achieved one-half hour after IM and 2 to 6 hours after oral administration, and for chlorpromazine, one-half hour after IM and one and one-half to 3 hours after oral administration. Antipsychotic medications are absorbed somewhat faster when administered as elixir rather than pill form. Diazepam, in contrast to haloperidol and chlorpromazine, is absorbed more completely, with less variability, and more quickly after oral than IM administration. Peak plasma levels are achieved one-half hour after oral and 1 hour after IM administration. Peak plasma levels of diazepam are obviously achieved most quickly by the intravenous route. It should be noted that chlordiazepoxide, closely related to diazepam, is notorious for poor absorption after IM injection. Thus rapaid and reliable sedation and calming require intravenous or oral administration of diazepam, or IM administration of haloperidol, chlorpromazine, or other antipsychotic medications. Because diazepam, haloperidol, and chlorpromazine are highly lipid soluble, they are taken up quickly by the brain, which contains a high proportion of lipids. The main mechanism of inactivation for all three drugs is enzymatic degradation in the liver. However, a significant proportion of metabolites of chlorpromazine and diazepam are pharmacologically active. Diazepam is converted to desmethyldiazepam which has a plasma half-life of 2 to 4 days, even longer than the plasma half-life of diazepam of 1 to 2 days. The plasma half-life of haloperidol ranges from 10 to 38 hours, and that of chlorpromazine is about 6 hours. Because of the high lipid solubility of these drugs, they can be sequestered in fat tissue, including brain, and their tissue half-lives, and hence clinical effects are much longer than plasma half-lives, on the order of days.

The optimal amount of medication is best titrated by using clinical endpoints. Within an hour of initial administration of diazepam or antipsychotic, the peak absorption and peak clinical effect can begin to decline. If the desired clinical effect has not occurred, then repeat administration of the same or higher dose may be needed. If the desired clinical effect has begun to wear off, repeat administration can be helpful.

A useful plan in an emergency room with an agitated psychotic patient is IM haloperidol 10 mg initially and then 5 mg IM every hour until significant improvement occurs, or the patient is asleep, or worrisome side effects occur (Donlon et al., 1979). Sleep can be an extremely helpful endpoint. As long as the patient is still awake, it is unlikely that an excessive amount of medication has been given. If the patient does fall asleep, then the medication should be held until he has awakened. The sleep is usually of short duration and therapeutic. With a potentially violent and assaultive patient, it is better to err on the side of overmedication than undermedication in the emergency situation.

In treating psychiatric emergencies with repeated doses of med-

Table 18.4
Pharmacokinetics of Haloperidol, Chlorpromazine, and Diazepam

	Haloperidol (Haldol)	Chlorpromazine (Thorazine)	Diazepam (Valium)
Absorption	IM › PO	IM › PO	PO › IM
Peak plasma level	1/2 hour IM 2–6 hours PO	1/2 hour IM 1 1/2–3 hours PO	1 hour IM 1/2 hour PO
Lipophilic	Yes	Yes	Yes
Inactivation	Liver	Liver	Liver
Active metabolites	?	Yes	Yes
Plasma Half-life	10–38 hours	6 hours	1-2 days
Tissue Half-life	Days	Days	Days

ication, the pharmacokinetic concept of a "loading dose" is helpful. When a drug is given in a fixed daily dosage, a certain length of time is required to build up to steady-state conditions (Levy and Gibaldi, 1975). (see Figure 18.1). Steady-state conditions are reached when the daily elimination of the drug equals the daily dose. At steady-state, relatively constant tissue levels of the drug are maintained. The longer the half-life of a drug, the longer it takes to establish a steady-state with a fixed daily dose. For drugs with long half-lives, such as chlorpromazine, haloperidol, and diazepam, it takes at least a week to reach steady-state in plasma, and longer in brain tissue where the half-life is longer. Plasma and tissue levels at steady-state on a therapeutic medication regime define the therapeutic levels. If, over the course of the first day of treatment, a medication is administered in an amount that would be a daily therapeutic dosage with chronic use, then therapeutic levels would be achieved only transiently at best. For an hour or two after each administration, plasma levels might be as high as they would be at steady-state, and will then fall below this therapeutic level.

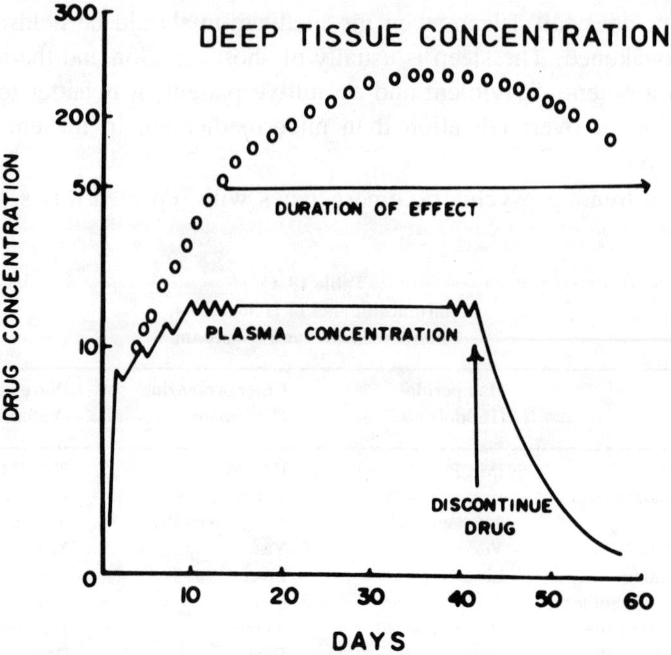

Figure 18.1 Relative concentration of drug in plasma and "deep" compartments in which drug is not metabolized.

In order to reach therapeutic steady-state tissue levels more quickly, a "loading dose" can be administered. A "loading dose" is the amount of medication, higher than the usual daily therapeutic dose, that quickly builds a steady-state drug level that can then be maintained by daily administration of the daily therapeutic dose. The classic example in medicine of a "loading dose" is the use of a "digitalizing" dose of digitalis in acute congestive heart failure. Most psychotropic medications have long half-lives and can be considered to be similar to digitalis for some pharmacokinetic purposes.

Some clinicians have administered haloperidol in a cumulative dose of up to 100 mg in the first 24 hours of acute psychotic episodes (Donlon et al., 1979). This procedure allows therapeutic steady-state tissue levels to be achieved quickly, and is associated with marked clinical improvement within the first 24 hours. This seems to be a relatively safe procedure in a hospital setting. However, whether this allows haloperidol to exert its specific antipsychotic effects faster, or reduces the total time needed to effectively treat the patient with an acute psychotic episode has yet to be established. One does not need to use a full loading dose over the first 24 hours to make use of this principle. The important point is that the carefully monitored use in the first 24 hours of an amount of diazepam, chlorpromazine, and haloperidol in excess of the usual daily therapeutic dose is on sound pharmacokinetic and clinical grounds.

The metabolism of these medications points to several clinical situations in which lower doses should be used. Because the liver is the site of inactivation of diazepam and chlorpromazine and haloperidol, patients with liver disease may have impaired ability to inactivate these compounds and should receive lower doses initially. An alternative to diazepam in patients with impaired hepatic function is oxazepam (Serax) 10–30 mg orally. Oxazepam is not inactivated in the liver but is excreted by the kidney. Elderly patients often metabolize drugs more slowly and are in addition more sensitive to the therapeutic effects and side effects. For these reasons, very small doses of psychotropic medications should be used initially in the elderly. For example, an initial dose of 2 mg of diazepam or 1 mg of haloperidol might be useful. Again, the optimal amount of medication must be determined by titration against clinical endpoints. The elderly should not be denied the advantages of pharmacotherapy simply because of their age.

What are the practical requirements that enable one to treat agitated or violent patients pharmacologically? These patients may be disoriented, paranoid, hostile, and impulsive. They are often unwilling or unable to consent or assent to administration of medication, and sometimes will be physically resistive. The treating physician must be familiar with the laws in his state governing the administration of medication to patients against their will. Depending on whether the patient is considered competent to refuse medication or is voluntary, in the process of being certified, certified, or committed, guidelines may vary. In general, medication can be administered against a patient's will in psychiatric emergencies where the patient is considered to be an imminent danger to himself or others.

Forcible administration of medication usually involves subcutaneous or IM injection into the upper arm or buttock. Chlorpromazine should always be given IM into the buttock. In our experience, a minimum of two or three people who are trained, able, and willing to physically restrain a patient are needed, in addition to the person giving the injection. A useful technique is to assign each of four staff members to restrain one of the patient's limbs. Bed restraints may be needed temporarily while the medication takes effect. In a potentially resistive and violent patient, it is best to assemble the staff before telling the patient he will need an injection. It is always good practice to explain the need for medication to the patient and give him the opportunity to accept treatment voluntarily. However, if in an emergency the patient does not agree to the medication, the physician should make it very clear that the patient has no choice. A show of overwhelming force and numbers will often have a calming effect on the patient and secure compliance without the patient having to be physically restrained. Some patients will agree to take medication orally rather than be forced to receive an injection. Depending on the urgency of the clinical situation, this can be acceptable. Chlorpromazine and haloperidol are available as elixirs, which are more difficult for a patient to hide or "cheek" without actually swallowing than pills.

Follow-Up Care

The final task of the clinician in treating psychiatric emergencies is helping to arrange follow-up treatment. Depending on the nature of the referral, more or less aggressive and definitive pharmacological treatment can be prescribed from the emergency setting. Referral can be to a hospital inpatient unit, to outpatient care that the patient seems likely or unlikely to follow through, or to the inpatient or outpatient care of the clinician treating the emergency.

For patients with schizophrenic or schizophreniform psychosis, after management of the acute symptoms, hospitalization is usually indicated. Although choice of medication is usually best left to the physician who will care for the patient, the medication used in the emergency situation can sometimes establish guidelines for further treatment. Choice of particular antipsychotic medication should be based on previous response of the patient and spectrum of side effects. The dosage of medication needed initially in the hospital can be estimated from the amount needed to control agitation and psychosis in the emergency situation. Patients with acute manic episodes usually need hospitalization and institution of lithium treatment once the more flagrant symptoms are under control with antipsychotic medication.

Patients with major depressions can be treated sometimes as outpatients depending on the patient's suicidality, vegetative symptoms, and family supports. Antidepressants take at least several weeks to work, and it is usually best to leave the decision about using antidepressants to the physician who will follow the patient. If there is a possibility that the symptoms reflect a minor depressive syndrome with reactive and neurotic elements that might not require antidepressants, it can be important to withhold antidepressants initially. Sleeplessness is a common complaint in depression and sometimes can become a psychiatric emergency. Flurazepam, 15–30 mg at bedtime, is a safe treatment in uncomplicated cases. For depression with severe agitation or psychotic elements, a sedating antipsychotic such as chlorpromazine or thioridazine 25–100 mg at bedtime can be helpful. If the emergency physician plans to follow the patient himself, and can follow the patient closely, then a tricyclic antidepressant can be started with a nighttime dose that sometimes improves insomnia within the first few nights. In writing outpatient prescriptions for patients initially seen because of a psychiatric emergency, it is prudent not to prescribe an amount of medication that could be lethal in an overdose. Depressions are treatable in most cases and, if there is any question about a depressed patient's suicidality or ability to function as an outpatient, a short hospitalization should be strongly considered.

For patients seen in an emergency situation because of anxiety states, a small amount of diazepam or flurazepam may be prescribed for future use, so long as this does not interfere with the patient's follow through on referral to the appropriate psychotherapeutic treatment. For uncomplicated insomnia, flurazepam 30 mg has been shown to induce and maintain sleep. In contrast to barbiturates and barbituratelikc hypnotics, flurazepam maintains the improvement over 2 to 4 weeks (Kales, Allen, Scharf, et al., 1970).

REFERENCES

Baldessarini, R. J. (1977), *Chemotherapy in Psychiatry*. Cambridge, MA & London: Harvard University Press.

Byck, R. (1975), Drugs used in the treatment of psychiatric disorders. *The Pharmacological Basis of Therapeutics*, eds. L. S. Goodman & A. Gilman. New York: Macmillan.

Cressman, W. A., Bianchine, J. R., Slitnick, V. B., et al., (1974), Plasma level profile of Haloperidol in man following intramuscular administration. *Eur. J. Clin. Pharmacol.*, 7:99–103.

DiMascio, A., Shader, R. I., & Giller, D. R. (1968), Behavioral toxicity. In: *Drug Side Effects*, eds. A. DiMascio & R. I. Shader. Baltimore, MD: Williams & Wilkins.

Donlon, P. T., Hopkin, J., & Tupin, J. P. (1979), Overview: Efficacy and safety of the rapid neuroleptization method with injectable Haloperidol. *Amer. J. Psychiat.*, 136:273–278.

Drugs for Psychiatric Disorders (1976), *Medical Lett.*, 18:89–96.

Forsman, A., & Ohman, R. (1976), Pharmacokinetic studies on Haloperidol in man. *Curr. Ther. Res.*, 30:319–336.

Hillestad, L., Hansen, T., Melson, H., et al., (1974), Diazepam metabolism in normal man. I. Serum concentrations and clinical effects after intravenous, intramuscular, and oral administration. *Clin. Pharmacol. Ther.*, 16:479–484.

Hollister, L., Curry, S. H., Derr, J. E., et al. (1970), Studies of delayed action medication. V. Plasma levels and urinary excretion of chlorpromazine in four different dosage forms given acutely and in steady-state conditions. *Clin. Pharmacol. Ther.*, 11:49–59.

Kales, A., Allen, C., & Scharf, M. B., et al. (1970), Hypnotic drugs and their effectiveness. *Arch. Gen. Psychiat.*, 12:226–232.

Klein, D. F. (1964), Delineation of two drug-responsive anxiety syndromes. *Psychopharmacologia*, 5:397–408.

——— Davis, J. M. (1968), *Diagnosis and Drug Treatment of Psychiatric Disorders*, Baltimore, MD: Williams & Wilkins.

Levy, E., & Gibaldi, M. (1975), Determinants of drug concentration and activity, *Concepts in Biochemical Pharmacology* (*Hand xp. Pharm. XXVIII/3*), eds. J. R. Gillete & J. R. Mitchell. New York: Springer.

Spitzer, R. L., Endicott, J., & Robins, E. (1975), Research diagnostic criteria. *Psychopharmacol. Bull.*, 11:22–25.

Commentary

Jonathan M. Himmelhoch, M.D.

"If your grandmother had wheels, she'd be a streetcar." Such was my mother's laconic reply to the myriad, crazy ideas of her three children, who were forever hatching schemes based on false assumptions. Extein's chapter, "Psychopharmacology in Psychiatric Emergencies," is admirable in every respect except that it is based on a false assumption, namely, that actual psychiatric illness accounts for the majority of psychiatric emergencies. Extein presents accurate, up-to-date, and useful information about rapid neuroleptization, the use of minor tranquilizers, and the role of other "diagnostic-specific" treatments for acutely ill psychiatric patients. Showalter and Thornton (1977) and Boehnert and Lovejoy (1985) present additional basic information about the tricyclics and benzodiazepines. Extein's section on pharmacokinetics is particularly important and gives the student actual pharmacological bases for treatment design, in place of the hit-or-miss polypharmacy that too often serves as so-called "emergency" treatment. However, intoxication with and/or withdrawal from the many intoxicants and euphorigens man has developed for himself (alcohol, sedatives, narcotics, anticholinergic substances, psychomotor stimulants, psychotomimetics, and so on) are the most common causes of the agitated, aggressive, psychotic, and/or euphoric behavior that presents in emergency situations. When medically or neurologically caused delirium and dementia are added to drug-related pathology, it can be safely stated that psychiatric pathology accounts for less than 40 percent of psychiatric emergencies presenting to the average emergency room. Suspicion of substance abuse and/or of medical–neurological illness, therefore, is the operating basic assumption of good emergency psychiatric care.

Extein only gives passing attention to this epidemiologic reality in his review. Nevertheless, it has far-reaching implications for the safe and effective use of pharmacologic agents in the treatment of psychiatric emergencies. It becomes critically important to obtain and understand medical, neurological, and toxicological parameters, whether they are as basic as vital signs, or as subtle as small pupillary changes, or changes in vestibular response to cold water. Three case examples bring out the importance of this basic assumption of psychiatric emergency management into stark relief:

Case Example

1. A 19-year-old, black, single female is brought into the emergency room by three girl friends, in the midst of a violent, psychotic rage. Little is comprehensible except that she is angry at her boyfriend. She scratches a nurse and the psychiatric resident is inveigled to give her 100 mg IM Thorazine. Meanwhile, her three girl friends disappear into the night. The patient's blood pressure rapidly drops to zero over zero and she stops breathing. The senior psychiatrist is called. He has an anesthesiologist intubate her and support her blood presure with IV sympathomimetics. The police are called to find and bring back the patient's three friends. They arrive an hour later and reveal that the patient had ingested three 8-ounce bottles of paregoric and one 12-ounce bottle of rubbing alcohol to "get even" with her unfaithful boyfriend. The patient is treated with narcotic antagonists and begins to breathe spontaneously. After 4 hours she can support her own blood pressure.

Case Example

2. A 45-year-old, separated, male alcoholic comes to the emergency room intoxicated and physically aggressive. He is beginning to go into withdrawal. Emergency room treatment with Librium *per os* stabilizes him and he willingly admits himself to the local mental health center. In the middle of the night he pinches the night nurse's bottom. She calls the on-call resident and insists that the patient be given IM Thorazine because "he is psychotic." The resident refuses but recants when pressured by his senior supervisor. The patient is found dead on morning rounds.

Case Example

3. A known client of a local alcohol program is brought in, seemingly inebriated, by her family, who also have been drinking. Her emergency room cubby stinks of alcohol, so the medical triage officer calls the psychiatrist. By the time the psychiatrist examines the patient, her family has left and she is nearly unconscious. Moreover, there is no alcohol on her breath and little residual odor in the emergency room cubby. Her admission temperature is noted to be 96° Fahrenheit. The medical staff is requested to do a "stat" blood sugar (both by glucostick and in the lab). After a brief argument, the resident tests her blood with a glucostick and finds her blood sugar to be unrecordable. Forty millimeters of intravenous, 50 percent dextrose produce a dramatic recovery of consciousness. Laboratory glucose returned and is recorded at 6 mg percent.

The first two cases show clearly the danger of reflex use of parenteral chlorpromazine. Indeed, the hypotensive effects of this parenteral drug are so marked, particularly in the intoxicated and/or the medically ill, that it is *too dangerous* for any psychiatric emergency where diagnosis, drug status, and medical status are not fully understood. The third case demonstrates the need for thorough evaluation and for a medically well-grounded knowledge of the causes of altered states of consciousness. Together the cases emphasize that it is effective information gathering, above all else, that is the sine qua non of the good management of psychiatric emergencies. Accurate information gathering requires the clinician's suspended involvement, his moral neutrality, a modulated affect that does not overstimulate, gentle questioning in place of the third degree, the accurate indentification of one's own feelings as a barometer of the patient's, and, above all, *the use of all sources of information*. Psychopharmacological interventions can only be effectively used in the framework of accurate clinical information. It is only at this stage that the clinician can begin to use the excellent information provided in Extein's chapter.

References

Boehnert, M. T., & Lovejoy, F. H. (1985), Value of the QUS duration versus the serum drug level in predicting seizures and bentricular arrhythmias after an acute overdose of tricyclic antidepressants. *N. Engl. J. Med.*, 313:474–479.

Showalter, C. V., & Thornton, W. E. (1977), Clinical pharmacology of phencyclidine toxicity. *Amer. J. Psychiat.*, 134:1234–1238.

Annotated Bibliography

Linden, R., Davis, J. M., & Rubinstein, J. (1982), High vs. low dose treatment with antipsychotic agents. *Psych. Annals,* 12:769–781.

A review of the literature comparing high to low dose treatment with neuroleptics. The studies reviewed consistently failed to show either short-term or longer term benefit in the use of doses of antipsychotics greater than 300 mg of chlorpromazine—despite the variability in individual responses. It appears that depressed patients are often undermedicated while schizophrenics receive doses of medication at higher levels than what appears warranted from the findings of clinical research. The authors point to the term "rapid tranquilization" as illustrating the assumed special properties of the major tranquilizers.

Donlon, P. T., Hopkin, J., & Tupin, J. P. (1979), Overview: Efficacy and safety of the rapid neuroleptization method with injectable haloperidol. *Amer. J. Psychiat.,* 136:273–278.

An important contribution to the growing literature on the efficacy and safety of rapid neuroleptization. The authors review the published reports on injectable haloperidol in acute psychotic states and particularly those on the rapid neuroleptization technique. They focus on both medical and nonmedical factors that must be carefully considered when assessing the effectiveness of the rapid titration method in the treatment of schizophrenic and related disorders.

19

Admission Decisions and Multiaxial Diagnosis

Juan E. Mezzich, M.D., Ph.D.,
Karen J. Evanczuk, R.N., Ph.D.
Reba J. Mathias, R.N., and
Gerald A. Coffman, M.S.

Admission into the hospital is one of the most crucial decisions in the care of psychiatric patients. It involves removal of the patient from his family and community into a typically highly controlled and supervised setting where intensive diagnostic studies and therapeutic interventions are conducted. The alternative to hospitalization is referral to ambulatory care services, which, during the past decade, have grown in availability and differentiation.

A number of studies have attempted to identify variables that are determinant or predictive of the decision to hospitalize. Reflecting the complexity of the process underlying this decision, variables investigated have included the patient's demographic identification (Jones, Kahn, and Langsley, 1965; Tischler, 1966; Baxter, Chodorkoff, and Underhill, 1968; Mendel and Rapport, 1969; Hanson and Babigian,

This chapter was first published in *Archives of General Psychiatry* (1984), 41:1001–1004, and is reprinted by permission.

1974), history of previous psychiatric treatment (Hanson and Babigian, 1974; Mendel and Rapport, 1969; Feigelson, Davis, Mackinnon, Shands, and Schwartz, 1978), psychiatric syndromes (Tischler, 1966; Baxter et al., 1968; Hanson and Babigian, 1974; Goodman, Streiner, and Woodward, 1974; Rose, Hawkins, and Apodaca, 1977; Feigelson et al., 1978; Johnson, Klingler, and Giannetti, 1979; Meyerson, Moss, Belville, and Smith, 1979), severity of psychopathologic symptoms (Jones, et al., 1965; Tischler, 1966; Streiner, Goodman, and Woodward, 1975; Feigelson et al., 1978), dangerousness of the patient (Wood, Rakirsin, and Morse, 1965; Tischler, 1966; Baxter et al., 1968; Hanson and Babigian, 1974), availability of social supports (Tischler, 1966; Mendel and Rapport, 1969; Streiner et al., 1975), background of the clinician (Baxter et al., 1968; Mendel and Rapport, 1969; Cohn, 1973; Streiner et al., 1975; Feigelson et al., 1978; Meyerson et al., 1979; Clavelle and Turner, 1980), and institutional concerns (Feigelson et al., 1978; Streiner, 1975).

Several of these variables reflect components of a comprehensive diagnostic formulation, which is one that includes syndromic considerations but goes beyond them. Such a comprehensive approach is implemented in the multiaxial diagnostic model (Mezzich, 1979, 1980). This model describes the patient's condition according to separate aspects or variables, termed "axes," such as psychiatric syndromes, concomitant physical disorders, psychosocial stressors, and adaptive functioning. The separate rating of various clinical aspects in a multiaxial system offers the possibility of identifying specific aspects useful for particular purposes or clinical decisions. This involves the ability to ask, for example, which axes of a given multiaxial system are most strongly related to making inpatient versus outpatient dispositions.

Addressing this question appears particularly important when one considers the current interest in multiaxial diagnosis and its perspectives. A number of systems have been proposed since 1947 (Essen-Möller and Wohlfahrt, 1947), especially in the past decade in various parts of the world (Strauss and Helmchen, 1982), with one example of these systems being the DSM-III (American Psychiatric Association, 1980). A crucial question for the development of future standard diagnostic systems (i.e., DSM-IV, tenth revision of the *International Classification of Diseases*) involves the selection of specific axes, which should be based in part on their demonstrated usefulness for making important clinical decisions.

The objective of this study was to assess the relative value for making admission decisions afforded by the five various diagnostic axes of the DSM-III: (1) clinical psychiatric syndromes; (2) personality and specific developmental disorders; (3) physical disorders; (4) overall severity of psychosocial stressors; and (5) highest level of adaptive functioning in the past year, and a sixth axis involving current adaptive functioning. The study was based on the multiaxial diagnoses and admission decisions made for all new patients who came for care during a 6-month period at a comprehensive psychiatric facility. Several nondiagnostic variables relevant to the dispositional process were also studied; those findings are reported elsewhere (Mezzich, Evanczuk, Mathias, and Coffman, 1984).

METHODS

Clinical Setting and Evaluation Process

This study was conducted at the Western Psychiatric Institute and Clinic (WPIC) of the University of Pittsburgh, a large, comprehensive, urban-based university psychiatric facility that also serves as a community mental health center. It admits approximately 1,600 inpatients and has over 100,000 outpatient visits per year. This psychiatric population belongs to all age groups, and it experiences a wide variety of forms and levels of psychopathologic symptoms; it is served through specialized child, adolescent, adult, and geriatric clinical programs.

The immediate setting of the study was the Diagnostic and Evaluation Center, a 24-hour-a-day, 7-day-a-week walk-in clinic and the main entry point for inpatient and outpatient care at the WPIC. Its major functions are to provide psychiatric evaluations, emergency care, and clinical dispositions.

Patient evaluations are typically conducted by an initial interviewer (a psychiatric resident or a nurse clinician specially trained in psychiatric assessment) and a supervising faculty psychiatrist. The initial interviewer reviews any pertinent records and interviews the patient and accompanying persons according to the Initial Evaluation Form, (Mezzich, Dow, Rich, Costello, and Himmelhoch, 1981), a semistructured assessment procedure having mutually complementary narrative and standardized components. The initial interviewer then presents the case, including a full multiaxial diagnostic formulation, to the faculty psychiatrist, who conducts a brief complementary interview of the patient to clarify any pending issues and the diagnosis. Finally, a disposition decision is made.

The diagnostic formulation is organized according to a format (Mezzich, Coffman, and Goodpastor, 1982) that facilitates the implementation of all five axes of the DSM-III, as well as a sixth axis used in our setting to deal with current functioning at work or school, with family, and with other persons or groups (each measured on a five-point scale, where "1" is equal to "superior" and "5" is equal to "markedly impaired"). Completed initial evaluation forms are regularly reviewed by a senior unit clinician and their standardized components are computerized by a systems specialist, as part of WPIC's clinical information system (Mezzich, Dow, and Coffman, 1981).

Patient Population

The subjects of this study were all of the 745 new patients who came for examination and care at WPIC's Diagnostic and Evaluation Center from August 1, 1980 through February 15, 1981, who were either admitted to inpatient care (54 percent) or assigned to an outpatient program (46 percent) at the WPIC. Not included in the study were 366 new patients who came for examination during the above-mentioned period but were referred to either their own community mental health centers or other facilities outside the WPIC, and for whom there was no control or information on their eventual inpatient or outpatient arrangements.

Of the 745 study patients, 133 (18 percent) were 19 years of age or less, 544 (73 percent) were 20 to 59 years of age, and 68 (9 percent) were 60 years of age or more. Four hundred (54 percent) were male and 345 (46 percent) were female. Regarding marital status, 412 (55 percent) were single, 151 (20 percent) were married, 83 (11 percent) were divorced, 50 (7 percent) were separated, and 49 (7 percent) were widowed. Five hundred twenty-two (70 percent) were white, 213 (29 percent) were black, and 10 (1 percent) belonged to other minorities.

As will be seen later, this patient population presented a wide diversity of forms and levels of psychopathologic conditions.

Data Analysis

A correlation coefficient was computed to evaluate the relationship between each of the diagnostic variables and inpatient–outpatient disposition. As a preliminary step, each of the broad diagnostic categories in the DSM-III Axes I, II, and III was defined as a dichotomous variable ("1" stood for "present as either first, second, third, or fourth diagnosis"; "0" stood for "absent"). For example, if a patient had a diagnosis of schizophrenic disorder, the corresponding dichotomous variable was given a 1; otherwise the variable was given a 0. Similarly, for the inpatient–outpatient disposition variable, a patient was assigned a 1 if he was admitted to the hospital and a 0 if he was referred to outpatient care. The DSM-III Axes IV and V (each measured on a seven-point scale) and our sixth axis on current functioning (measured on a five-point scale) are quantitative variables, so no transformations were needed for the computation of correlation coefficients. The statistical significance of the resulting correlation coefficients was assessed via *z*-transformations.

The combined contribution of the various diagnostic variables to predict or explain inpatient versus outpatient disposition was assessed through stepwise multiple regression analysis (Nie, Hull, Jenkins, Steinbrenner, and Bent, 1975). This technique first selects the variable with the highest univariate correlation with the criterion, and then, at each step, enters the variable that adds more to the predictive power of the equation developed up to that point. Through this procedure, a subset of variables was selected, and their respective regression coefficients, which maximize for the patient sample the multiple correlation coefficient (R), were calculated.

Results

The findings of this study are presented first in terms of the relationship between individual diagnostic variables and inpatient versus outpatient disposition, and then regarding the combined relationship of diagnostic variables to admission decisions.

Table 19.1 presents the relationship between individual diagnostic variables and clinical disposition. Exhibited first are the number and percentage of patients in each diagnostic category assigned to either inpatient or outpatient care, and then the mean and SD of each quantitative axis among hospitalized and nonhospitalized patients. The last column shows the correlation coefficients between each diagnostic variable (categorical or quantitative) and inpatient–outpatient disposition.

Regarding the list of psychiatric disorders encompassed in the DSM-III Axes I and II, broad diagnostic categories at least partially involving psychotic syndromes (psychotic disorders not elsewhere classified, organic mental disorders, and, to a lesser extent, schizophrenic disorders) tended to be associated with inpatient disposition. Nonpsychotic conditions (anxiety disorders, adjustment disorders, personality disorders, and conditions not attributable to a mental disorder) tended to be associated with outpatient referral. To clarify the importance of psychosis for admission decisions suggested by these findings, all psychotic diagnoses (organic mental disorders with delusions or hallucinations, schizophrenic disorders, paranoid disorders, affective disorders with psychotic features, pervasive developmental disorders, and psychotic disorders not elsewhere classified) were grouped together and were found to have the strongest positive correlation with inpatient disposition.

The computation of correlation coefficients between individual diagnostic variables and disposition is pertinent to the following question: For a whole psychiatric population, which variables from a group of descriptors of the patient's condition (e.g., the presence of an affective disorder, the severity of psychosocial stressors, the degree of adaptive functioning) are most useful in making an inpatient versus outpatient disposition? This question, in fact, is the central one underlying the present study, which attempts to compare the value of various categorical and quantitative axes to make hospitalization decisions. Additionally, one may consider the following question: How likely is it that patients with diagnosis "x" (versus those with diagnosis "y," "z," etc.) will have an inpatient (or outpatient) disposition? In this case, the most relevant statistic is the percentage of patients with a given diagnosis who have an inpatient (or outpatient) disposition.

Axis III broad diagnostic categories used for 5 percent or more of the patients included endocrine disorders, neurologic disorders, cardiovascular disorders, and ill-defined conditions. None of these categories nor a global positive diagnosis on this axis was significantly associated with psychiatric hospitalization.

Table 19.1
Patient Distribution and Summary Data According to Diagnostic Variables[a] and Inpatient and Outpatient Disposition

Diagnostic variables	Inpatient disposition, n (%) (N = 402 [54%])	Outpatient disposition, n (%) (N = 343 [46%])	Correlation between diagnostic variable and inpatient disposition, r
Axis I: Clinical psychiatric syndromes			
Disorders of infancy, childhood, and adolescence	48 (64.9)	26 (35.1)	.07
Organic mental disorders	37 (80.4)	9 (19.6)	.14[b]
Substance use disorders	71 (63.4)	41 (36.6)	.08
Schizophrenic disorders	59 (61.5)	37 (38.5)	.06
Affective disorders	110 (59.5)	75 (40.5)	.06
Psychotic disorders not elsewhere classified	40 (81.6)	9 (18.4)	.15[b]
Anxiety disorders	5 (20.8)	19 (79.2)	−.12[b]
Adjustment disorders	26 (28.0)	67 (72.0)	−.20[b]
Other psychiatric disorders[c]	9 (32.1)	19 (67.9)	−.09
Condition not a mental disorder	16 (30.8)	36 (69.2)	−.13[b]
Deferred or no diagnosis	54 (48.6)	57 (51.4)	−.04
All psychotic disorders[d]	127 (70.2)	54 (29.8)	.18[b]
Axis II: Personality disorders	52 (39.7)	79 (60.3)	−.13[b]
Axis III: Physical disorders, positive diagnosis on this axis	151 (57.9)	110 (42.1)	.06

Table 19.1 (cont.)

	Inpatient disposition, mean score ± SD	Outpatient disposition, mean score ± SD	r
Axis IV: Overall psychosocial stressor severity	4.1 ± 1.0	3.9 ± .09	.12[b]
Axis V: Highest level of adaptive functioning during past year[e]	4.3 ± 1.0	3.7 ± 1.1	.27[b]
Axis VI: Current functioning[e]			
At work and/or school	4.3 ± 0.9	3.3 ± 1.2	.40[b]
With family	4.1 ± 0.9	3.3 ± 1.0	.40[b]
With other persons and groups	4.1 ± 0.9	3.2 ± 0.9	.44[b]
Average current functioning[f]	4.2 ± 0.8	3.3 ± 0.9	.45[b]

[a]Diagnostic categories mentioned as primary, secondary, tertiary, or quarterary diagnoses and diagnostic dimensions.

[b]The statistical significance of the correlation coefficients as being different from zero is $p < .001$.

[c]Includes the following infrequently used DSM-III Axis I broad categories: paranoid disorders ($n = 6$), factitious disorders ($n = 1$), somatoform disorders ($n = 4$), dissociative disorders ($n = 2$), psychosexual disorders ($n = 8$), disorders of impulse control ($n = 5$), and unspecified psychiatric disorders ($n = 2$).

[d]Includes all DSM-III categories considered to represent psychotic diagnoses, i.e., organic mental disorders with delusions or hallucinations, schizophrenic disorders, paranoid disorders, affective disorders with psychotic features, pervaslve developmental disorders, and psychotic disorders not elsewhere classified.

[e]A higher score indicates greater impairment in functioning.

[f]Average of current functioning at work and/or school, with family, and with other persons and groups.

Clearly, the diagnostic variables most strongly associated with hospitalization were those involving adaptive functioning. These included the DSM-III Axis V (highest level of adaptive functioning in the past year), and, even more prominently, our sixth axis, current functioning at work and/or school, with family, and with other persons and groups. The correlation coefficient for Axis V (.27) was significantly higher ($p < .001$) than those for the diagnostic variables corresponding to the first four axes of the DSM-III. In turn, the correlation coefficient obtained for average current functioning (.45) was significantly higher ($p < .001$) than those for all five axes of the DSM-III.

Given the high dispositional value noted for both aspects of adaptive functioning (highest level in the past year and current level), the relationship between these two variables was then examined. Table 19.2 displays the cross-tabulation of 974 patients by both aspects of adaptive functioning. The remaining 137 patients were not included in the cross-tabulation, as they had "unspecified" ratings in Axis V or VI. To facilitate the appraisal of patterns, the seven levels of Axis V were collapsed into three and the five levels of Axis VI into two levels. It can be seen that all patients having the poorest ratings in Axis V also had the poorest ratings in Axis VI. Patients having the best ratings in Axis V tended to have the best ratings in Axis VI, but 27 percent of them had the poorest ratings in Axis VI. The correlation coefficient computed between Axes V and VI (with all of their levels considered in full) was .60.

The question then arose of the impact on admission decisions of

Table 19.2
Cross-Tabulation of Patients by Axis V (Highest Level of Functioning in Past Year) and Axis VI (Current Functioning)

	Axis VI	
Axis V	**Superior, adequate, or slightly impaired**	**Moderately or markedly impaired**
Superior, very good, or good	228	83
Fair or poor	191	398
Very poor or grossly impaired	0	74

the degree of worsening in adaptive functioning from its highest level in the past year to its current level. For each patient, the degree of worsening was computed as the difference between the standardized scores of average current functioning and the highest level in the past year. This degree of worsening had a correlation of .20 with hospitalization decisions, which, when compared with the dispositional correlations for all diagnostic axes and categories listed in Table 19.1, was only lower than those for Axes VI and V.

Next, the dispositional value of average current functioning was examined for specific groups of patients, as defined by their Axis I diagnoses. Correlation coefficients computed between current functioning and inpatient–outpatient disposition within particular diagnostic groups achieved statistical significance ($p < .001$) among patients with the following disorders: schizophrenic (.50), adjustment (.49), substance use (.32), those of infancy, childhood, and adolescence (.32), and affective (.31).

Table 19.3 summarizes the stepwise multiple regression analysis aimed at predicting inpatient versus outpatient disposition with a linear combination of diagnostic variables. The first variable entered into the equation was current functioning, which was expected, given that it had the highest univariate correlation with hospitalization. Three other diagnostic variables, all dealing with psychiatric syndromes, were then gradually added to the equation; but their total contribution raised the multiple correlation coefficient from .453 to only .482.

COMMENT

One of the findings of this study was that psychotic disorders, as defined in the DSM-III, tended to be associated with admission decisions, while nonpsychotic disorders were associated with outpatient referrals. This is in line with literature reports that showed that psychoses (Tischler, 1966; Baxter et al., 1968; Goodman et al., 1974; Hanson and Babigian, 1974; Rose et al., 1977; Feigelson et al., 1978; Johnson et al., 1979; Meyerson et al., 1979) were the psychiatric diagnoses most frequently associated with hospitalization, while neuroses (Tischler, 1966; Hanson and Babigian, 1974; Johnson et al., 1979), situational disturbances (Hanson and Babigian, 1974; Meyerson et al., 1979), and personality disorders (Tischler, 1966; Goodman et

Table 19.3
Summary of Stepwise Multiple Regression Analysis Aimed at Predicting Clinical Disposition (1 = Inpatient; 0 = Outpatient) with a Set of Diagnostic Variables

Entered diagnostic variables	Multiple *R*	*F* Value to enter	Final regression coefficients
Average current functioning[a]	.453	181.4	.23
Personality disorders	.468	12.4	−.14
Adjustment disorders	.475	6.0	−.13
Condition not a mental disorder	.482	6.5	−.16

[a]A higher score indicates greater impairment in functioning. The regression constant for the final regression coefficients is −.27.

al., 1974; Hanson and Babigian, 1974; Meyerson, 1979) were associated with outpatient disposition.

Of perhaps even greater interest in regard to Axis I diagnoses were the following two points. First, the highest correlation among Axis I categories obtained for the special grouping of all psychotic disorders suggests that the presence of psychosis is a factor that is useful to consider systematically in disposition decisions. The very high percentage of inpatient dispositions made for patients with psychotic disorders not elsewhere classified (who almost always presented florid psychotic symptoms) also bears this out. The second point refers to the positive relationship found between inpatient disposition and both "organic mental disorders" and "psychotic disorders not elsewhere classified" (70 percent of which corresponded to "atypical psychosis," which is most frequently used in our setting to indicate psychosis of unspecified type). This suggests that another construct related to hospitalization is the need to clarify the nature of the patient's condition (the organic factors involved, in one case, and the type of psychosis, in another).

The main findings of the study were related to its basic objectives; that is, the comparison of the relevance of various diagnostic axes to inpatient versus outpatient disposition. By far, the variables with the highest correlations with admission decisions were those involving current adaptive functioning, followed by the highest level of functioning in the past year. The degree of worsening from the highest level in the past year to the current level of functioning was also noted to be positively correlated with hospitalization, but not as highly as the above-mentioned functioning variables. The dispositional value of current functioning was noted not only for the generality of psychiatric cases but also for cases that had certain Axis I diagnoses (for example, schizophrenia) already specified. Furthermore, the results of the multiple regression analysis suggested that other diagnostic axes appear to add little to the predictive or explanatory power provided by current functioning for such a crucial clinical decision. These findings point out the importance of systematically taking into consideration the assessment of adaptive functioning during the dispositional process.

Of course, in addition to the diagnostic variables reported here there are probably several others that importantly influence admission decisions, such as the dangerousness of the patient, certain demographic variables, the history of previous psychiatric hospitalization, and the background of the clinician. A study of several of these variables is reported elsewhere (Mezzich et al., 1984).

From the viewpoint of diagnostic models, it should be noted that the separate rating of various key clinical aspects required by multiaxial diagnosis allowed the comparative assessment of their value for admission decisions, as well as the identification of adaptive functioning as the most important one for this purpose. Further research on the comparative usefulness of various diagnostic axes for several clinical decisions, and for the prediction of course and outcome, should contribute to strengthening the empirical base for the development of improved diagnostic systems.

REFERENCES

American Psychiatric Association (1980), *Diagnostic and Statistical Manual of Mental Disorders*, 3rd ed. (DSM-III). Washington, DC: American Psychiatric Press.

Baxter, S., Chodorkoff, B., & Underhill, R. (1968), Psychiatric emergencies: Dispositional determinants and the validity of the decision to admit. *Amer. J. Psychiat.*, 124:100–106.

Clavelle, P. R., & Turner, A. D. (1980), Clinical decision-making among professionals and paraprofessionals. *J. Clin. Psychol.*, 36:833–838.

Cohn, J. B. (1973), The physician's condition versus the patient's in deciding hospitalization. *Hosp. Commun. Psychiat.*, 13:492–493.

Essen-Möller, E., & Wohlfahrt, S. (1947), Suggestions for the amendment of the official Swedish classification of mental disorders. *Acta Psychiat. Scand.*, Suppl., 47:551–555.

Feigelson, E. B., Davis, E. B., Mackinnon, R., Shands, H. C., & Schwartz, C. C. (1978), The decision to hospitalize. *Amer. J. Psychiat.*, 135:354–357.

Goodman, J. T., Streiner, D. L., & Woodward, C. A. (1974), End Results Analysis of Mental Health Services: The Effects of Psychiatric Hospitalization, Final Report. Ontario provincial grant, PR-167.

Hanson, G. D., & Babigian, H. M. (1974), Reasons for hospitalization from a psychiatric emergency service. *Psychiat. Quart.*, 48:336–351.

Johnson, J. H., Klingler, D. E., & Giannetti, R. A. (1979), A study of mental status and anamnestic factors related to the decision for inpatient or outpatient treatment. *J. Clin. Psychol.*, 35:844–850.

Jones, N. F., Kahn, M. W., & Langsley, D. G. (1965), Prediction of admission to a psychiatric hospital. *Arch. Gen. Psychiat.*, 12:607–610.

Mendel, W. M., & Rapport, S. (1969), Determinants of the decision for psychiatric hospitalization. *Arch. Gen. Psychiat.*, 30:321–328.

Meyerson, A. T., Moss, J. Z., Belville, R., & Smith, H. (1979), Influence of experience on major clinical decisions. *Arch. Gen. Psychiat.*, 36:423–427.

Mezzich, J. E. (1979), Patterns and issues in multiaxial psychiatric diagnosis. *Psychol. Med.*, 9:125–137.

——— (1980), Multiaxial diagnostic systems in psychiatry. In: *Comprehensive Textbook of Psychiatry*, 3rd ed., eds. H. I. Kaplan, A. M. Freedman, & B. J. Sadock. Baltimore, MD: Williams & Wilkins.

——— Coffman, G. A., & Goodpastor, S. M. (1982), A format for DSM-III diagnostic formulation: Experience with 1,111 consecutive patients. *Amer. J. Psychiat.*, 139:591–596.

——— Dow, J. T., & Coffman, G. A. (1981). Developing an efficient clinical information system for a comprehensive psychiatric institute: I. Principles, design and organization. *Behav. Res. Meth. Instrum.*, 13:459–463.

——— ——— Rich, C. L., Costello, A. J., & Himmelhoch, J. M. (1981), Developing an efficient clinical information system for a comprehensive psychiatric institute. II. Initial evaluation form. *Behav. Res. Meth. Instrum.*, 13:464–478.

——— Evanczuk, K. J., Mathias, R. J., & Coffman, G. A. (1984), Symptoms and hospitalization decisions. *Amer. J. Psychiat.*, 141:764–769.

Nie, N. H., Hull, C. H., Jenkins, J. G., Steinbrenner, K., & Bent, D. (1975), *Statistical Package for the Social Sciences*, 2nd ed. New York: McGraw-Hill.

Rose, S. O., Hawkins, J., & Apodaca, L. (1977), Decision to admit: Criteria for admission and readmission to a VA hospital. *Arch. Gen. Psychiat.*, 34:418–421.

Strauss, J. S., & Helmchen, H. (1982), Multiaxial diagnosis. Paper presented at the International Conference on Diagnosis and Classification of Mental Disorders and Alcohol and Drug-Related Problems, Copenhagen, April 13–17.

Streiner, D. L., Goodman, J. T., & Woodward, C. A. (1975), Correlates of the hospitalization decision: A replicative study. *Can. J. Pub. Health*, 66:411–415.

Tischler, G. L. (1966), Decision-making process in the emergency room. *Arch. Gen. Psychiat.*, 14:69–78.

Wood, E. C., Rakirsin, J. M., & Morse, E. (1965), Resident psychiatrist in the admitting office: A man in conflict. *Arch. Gen. Psychiat.*, 13:459–463.

Commentary

Jack A. Wolford, M.D.

In chapter 19, Mezzich and his co-workers have shown a continuing way to look at and test both the value and utility of DSM-III and its multiaxial components. Mezzich is a nationally recognized expert in multiaxial diagnosis, and he and his colleagues have published extensively in this field. They are careful and sound investigators who do not make excessive claims or careless deductions regarding their findings. They state that admissions are more likely for persons who on Axis I have a psychotic disorder. A subgroup of organic psychosis and psychosis of unspecified type that require further assessment were noted and highly correlated with admission. Further assessment needs, coupled with florid symptoms, is an extremely important criterion for admission. Surprisingly, the diagnosis of schizophrenia was somewhat less correlated with inpatient admission than others. It would be helpful to have had a breakdown between acute and chronic schizophrenia and persons with schizophrenia who were well known to the system. Patients with acute schizophrenia would almost always be admitted whereas the person who has chronic schizophrenia and is known to the people in the emergency room may have other alternatives.

It comes as no surprise that adaptive functioning correlated the highest with admission to the hospital. DSM-III, Axis V, which is the "Highest Level of Adaptive Functioning in Past Year" had a correlation coefficient higher than Axes I through IV. The authors discuss a sixth axis that is used in the Western Psychiatric Institute and Clinic. This axis relates to "current functioning at work and/or school, with family and with other persons and groups." They found the highest correlation for this group. Elsewhere, the authors have written on symptoms and hospital decisions, "Self neglect; thought process disorganization; impulsivity; suspiciousness; violent behavior; bizarre behavior; recent intellectual impairment; hostility; delusions of reference, jealousy, or grandiosity; and lack of insight" (Mezzich, Evanczuk, Mathias, and Coffman, 1984) were identified as symptoms particularly associated with hospitalization. When these plus those related to dangerousness to self or others appeared in clusters, they were highly correlated with the decision to hospitalize. There can be no question that these symptoms are also related to Axis V, and particularly Axis VI, in that they would certainly interfere with "current functioning at work and/or school, with family and with other persons and groups."

Both papers suggest that there are other variables, such as demographic ones, the history of previous psychiatric hospitalization, support systems available, the background of the clinician and institutional beds available that help determine the decision to hospitalize.

We would agree that the decision to admit to an inpatient unit is a complex and important one since it has many implications for the person admitted. We are all looking for a perfect decision-making process regarding admission. Mezzich and his collaborators teach us that there is actually no easy checklist to replace a careful evaluation of the total person and his or her environment by knowledgeable mental health clinicians who have been taught to synthesize data. They also teach us, however, that there are guidelines that show some consistency from patient to patient that help in teaching and decision making.

References

Mezzich, J. E., Evanczuk, K. J., Mathias, R. J., & Coffman G. A. (1984), Symptoms and hospitalization decisions. *Amer. J. Psychiat.*, 141:764–769.

Annotated Bibliography

Mezzich, J. E., Evanczuk, K. J., Mathias, R. J., & Coffman, G. A. (1984), Symptoms and hospitalization decisions. *Amer. J. Psychiat.*, 141:764–769.

Using a semistructured evaluation of all 1,463 new patients presenting during a one-year period and either admitted to inpatient care or assigned to an outpatient program at the Western Psychiatric Institute and Clinic, Pittsburgh, Pennsylvania, the authors systematically assessed the relationship between various aspects of the patient's symptoms and hospitalization decisions. The individual symptoms correlating the highest with admission to the hospital were self-neglect, disorganized thought process, and impulsivity.

Friedman, S., Margolis, R., David, O. J., & Kesselman, M. (1983), Predicting psychiatric admission from an emergency room: Psychiatric, psychosocial, and methodological factors. *J. Nerv. & Ment. Dis.*, 171:155–158.

A report on a cross-validated multiple regression analysis of determinants of hospitalization on 238 patients presenting for care at an inner-city municipal hospital. The analysis revealed two determinants of hospitalization—severity of schizophrenic symptoms and active suicidal and/or homicidal ideation.

Hoehn-Saric, R., Hatcher, M. E., & Weiskopf, C. (1980), Disposition of psychiatric emergency patients: Patient characteristics associated with hospitalization. *Ann. Emerg. Med.*, 9:605–609.

A report on those characteristics of psychiatric patients seen in a general emergency department which are associated with subsequent hospitalization. The data obtained by psychiatric residents and nondoctoral psychiatric workers revealed that for psychotic patients overall severity of illness, difficulties in management, as well as lack of preceding psychiatric treatment were related to hospitalization. For the nonpsychiatric patients, hospitalization appeared more often related to the degree of depression and solitary living conditions than to the severity of symptoms.

Feigelson, E. B., Davis, E. B., Mackinnon, R., Shands, H. C., & Schwartz, C. C. (1978), The decision to hospitalize. *Amer. J. Psychiat.*, 135:354–357.

An explanation of determinants of psychiatric hospitalization. Using four Manhattan general hospitals, the authors found that although the nature and severity of a patient's problem played the most important role in the decision to hospitalize, the facility, including its composition and makeup, was also a determining factor.

Apsler, R., & Bassuk, E. (1983), Differences among clinicians in the decision to admit. *Arch. Gen. Psychiat.*, 40:1133–1137.

A review of the effects for and difficulties in elucidating the nature of the decision process in admitting patients for psychiatric treatment. Of special interest in that this study examined individual differences among clinicians involved in this decision-making process.

20

Psychiatric Consultations in the Emergency Room

Jose M. Albornoz-Ruiz, M.D.

> "My worthy friend, gray are all theories and green alone life's golden tree."
> —Mephistopheles, impersonating Faust to a student
>
> (*Faust*, Act I, Scene 4)

Psychiatric consultations in the emergency room are an expanding modality of professional practice for the modern psychiatrist. It would be difficult to trace this form of psychiatric intervention to its beginnings with any degree of accuracy, but it is probably safe to say that it developed in connection with the community psychiatry movement in the sixties. At any rate, gone are the days of the alienist, secluded in his country clinic, student and lord of the social outcasts of preceding centuries. Advances in psychiatry and irreversible changes in modern societies have placed the new psychiatrist astride the scientific progress in the physiological and biochemical workings of the mind as a function of the brain, away from jargon and mysticism. Yet, the Freudian

This chapter was first published in the *Maryland State Medical Journal* (1972), 21:53–60, and it is reprinted by permission.

warning that things psychological must be apprehended through psychological means remains as true as ever.

Therefore, in approaching the problem of psychiatric consultations in an emergency room, it appears desirable to make some general considerations to achieve a proper frame of reference in which the elaboration of fact, theory, technique, and opinion may produce insights of genuine clinical value. The concepts and ideas expressed in this monograph represent the experience of four years of doing psychiatric consultations in the emergency room, first at Sinai Hospital of Baltimore between 1966 and 1968, and then at Baltimore County General Hospital since 1969 to the present.

A perusal of the literature on the subject will show that in the absence of such context an inevitable emphasis results in statistical tabulations of limited value, or in overstructured versions about how to adapt or incorporate accepted psychiatric tenets into working techniques for management. It would appear that in either case a somewhat overwrought effort to make the clinical material into a scientific model results in an implied denial of the simple fact that a psychiatric consultation in an emergency room is not so much a scientific performance as it is a clinical act. The consultation is a highly visible example of the difference between medical technology as a body of scientific knowledge and medical practice as an age-worn Hippocratic art. The remarks of a geneticist seem a fitting keynote to this article. Dr. McKusick (1971) states that

> to the practicing clinician the question of whether a particular pathologic constellation is filed in the proper conceptual pigeonhole would appear as little relevant as the subtle taxonomic distinction between *Pinus strobus* and *Pinus sylvestris* would be to a practicing lumberman or carpenter.

Nowhere would this consideration find more appropriate application than in the context of the psychiatric consultation in an emergency situation, where the uncertain and vague nosology of psychiatric disorder must be used for a guideline in defining prognosis and treatment, without the benefit of an extended evaluation and with none of the externals that allow for a thoughtful and relaxed approach in the office situation. On the other hand, no rational intervention will be possible in the absence of a well-informed and scientifically grounded decision-making process. In its ultimate essence, the consultation in the emergency room must be at the same time a psychotherapeutic intervention, and psychotherapy is "an informed transaction that has a state-of-the-art and a technology." To intervene in such a situation without a keen awareness of such factors is truly "a travesty of decent psychiatric service" (Garber, 1971).

Studies carried out to determine the significance of psychological distress in medical patients have shown that "the doctor is not always sought as a medical expert, but also as a substitute affiliation in times of emotional loss, as an authority to sanction decisions which a person cannot make himself, as a confidant in a variety of situations, and as a mediator in many others" (Stoeckle, Zola, and Davidson, 1964). This is particularly apparent in the emergency room, where the failure to identify these parameters in a crisis is an ever-present possibility, resulting in inadequate care if not in more serious and even fatal outcomes. In this context it is important to emphasize the concept of Parsons, who regards illness as a social role that defines appropriate behavior and obligations toward oneself and others, thereby acquiring a conceptual meaning well beyond what can be encompassed in a biological medical diagnosis.

In a very general manner, the psychiatric consultant in an emergency room would do well by substituting the question of "what disease does this patient have" with that of "what is the matter with this person," giving proper weight to the fact that "linguistic transaction is in fact a system of mutual expectations" (Elkes, 1970). Therefore, more than a semantic game, it is the substitution of the aseptic language of scientistic—rather than scientific—medicine for that of the genuinely humanistic clinician that is achieved. In the language of the psychiatrist it could be said that by so doing the groundwork is laid for adequate structuring of the situation. In this new frame of reference there is no room for the all-too-familiar pronouncement "there is nothing the matter with him"; what remains is the difficult challenge of defining the patient's ailment in terms relevant to his own idiosyncratic way of expressing his needs. At this point, then, it becomes quite apparent that the consultation situation is a highly fluid, subjective, and unpredictable transaction in which factors other than the actual quality and nature of the patient's presenting psychopathology play a definitive role.

Any individual who reaches the psychiatrist goes through four milestones as he follows his path down to the psychiatrist. First, there has to be the abnormal behavior, and then there has to be the perception of his behavior as being abnormal. Then, there has to be an evaluation of this perceived behavior as either delinquent or disturbed (Hollingshead, 1957). This would appear as the most likely explanation for the variation in statistical figures as to frequency of psychiatric cases in emergency rooms, from 2.5 percent to 6 percent of the total visits for a given period of time according to different surveys (Beaver, Sordo, and Wheltle, 1969; Watson, 1969). What and whether to name a symptomatic constellation as a psychiatric disorder in that setting may depend not only on degree of psychiatric sophistication of the attending physician, but also on the degree of tolerance and receptivity to questionable forms of communication, both verbal and nonverbal, and on value judgments which even nowadays include a certain notion that a psychiatric intervention is both unthinkable or unacceptable to patients and/or doctors alike.

In the terms of a widely read book (Laing, 1967),

> The person labeled (as a psychiatric patient) is inaugurated not only into a role but into a career of patient by the concerted action of a coalition or a conspiracy of family, general practitioner, mental health officer, psychiatrist, nurse, psychiatric social worker, and fellow patients.

It is beyond the scope of this presentation to examine the merits of such a position which is quoted only to emphasize further the peculiar dimensions of the consultation in an emergency room. The consultant must, therefore, encompass in his conceptual frame of reference a total outlook that allows for the synthesis of all the truly relevant factors—medical, social, emotional, and symbolic—conducive to effective grasp of the patient's situation and to appropriate management and recommendations. As a clinician, he should be aware that he must somehow find his way into the patient's underlying and sometimes unspeakable needs. As a consultant he has to realize that his intervention ought to result in an expeditious and useful resource to the emergency room staff. As a scientist he will do well in reminding himself about the inevitable limitations of the art.

Psychopathological Variables

I will now attempt a review of some of the situations under which psychiatric consultations are likely to be requested in an emergency room. The review is not intended to be exhaustive, because such situations actually encompass the total spectrum of psychiatric disorders from mental retardation to adjustment reactions of late life. Rather, it means to bring out some of the psychodynamic constellations that are more frequent and more troublesome to the consultant. It will be followed by a theoretical construct of my own regarding the dynamics of the consultation process and some of the pitfalls that should be avoided if the consultation is to have the desired impact.

Before getting on with the description of the phenomenological and dynamic issues involved in the consultation, it may be well to remember that in many cases the whole thing turns into a rather routine matter in which the psychiatrist simply endorses and confirms diagnoses and dispositions already made by alert and well-informed colleagues. Every emergency room has its "repeaters" who simply show up to secure medical certificates and transportation to mental health facilities in the course of situations that may appear urgent and critical to almost everyone except the patient himself, for whom the whole proceedings are a familiar, commonplace manifestation of a life-style. These may actually represent a pitfall for the unexperienced psychiatrist who, in his eagerness to be "involved," may generate friction and interference in the emergency room.

Following is a descriptive analysis of some of the most frequently encountered situations.

Self-destructive Behavior

Self-destructive behavior is a manifestation of anger turned upon the self. Anger is a very primitive emotional reaction in people that is better observed in its most uncontrolled fashion in the preschool child when he is having a tantrum; the physiological and behavioral responses in an angry child are a matter of everyday experience; the expression of the face, the extreme agitation of the limbs, the more or less destructive responses toward the environment are readily apparent. In the child, however, the actual physical possibilities for destruction and damage are so limited that no one gets scared. The child will be brought under control by a variety of means of coercion without responses of guilt in the parent. However, when an explosion of rage occurs in the chronological adult, the possibilities for injury and damage increase in direct proportion with the physical power of the person so afflicted, and the fear and counterforce generated in the persons that surround him. In general, anger gives an illusion of power, based on the shift from passivity and helplessness to activity.

On the other hand, an angry outburst, regardless of pejorative labeling as immature, neurotic, or psychotic, is a source of power as a matter of fact. An angry person can modify a situation by virtue of the coercive effects of his rage on the environmental situation, but there is always the possibility of a devastating retaliatory blow. This gives the phenomenon of anger a socio-psychological dimension different and separate from its meaning as a simple psychological defense mechanism. It is precisely because of this that sometimes a paradoxical compromise is achieved in which this powerful emotion is discharged against the self rather than against others, sometimes with unpredictable results. Two clinical configurations are common.

The Suicidal Gesture. As the name implies, there is no element of true suicidal intent. These patients, in discharging their anger upon themselves, are not trying to kill themselves and do not mean to kill themselves. However, in the emergency room situation, they are assumed to be suicidal because of their self-assaultive behavior. Although a number of techniques have been developed to assess the lethality of self-directed aggression (Peck, 1971), none of them can substitute for the skill of the experienced clinician. However, there are certain features that can be helpful in the differential diagnosis. The suicidal gesture usually occurs in young people. The patient is angry and frustrated and will freely acknowledge that fact as well as the reasons for his resentment.

Suicidal behavior often is impulsive, poorly planned and executed, and there is usually a clear-cut target to the aggressive feeling. There is usually a clear manipulative intent. These are people whose family structure is usually intact; they show a reasonable level of achievement and vocational adjustment; and more often than not, they express regrets and shame about their sudden loss of self-control. This group also includes the mislabeling of accidental overdoses in people who may have used an excessive amount of medication by mistake when trying to sedate themselves, and who are whisked to the emergency room by an anxious relative or a well-meaning neighbor.

The Suicidal Attempt. Before setting down some guidelines for the identification of the true suicidal syndrome, it is important to emphasize the relativity of all generalizations in this particular context. Beall (Arneson, 1971), in a comprehensive review of the dynamics of suicide, points out that "suicide is not limited to depressive disorders, nor do all depressives commit suicide" in what amounts to be a clear refutation of commonly held notions. Several observations about the patient may contribute to a better assessment of the suicidal potential. The presence of a psychotic disturbance may result in suicide in a person who is in no position to measure the consequences of his actions, making the event a genuine accidental death.

Disturbances in thought process may be apparent in a number of ways, such as irrelevance or incoherence in the semantic component of the communication, or abnormalities in the behavioral and affective component. While the former are readily apparent to the nonpsychiatrist, the latter may be ambiguous and easy to miss. The patient may show inappropriate responses to the doctor, who may be belittled or criticized by the patient for no apparent valid reason. An attitude of hopelessness may find expression in a peculiar disregard for the presence and activities of others. Unabashed, open admissions of guilt suggest a dangerous collapse of the usual mechanisms of denial, suppression, and projection by which this most painful emotion is usually controlled. A previous and extended psychiatric history should always be a source of concern. Older patients and displaced persons without interested relatives are a grave risk. Also, the self-assaultive behavior of the true suicide is truly lethal and often bizarre because of hidden symbolic connotations in which the suicidal act is an act of expiation or the symbolic murder of an internalized other.

Altered States of Consciousness

These are situations in which the patient is confused and disoriented as to time, place, and person. There is no question to peculiar, idiosyncratic symbolism here. While confusion and disorientation may emerge in the context of a psychogenic disorder in the generally accepted sense of the term, more often than not they are related to severe metabolic disturbances in the central nervous system. From this viewpoint, mental status has been considered "one of the clinical barometers of cardiac function" (Lunde, 1971), and, indeed, it is one of the most sensitive indicators of the breakdown of homeostasis in many different kinds of systemic illnesses. Here the critical challenge to the psychiatric consultant is that of recognizing the associated medical disorder, perhaps missed by a hasty colleague who may have felt that this was a psychiatric case because of the mental status findings.

In this context, it may be helpful to remember that confusional states related to depressive-hysterical neurosis, particularly in cases associated with borderline mental retardation, are quite similar to those seen in patients with cerebral ischemia, whether central or peripheral in origin. This is particularly important when dealing with the elderly, in whom cerebral circulatory changes are more common but, of course, do not rule out or exclude an underlying psychogenic disturbance. The possibility of a toxic state associated with drug abuse must also be considered, particularly in younger people. Special attention should be given to states of confusion with clear sensorium, rather characteristic of the Korsakoff syndrome in patients with long-standing histories of alcoholism. States of altered consciousness related to epilepsy are often easily recognized on the basis of the clinical history.

Assaultive and Belligerent Behavior

This type of situation presents many complicated variables to the consultant. The unrestrained expression of anger toward others usually has ethical and legal connotations. It is a relief to the collective conscience of society to label violent, morally unacceptable behavior as "sick" behavior. This pejorative approach finds paradigmatic expression in patients that are taken to the emergency room following an explosion of anger in the context of a marital argument or some other similar situation. In naming the angry outburst "sick," a smokescreen is cast over the ethical and legal issues involved; thus labeling serves as a rationalization for everyone concerned. It would appear as though some states of rage are holy, while others are just "sick." From a psychiatric viewpoint, however, the phenomenon can be looked at only for what it is, and for what it means to the patient and to others, especially from the viewpoint of dangerousness to life, limb, and property.

Paranoid states are commonly seen in this connection. While the psychiatrist has little difficulty in recognizing this disorder, these cases are likely to present many problems to the staff in an emergency room. The paranoid patient often shows no gross indication of confusion and his communication can appear to the inexperienced observer as objective and to the point. Quoted from a medical record is this statement, "This lady is paranoid enough to realize that she is not that crazy." It is said in psychiatric circles that a paranoid person is one who has all her facts right and all her conclusions wrong. This is generally so because of the way in which she integrates her experience in terms of her own subjective feelings and needs. The French used to call this disorder "folie raisonante" precisely because of the inner consistency of the patient's logic. It is for the consultant to decide whether such a state is a manifestation of an underlying schizophrenic disorder, or the expression of an anxious state in a paranoid personality. There are usually other parameters that allow for the distinction.

Instances of violent behavior are also seen in cases of alcoholism and epilepsy but in such cases the history is clear-cut and helps a great deal in the differential diagnosis. Aggressive behavior in the mentally retarded usually presents no diagnostic problems.

At any rate, I am under the impression that in most cases aggressive and assaultive behavior is actually reactive behavior, directed toward the meaningful other in the patient's life, and tends to subside as soon as the patient recognizes the therapeutic intent in the environment.

Odd and Unconventional Behavior

Not infrequently the consultant gets called about patients who seem to act strangely around the emergency room, or who may have been referred to the emergency room from other areas of the hospital. They do not seem able to state a complaint or make unusual requests. This type of mental disturbance is often seen in connection with chronic psychotic conditions or hysterical dissociative states. Although they represent no acute emergency as such, they are often turned into one because of the lack of sensitive management. Proper recognition of the situation for what it is results in significant gains for the emergency room staff in terms of avoiding unnecessary tests and waiting, and expediting the referral of the patient to the proper sources of care.

CONSULTATION PROCESS

Turning our attention to the group process in the consultation, it seems important to bring out several points. "To leave the conceptualization of the consultation process to the private discovery of the resident, without supervision and guidance, makes as little sense as to say to him to conduct group or individual psychotherapy without learning the appropriate theoretical framework'' (Mendel, 1967). The psychiatric consultant should be aware that he, as a person and as a professional, is a very substantial factor in what develops. If he manages to do what is appropriate, the issues raised and the emotions aroused around the consultation situation will come to an orderly resolution, without undue harassment or discomfort in the majority of cases. It is important not to feel obliged to respond to the occasional needle or wisecrack of the nonpsychiatric staff whose motivations are not the case to explore at the time of the consultation. Nor is the consultant to become an unsolicited teacher to the colleague whose attention is usually taxed with other responsibilities in the emergency room area. He must, indeed, recognize the mistakes that might have been made in the management of the situation prior to his arrival for the purpose of allaying anxieties and hostilities that may interfere with his duty to the patient and to the staff he is supposed to consult for.

I have classified the consultation process in a four-stage manner, which I believe reflects the natural course of events in nearly every occasion as follows: (1) evaluation and structuring, (2) first impact, (3) confirmation, (4) resolution.

Stage I—Evaluation and Structuring

The consultant must become thoroughly conversant with the facts of the situation prior to seeing the patient. A review of the emergency room protocol saves a lot of unnecessary questions and allows the synthesis of observations and comments from the emergency room staff members; that provides sufficient guidelines as to what to look for in the interview. Then, as the interview begins at the bedside, it is important to remember that the patient be given the opportunity to set the pace; as opposed to the office situation, the patient should be allowed to structure the interview. At this particular time ''the equanimity, calmness, and composure of the physician is his single most valuable asset '' (Zunin and Barr, 1971). It should be remembered that in his particular predicament, the patient is truly regressed, in a volatile emotional state, and quite unable to tolerate any frustration.

In addition, he may be reluctant to talk because of previous mismanagement by the emergency room doctor who through paternalistic, jocular, or overanxious approaches may have led the patient into a defensive withdrawal. Regressed as he may be, the patient fortunately can still mobilize his own ego resources. He has his own experience and knowledge and is quite capable of detecting untoward attitudes in the doctor that may interfere with his responding to the situation in the way that may be desired. The point is cogently illustrated by a remark made by a patient who once told me, "If nothing else, all these years of psychiatric problems have taught me to recognize a friend when I see one." One minor, if significant, manifestation of concern and interest by the consultant has to do with recommending, in agreement the attending staff, the removal of IV fluids, urethral catheters, tight restraints that might have been very well advised several hours before, but which by the time of the consultant's arrival amount to nothing other than mild forms of torture that usually are permitted to last longer than necessary.

Another point has to do with management of relatives. It must be kept in mind that very often a hidden drama—sometimes a comedy—is under way, and that much of what the patient says and does is intended to be seen and heard by the relative. Therefore, it is important to separate them during the interview, carefully avoiding to take sides in any controversy. The consultant must not be afraid of the patient. Talking to people who have been through the painful and bewildering experience of undergoing a psychotic state, I know the impact of the reassurance of an understanding doctor who is capable of responding to the vestiges of rationality left in the patient without being overwhelmed by the uncertainties and fear of everybody else around him. The feelings and working habits of the emergency room staff must be kept in mind. The emergency room can become, at times, the setting of frantic activity that creates a hectic atmosphere where the pipe of the psychiatrist becomes curiously irrelevant if not downright offensive to the rumpled and harassed staff.

Stage II—First Impact

As with any other theoretical scheme, this one attempts to present separately things that are actually developing simultaneously or in very close succession. For the patient, the information that he is going to be seen by a psychiatrist often amounts to the equivalent of a subcutaneous injection of adrenaline, particularly when it happens for the first time. In some cases, it begins with the awed, avoiding response of a staff doctor or nurse who, after a couple of sentences to the patient, blurts out a pronouncement that the patient must be seen by a psychiatrist, in what amounts to the patient as a crude verdict of insanity. Or he can sense that his complaints or requests are being questioned, ignored, or misunderstood. But even when the staff is sensitive and tactful, and when the patient seems to be thoroughly rational, he still seems to feel that his rationality is put to test, to say the least. The consultation is accepted in the spirit of a veritable defeat.

As for the relative, he may be loath to the inevitable questions and confrontations that may be expected when the consultation takes place. Depending on the situation and what it means to the patient, he may respond by becoming even more agitated, angry, or confused. Conversely, he may settle and calm down in those cases in which he feels a desperate need for someone who will understand. From a certain viewpoint, it would be highly desirable if the doctor in charge could envision the patient's mental status with the same degree of objectivity that he looks at his electrocardiogram. This, however, is not possible because the patient's emotions create around him a great degree of affective resonance that interferes with the professional's critical faculty in a way that could be appropriately compared with the effects of a highly charged electromagnetic field on a radio signal.

In the context of this first impact, it is important to realize that the cubicle in which a patient is observed in an emergency room is an almost ideal place to carry out acts of self-assault. There are often pieces of tubing, first-aid trays, and other implements that can be easily used as weapons. I still remember the case of a young woman who, while being restrained, removed a pair of scissors from the uniform pocket of one of the staff nurses. She later attempted to use them against the personnel when the time came to transfer her to a psychiatric hospital. Fortunately no one was hurt. It is, therefore, important to remind the nursing personnel that if the patient is suspected of being psychotic or appears confused, he must be maintained under direct and continuous visual supervision until the situation is under control. This is a fundamental aspect of the consultation.

The control of the patient's response during this stage begins with proper reassurance. Very often, the patient's recognition that what is being done is helpful and relevant to his needs prompts him to mobilize the healthiest aspects of his personality in order to help his helpers. However, sometimes it does not work that way, particularly when the patient is very sick or drunk. In those cases, the consultant must be able to take command of the situation, without guilt, without embarrassment, and without hesitation. It would be apparent that the consultant's source of authority in such situations is particularly strong, on a twofold basis—transferentially, because the patient, regressed as he is, responds to him as if he were his father, and actually because for the time being the consultant is the person in charge. In such instances it is appropriate to demand that the patient behave, and it is no surprise to the well-trained psychiatrist that even violent and psychotic patients show an abrupt change of attitude and a more cooperative disposition. This depends, basically, on the character and forcefulness of the psychiatrist, but chances are that somewhere along the line the patient will hook on, so to speak, to the therapeutic intention. I believe that, except for very rare cases, a patient's assaultive behavior toward the doctor is related to errors in the doctor's technique. At the time of this kind of crisis the patient's self-esteem is at a very low ebb and even trivial acts of tactlessness may be construed in the patient's mind as offensive or unacceptable, with unpredictable consequences.

Stage III—Confirmation

After the psychiatric consultation reaches the point of offering the first alternatives—discharge from the emergency room with extended evaluation later on, hospitalization, certification, etc.—the human drama that is unfolding, it is hoped under the guidance of the consultant, comes to a climax of sorts. Relatives and other interested persons may want to talk with the consultant to size up the implications of his determinations. The patient will want to see his relative. Brief conferences develop that may, from moment to moment, change the course of events. In short, a variety of psychodynamic forces are set into motion, which get further organized and systematized at a quickened pace in the minds of the patient, his relatives, or relative-surrogates, such as social workers, welfare workers, and others that may be directly involved in the outcome.

The consultant must answer many questions and study a number of alternatives. These situations are confusing precisely because everyone, the patient included, is right. The psychiatric consultant must then remain a flexible catalyst, an orchestra conductor as it were, whose hesitation and doubt must be shared with the patient and his family so that the crisis may come to a satisfying professional and human settlement. A dogmatic attitude in the consultant is a sure recipe for failure. I find it helpful to apply here a line of Hegelian dialectic, according to which the purpose of discussion and argument is to make explicit all that was implicit in the partial views. The consultant must remind himself at all times that there are usually underlying factors motivating the patient and his family that he probably does not know and cannot expect to know in the emergency room situation. In consideration of the high demands that the role places on the consultant, it seems advisable to have a rotating schedule where all available staff psychiatrists may participate. I do not believe that placing a professional person in charge of the management of crisis situations on a routine basis every day of the week is technically sound or psychiatrically defensible.

When psychopathology is truly severe and malignant, Stages I and III evolve without bringing about any significant change in the consultant's conception of what the problem is and what needs to be done. In such cases, it appears quite clear that the only course of action consists in ongoing evaluation and treatment in an inpatient psychiatric setting. Dynamically, this implies that the patient's ego resources are so inadequate that he cannot measure up to the demands of the crisis, and a total psychological breakdown ensues. On the contrary, in milder cases, the therapeutic aspects of the consultation—catharsis, clarification, redefinition, confrontation, support, and counseling—allow for the crisis situation to ease up, and a number of elective alternatives can be suggested for further implementation after the patient is released from the emergency room.

Stage IV—Resolution

This part of the process is concerned with the procedures evolved in cooperation with the emergency room staff for the purpose of securing rapid implementation of decisions made during the consultation. These have to be worked out with imagination and originality on the basis of the size and resources of the emergency room. The nursing staff ought to be conversant with all administrative steps necessary for psychiatric hospitalizations. Close liaison needs to be developed with psychiatric back-up facilities in the area. The consultant must stipulate clearly in his consultation note his recommendations, especially in reference to the use of medication while the patient remains in the emergency room area, and all other loose ends that may be involved with the case, such as manner of transportation if the patient is to be transferred out of emergency, or sources of referral and continuing care if the patient is to be discharged. In this connection, it is also important to educate the emergency room staff on the question of discharge against medical advice. It should be emphasized that in spite of every effort, the consultant seldom gets to the bottom of the story as it unfolds in the emergency room.

As far as the patient goes, in a large proportion of cases, the whole question of being the object of a psychiatric consultation is just an unthinkable and intolerable interference with his life. He is often supported in such a view by his family and relatives. He is just as confused as some doctors are by the dichotomy of what is "physical" and what is "mental," and he will simply refuse to cooperate in any way besides his perfunctory agreement to talk with the consultant. Such cases always present delicate quandaries of a legal nature, particularly when, in the consultant's opinion, a restriction of the patient's freedom is mandatory. In the more serious cases, this kind of situation requires the intervention of a court of law, and the consultant would do well in having very solid grounds before he orders or recommends the retention of a patient on the premises against his will. Sometimes we simply cannot help.

However, it is important to recognize that an otherwise neat professional intervention can be marred by inadequate follow-through by the emergency room staff. Lack of decisive, clear-cut follow-through, brings back elements of uncertainty and suspiciousness that may in fact destroy the therapeutic impact of the consultation. The fact that so many emergency rooms provide services to psychiatric patients without the benefit of having psychiatric consultations is to my mind sufficient empirical demonstration of the gradual overlapping of the functions of the physicians in charge with those of the psychiatric consultant when it comes to the management of the particular form of human suffering presented by psychiatric disorder. It is, indeed, a demonstration that common sense and compassion are by no means traits unique to the well-trained psychiatrist.

There is always a gradation of levels of care from the essential to the ideal. The patient can be trusted to produce his own original ways of coping with his conflict, which in the emergency room encompass the varying degrees of adequacy or inadequacy of services offered him in his moment of distress. Things will always work out, but for the practicing clinician it is the how and what of the emergent alternatives that define the relative merits of his intervention. The psychiatric consultant is presented with the challenge of helping people at a moment of their lives in which their need is understood by few people and properly handled by even fewer. An acceptable outcome against such odds is a highly gratifying experience.

SUMMARY

1. General considerations concerning psychiatric consultations in an emergency room as a newly emerging form of professional experience are made.

2. Some forms of psychopathology as they present in the emergency room settings are highlighted with some suggestions relative to management.

3. A theoretical scheme dividing the consultation process in four stages is advanced for the purpose of decreasing the unpredictability of what is discussed as a highly fluid and unpredictable transaction, full of potentials for miscarriage and inadequate management.

REFERENCES

Arneson, G. (1971), Spotting the "pseudocidal" patient. *Hosp. Physician,* 7:57–79.

Beaver, W., Sordo, J., & Wheltle, P. (1969), An in-depth analysis of the emergency department. *Maryland State Med. J.,* 18:63–68.

Elkes, J. (1970), Language and observation in psychiatry. In: *Hope, Psychiatry's Commitment,* ed. A. W. R. Sipe. New York: Brunner/Mazel, pp. 119–133.

Garber, R. S. (1971), Presidential address. *Amer. J. Psychiat.,* 128:33–43.

Hollingshead, A. B. (1957), Factors associated with prevalence of mental illness. In: *Four Basic Aspects of Preventive Psychiatry,* ed. R. H. Ojemann. State University of Iowa, pp. 29–58.

Laing, R. D. (1967), *The Politics of Experience*. New York: Pantheon Books, p. 84.

Lunde, D. (1971), Psychiatric aspects of heart transplant surgery. *Mod. Med.*, 39(3):121–124.

McKusick, V. (1971), The nosology of genetic disease. *Hosp. Pract.*, 6:93–101.

Mendel, W. (1967), A prescription for improving the psychiatric consultation. *Frontiers of Hosp. Psychiat.*, 4(4):1–2.

Peck, R. L. (1971), Perfecting a suicide prediction scale. *Hosp. Physician*, 7:53–55.

Stoeckle, V. D., Zola, I. K., & Davidson, G. E. (1964), The quantity and significance of psychological distress in medical patients. *J. Chronic. Dis.*, 17:959–970.

Watson, V. P. (1969), Psychiatric problems in accident departments. *Lancet*, 1:877–879.

Zunin, L., & Barr, N. (1971), How to handle psychiatric emergencies in a general hospital. *Resid. & Staff Physician*, 17:61–65.

Commentary

Paula T. Trzepacz, M.D.

There is a plethora of articles that address the specifics of differential diagnosis and management of psychiatric disturbances seen in the general hospital emergency room setting, but very few include any discussion of psychodynamic or systems issues. Albornoz-Ruiz's chapter is devoted to a discussion of such issues and is thus unique reading for psychiatrists. Maybe its most obvious weakness is related to its publication date of 1972; some of its terminology is outdated and the psychiatric nosology then was less well defined than it is now. However, these weaknesses seem to detract little from this material.

The general hospital emergency room is a busy setting with an unpredictable workload and a wide range of presenting patient problems. Although emergency room staff are trained to handle acute medical problems and trauma cases, not all cases are true emergencies and some may be mainly social. In addition, emergency room staff are usually not well versed or comfortable dealing with psychiatric problems. Physically ill patients may be mislabeled as psychiatric. General medical and psychiatric problems often coexist, particularly in the geriatric population. Psychiatric interventions are time-consuming and often require the integration of multiple resources. Thus, the general hospital emergency room staff usually is not geared toward the assessment of psychiatric problems.

In his introduction, Albornoz-Ruiz essentially describes the importance of what George Engel termed a *biopsychosocial* viewpoint in patient care. He mentions that the process of identification and referral of a patient for psychiatric consultation may be affected by time constraints, stigma, or the level of awareness of the emergency room staff regarding psychiatric problems.

Two major portions of this chapter address psychopathological variables and the consultation process. The former focuses on four types of situations that are frequently encountered in the emergency setting, while the latter describes four theoretical stages of a consultation process.

The first psychopathological variable addressed is self-destructive behavior. Anger is viewed as the important emotion that gives the illusion of power to an individual who otherwise feels helpless, and the expression of anger may in fact be powerful due to its coercive effects on other persons. Due to the threat of retaliation, anger may instead be directed against oneself, for example, in a suicide gesture wherein the patient's act is usually impulsive and/or manipulative without a clear intent to harm himself. A suicide attempt is differentiated from a gesture and may be lethal or have bizarre symbolic content. It is emphasized that suicide attempts are not limited to persons who have a major depressive disorder, contrary to a commonly held notion among nonpsychiatrists. The disorganized thought processes of a psychotic individual may increase the risk of suicide, but emergency room staff may not be perceptive of a thought-disordered state. Other traditional risk factors for suicide are not discussed.

Altered states of consciousness are discussed next. These essentially comprise the organic mental disorders, with delirium and drug intoxications/withdrawals most prevalent. Patients might be cognitively impaired or agitated and thus the elicitation of a proper history or the performance of a thorough physical assessment might not have been done by the emergency room staff. The presence of an organic mental disorder necessitates a search for underlying biological contributing factors and the consultant psychiatrist must interact with emergency room staff to educate them and advocate for appropriate medical care.

The third psychopathological variable is assaultive and belligerent behavior, which results from unrestrained anger toward others. Fear and pejorative perceptions of the patient might prevent the emergency room staff from making appropriate ethical and legal considerations.

By objectifying the violent act and discerning its meaning to the patient the consultant may simultaneously clarify relevant psychiatric symptoms such as paranoia. Because of factual correctness and cognitive clarity, emergency room staff may not recognize a paranoid patient's distorted conclusions. Often, the author states, violent behavior is the result of interpersonal conflicts with the patient's significant other and can be diffused by a therapeutic intervention.

Finally, "odd behavior" typified by bizarre actions or requests in the emergency room will culminate in a psychiatric referral. Such patients are often chronically psychotic or are histrionic. Certainly, the presence of organic mental disorders should not be overlooked either.

The process of consultation is viewed in four stages. The "evaluation and structuring" stage begins with a review of all information elicited by the emergency room staff, being alert for any possible mismanagement. An unstructured interview style is recommended for the initial patient contact. The patient's behavior may reflect, in part, his reaction to the emergency room staff. The author stresses the importance of interviewing the patient alone, although, in fact, it is crucial to also interview anyone who accompanied the patient to the emergency room.

The "first impact" stage comprises the multiplicity of coexisting events including the patient, the family, and the emergency room environment. The patient might feel that a psychiatric intervention implies that his original complaints are being ignored, or that he is insane. Reassurance and structuring are recommended strategies to help mobilize the patient's existing ego strengths. The family might become upset or might feel relief at the opportunity to be understood. The emergency room cubicle may need to be supervised if it contains implements that could be used as weapons. Preferably, a quiet room should be specifically designated for psychiatric patients.

The "confirmation" stage involves offering specific therapeutic interventions and/or discharge plans to the patients and also discussing these with family members, social workers, and so on. The author alludes to the cross-sectional nature of the assessment, and thus the clinicians may still not be privy to underlying factors that motivated the patient or family to go to the emergency room. Therefore, the consultant should avoid being dogmatic—unless there is a psychiatric emergency that requires he take control of this situation.

In the "resolution" stage administrative follow-through should occur to ensure a smooth transition for the recommended management and disposition of the patient. For example, the emergency room staff may not be as familiar with subtleties of the commitment process.

Though the chapter continues to be timely, I would have liked it to have a more in-depth analysis of the psychodynamic and systems factors that interrelate between the patient, the emergency room staff, and the consultant. The nurses and doctors in the emergency room have different needs and "agendas" regarding patient care, with attendant tensions arising. The emergency room is at the interface of the inpatient wards and the community, and thus there are other internal and external systems issues that were not addressed in chapter 20. Often the psychiatric consultant gets put in the middle of multilevel systems tensions, particularly when a patient is difficult to manage. There needs to be a clearer delineation of how much responsibility is appropriate for a psychiatric consultant in different types of situations and when this responsibility should shift back to the emergency room staff as the "primary" managing clinicians. The familiar dumping of a difficult patient may subvert proper medical attention or may preclude a valuable educational experience for the emergency room staff handling psychiatric problems.

Annotated Bibliography

Soreff, S. M. (1978), Psychiatric consultation in the emergency department. *Psych. Annals,* 8:61–66.

This paper describes a specific consultation liaison program in an emergency department. It is based on four components: comprehensive patient evaluation, referral planning and implementation, involvement with the community psychiatric treatment network, and liaison with the emergency department staff. This particular program encompasses permanent and substantial participation in the activities of the emergency department including formal and informal contacts with its entire staff, conducting of joint conferences, lectures on the department of emergency medicine, and commitment to psychiatric resident education in the emergency department.

Murphy, J. G., Fenichel, G. S., & Jacobson, S. (1984), Psychiatry in the emergency department: Factors associated with treatment and disposition. *Amer. J. Emerg. Med.,* 2:309–314.

An examination of psychiatric consultations regarding 246 patients seen in a general hospital emergency department, and factors associated with treatment and disposition. The foci of the review were dispositional decisions (admission, discharge, referral for psychiatric outpatient care, and so on). Psychiatric variables such as severity of symptoms, history of psychiatric hospitalization or outpatient treatment, and use of psychotropic medication were found to be associated with decisions made by both psychiatrists and nonpsychiatrists. Also, nonpsychiatric variables related to disposition decisions included patient's age, "rudeness," time of day, and month of presentation.

21

Planning for Psychiatric Emergencies

M. R. Eastwood, M.D.,
S. Stiasny, M.B.A.,
F. Cashman, M.D.,
S. K. Littmann, M.B., and
G. Voineskos, M.D.

The use of hospital emergency services has been increasing at an annual rate that exceeds that of the population's growth (Krass, 1977), and it has been suggested that "a fairly large segment of the public [in the United States] views the emergency room as a general treatment center rather than a place to go only in a real emergency" (American Hospital Association, 1976). While this may be true of the general medical emergency room, it is difficult to estimate the extent to which this is true of psychiatric emergency departments. This difficulty has largely been a problem of definition. Morrice (1968) suggested that a psychiatric emergency should be defined as "any situation which compels a person to seek *immediate* psychiatric treatment, or which impels his family, friends or an official agency to seek such treatment for him."

This chapter was first published in the *Canadian Medical Association Journal* (1979), 120:421–425, and it is reprinted by permission.

He endorsed Ungerleider's (1960) definition that "all patients whose condition warrants prompt psychiatric attention for whatever reason are designated emergencies" since most of those who present do have problems, although not necessarily urgent ones. Morrice argued that most psychiatric emergencies are social problems, and that patients are admitted to hospital as a second-best alternative to social and psychologic support at home.

Psychiatric emergency patients may have mental problems, physical symptoms, burdensome life events, failure to cope socially, or a combination of these difficulties. Of one group of 100 such patients most were physically well or had a physical condition that was being treated by the family physician (Eastwood, Mindham, and Tennant, 1970). Wilder, Plutchnik, and Conte (1977) found that of 314 such patients only 9 percent did not have a psychiatric disorder according to the Feighner criteria. A survey conducted in the United States indicated that family conflicts were the most common precipitants of psychiatric emergencies, and depression was the foremost presenting symptom; family physicians, relatives, and friends, and the patients themselves each accounted for one fifth of referral sources (Glasscote, Cumming, and Hammersly, et al., 1966). A Canadian center found that 80 percent of the patients using a crisis facility presented between 8 A.M. and 10 P.M. (Watters, Goodman, and Molnar, 1972).

While these data provide some idea of the psychiatric emergency situation, the contemporary picture is incomplete. Bartolucci and Drayer (1973) suggested that the average patient who goes to a psychiatric emergency department is seeking immediate treatment of his or her problems. Thus, with increased public awareness of mental health issues, the emergency department has become a pivotal and intense point for psychiatric care.

The Taylor report to the Ontario government recommended that hospitals assess the use by the community of their emergency services and organize the services so as to best meet the needs of the community (*Medical Post,* January 31, 1978, p. 1). An accurate description of the psychiatric, social, and demographic characteristics of patients who go to emergency rooms and an assessment of the frequency of this practice are important in the planning of emergency services. It is then possible to anticipate the patients' needs, whether serious or not, to decide when and by whom the patients should be seen, what type of staffing is required and how the personnel should be deployed. Undertaking such evaluations is a first step in the rationalization of the health care delivery system.

With this in mind, a survey of emergency patients was undertaken at the Clarke Institute of Psychiatry, Toronto, prior to the inception of a crisis unit in July 1977. The Clarke Institute of Psychiatry, a postgraduate teaching center, is one of eight teaching hospitals in downtown Toronto. The survey examined not only the characteristics of emergency patients, but also the frequency with which they used the emergency department over a 2-year period.

METHODS

For the purposes of this study an emergency was defined as the presentation to the outpatient department of a person without an appointment who was seeking immediate psychiatric attention or help at his or her own instigation or at that of others.

The study consisted of two parts: (a) from entries in the emergency logbook all emergencies at the institute between January 1, 1975 and December 31, 1976 were analyzed by the patient's sex and the time and date of the emergency, and (b) over a 3-month period (April to June 1977) a random sample of emergency patients presenting between 9 A.M. and 5 P.M. were interviewed by a research worker after they had been seen by a member of the clinical team. Each patient was assessed by means of the General Health Questionnaire (Goldberg, 1972) (used to determine whether a psychiatric disorder was present), a life events scale (Holmes and Rahe, 1967) (used to determine whether significant life events had occurred during the previous year) and a social adjustment scale (Weissman and Bothwell, 1976) (used to evaluate the coping skills of the patient). In addition, the patients were questioned about their use of medical and social services during the year prior to the emergency visit.

RESULTS

Emergencies during the 2 Years

Between January 1, 1975 and December 31, 1976 there were 8,912 psychiatric emergencies; 5,436 (61 percent) of the patients were male and 3,476 (39 percent) were female. The overall figures did not differ between the two years. Not all the patients were new: in 3,843 (43 percent) of the emergencies the patient already had a chart at the institute. Of the total, 1,279 patients (14 percent) were admitted from the emergency department as inpatients.

The daily number of psychiatric emergencies varied during the week: the peak number was on Monday, then the number declined for the rest of the week, except for Friday, when there was a small increase. In other words, the greatest number of patients appeared on Monday and the lowest number on Sunday. This trend, averaged for the 104 weeks, is shown in Figure 21.1. Daily inpatient admission figures were not directly related to emergency figures, since the mean number of admissions from the emergency department was 1.75 per day in general but 2.0 on weekend days. So, at the end of the week, while the number of emergencies declined, the number of admissions from the emergency department increased.

The daily number of psychiatric emergencies varied during the y ear as well: a significant peak in number occurred in August and significant troughs occurred in May and December. This trend, averaged by month for the 2-year period, is shown in Figure 21.2. The average daily number of emergencies ranged from 14.6 in August to

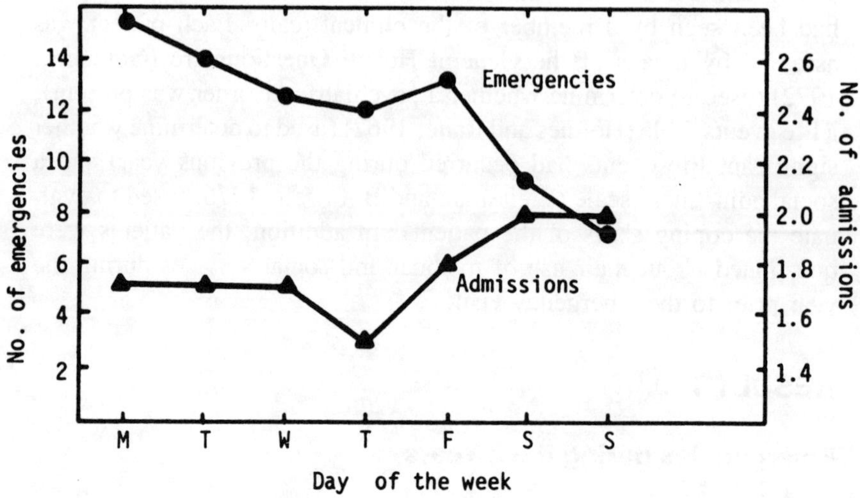

Figure 21.1 Average daily numbers of psychiatric emergencies and emergency admissions by day of the week, Clarke Institute of Psychiatry, January 1, 1975 to December 31, 1976.

10.2 in December. Average figures for August, May, and December were significantly different ($p < .05$) from those for the other months. The average daily number of inpatient admissions from the emergency department was 1.75, and the range was 1.36 in December to 2.37 in July. There was a close relation between the seasonal variation for numbers of emergencies and that for numbers of inpatient admissions. The proportion of emergency patients admitted was 12 to 18 percent.

There were more emergencies during the day (9 A.M. to 5 P.M.) than during the night 5 P.M. to 9 A.M.), the ratio being 1.4:1.0. For both males and females the ratio decreased during the week from 1.6:1.0 on Monday to parity on the weekend. The ratio did not significantly vary by month during the 2 years studied. The probability of a patient being admitted was 1:5 at night and 1:10 during the day.

Characteristics of Emergency Patients

General: Over a 3-month period (April through June 1977) 76 emergency patients chosen at random were examined in detail. Though small, this group appeared to be representative of the total daily emergency population. In addition to the 76 patients studied there were seven who refused to participate. A few of the questionnaire items could not be completed by the patients because of either acuteness of

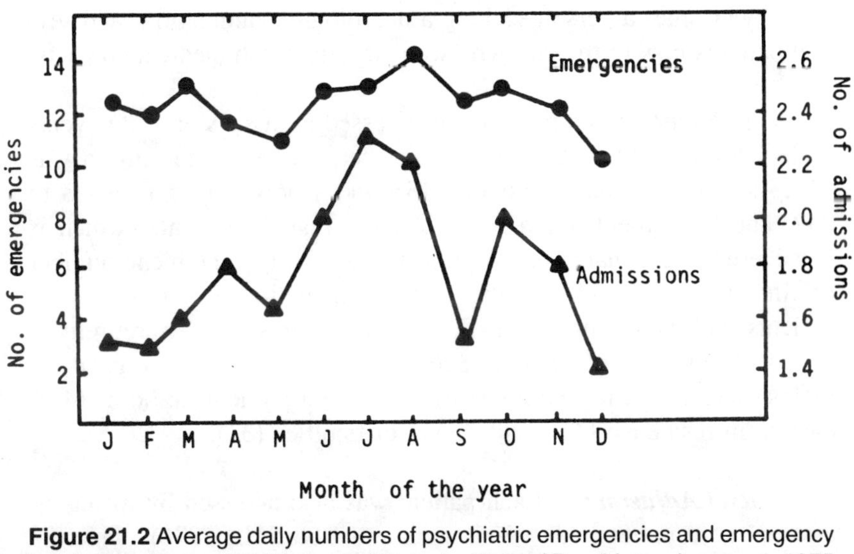

Figure 21.2 Average daily numbers of psychiatric emergencies and emergency admissions by month of the year, Clarke Institute of Psychiatry, January 1, 1975 to December 31, 1976.

illness or lack of time. The analyses were performed only on completed responses.

The group consisted of 45 males (59 percent) and 31 females (41 percent). The average age was 33 years and the median age 30 years. Of these patients 52 percent were single, 22 percent were married, and the rest were separated, divorced, or widowed. Most were Canadian-born or had immigrated to Canada early in life. The media number of years of education was 11; few had completed an undergraduate university program. Most were, or had been, employed in blue-collar occupations; 51 percent were presently unemployed. Most (82 percent) of the group had gone to the emergency department either of their own accord or on the advice of family and friends.

Mental Status. Each patient was administered the General Health Questionnaire. Scores of 5 and over indicated a high probability of there being a psychiatric problem. Of our sample 90 percent scored above the threshold; the mean score was 19. There were no differences in score between males and females. Since the patients were seen by any of the staff psychiatrists, residents, social workers, and nurses, it was not possible to allot diagnoses of the *International Classification of Diseases,* adapted to their disorders, although depressive symptoms predominated. Those with low scores included people with organic brain syndrome, a person seeking a neurologic examination, and several patients new to the city who were seeking fresh medical contacts.

Life Events. Each patient was assessed by means of a life events scale (Holmes and Rahe, 1967). The mean score for the group was 318.5 and the standard deviation 188; the scores ranged from 13 to 842, and 83 percent had a score of more than 150 points, which is considered a reasonable cutoff point for normality. The mean number of life events was 11 and the standard deviation 5.8. Only a few patients had experienced really important events such as retirement (3), death of spouse (1), marriage (1), divorce (1), or mortgage foreclosure (1); the most common events were arguments at home (43), change in residence (42), and sexual difficulties (34).

Social Adjustment. Each patient was also assessed by means of a social adjustment scale (Weissman and Bothwell, 1976), which is divided into the following categories: work function, leisure, extended family relations, marital relations, parental relations, family unit, and overall adjustment. The mean scores for our study group are compared in Table 21.1 with the scores elicited by Weissman and Bothwell (1976) from a group of depressed outpatients. The scores were comparable except that there were significantly more problems ($p < .05$) with extended families in our group than in Weissman and Bothwell's group. Their group was predominantly female.

Previous Use of Services. Each patient was questioned regarding the use of medical and social services during the previous year. The services were categorized as follows: hospitalization, consultations with doctors, centers for alcoholics, counseling, distress centers, financial assistance, manpower assistance, and others (probation and jail, for example). The range of responses is shown in Table 21.2.

The four measures for mental health for each patient were correlated. The extent of mental illness as indicated by the score on the General Health Questionnaire had a significant positive correlation with the scores for life events and social dysfunction ($r = 0.2432$ and 0.2760, $p < .05$) and a significant negative correlation ($r = -0.1973$, $p < .05$) with the previous use of medical and social services. The score for life events showed a significant positive correlation with the score for social dysfunction ($r = 0.2485$, $p < .05$) and the previous use of medical and social services ($r = 0.3092$, $p < .001$). However, social dysfunction was not significantly related to previous use of these services ($r = 0.0380$). There was no evidence from scattergrams of clustering of the scores.

Table 21.1
Social Adjustment Scores of Emergency Patients at the Clarke Institute of Psychiatry (group A) and Depressed Outpatients Studied by Weissman and Bothwell (group B)

	Mean (and standard deviation)		
Adjustment category	**Group A (n = 76)**	**Group B (n = 76)**	**Significance of difference[a]**
Work function	2.35 (0.74)	2.47 (0.71)	NS
Leisure	2.83 (0.78)	2.78 (0.66)	NS
Extended family relations	2.42 (0.85)	2.03 (0.59)	$p < .05$
Marital relations	2.71 (0.67)	2.47 (0.55)	NS
Parental relations	2.39 (1.13)	2.22 (0.80)	NS
Family unit	2.85 (0.97)	2.85 (0.81)	NS
Overall	2.63 (0.56)	2.48 (0.43)	NS

[a]NS = not significant

DISCUSSION

Our 2-year survey of psychiatric emergency patients showed variations between days and between months in the average daily number of patients. The average number declined during the week, except for a slight peak on Friday. This implies that patients may consider that more comprehensive care is given at the beginning of the week, that they may delay seeking help for problems arising on the weekend until the working week, or that their problems may not be randomly distributed over time. The finding that emergency patients were more likely to be admitted at night or on the weekend may also have several explanations, including the facts that patients are seen by residents rather than staff members at night, that no social or other support services are available then, and that problems seem particularly pressing at night. August was the peak month for daily numbers of emergencies, while May and December had the lowest numbers. This fluctuation could be due to social causes such as the absence on vacation of psychiatrists, general practitioners or family and friends in August, and happier spirits with the coming of summer and Christmas. Statistical analysis of the data showed that 40 percent of the variation in daily numbers was attributable to all these effects. Hence, staffing of the service can be planned accordingly; for example, more staff are needed at night.

Table 21.2
Proportions of Patients Using Medical and Social Services During the Year Prior to the Emergency

Service category	No. of instances of use; % of group				
	0	1–5	6–10	11+	Total
Hospitalization	68	32	—	—	100
Psychiatric consultation[a]	60	28	3	9	100
Consultation with general practitioners	15	69	8	8	100
Alcoholic centers	86	3	1	10	100
Distress centers	87	13	—	—	100
Finance (welfare)	51	11	6	32	100
Counseling	76	11	3	10	100
Manpower	72	25	3	—	100
Other (probation, jail)	93	4	3	—	100

[a] With both psychiatrists and general practitioners because of psychiatric problems

The 76 patients studied in detail were largely male, Canadian-born, of average socioeconomic status and unemployed. Most had had no prior contact with the hospital but were psychiatrically impaired. One in seven required hospital admission, and 90 percent scored above the cutoff point on the General Health Questionnaire. While there are no normative data for the social adjustment scale, the study group was comparable in maladjustment to a group of depressed outpatients. The only significant difference between the two groups pertained to relations with the nonmarital family, and here the study group showed more impairment. This is understandable in that the members of the study group were more likely to be unmarried and still living with the primary family. Many of the patients reported work problems, either being unemployed or having difficulty in coping with work. This raises the question of whether the illness or the work problem came first. Brenner (1973) demonstrated a significant correlation between the rates of admission to psychiatric hospitals and unemployment patterns in the past century. Therefore, under better economic conditions these patients might not have had comparable complaints. Since psychiatrists cannot deal with large-scale fiscal and social issues, they must decide how best to serve the medical and social needs of patients with employment difficulties under the current conditions.

While the lack of comprehensive data on health care delivery for the general population precludes any assessment of normal use of medical and social services, it appears that most of the study patients made limited use of such services apart from visits to general practitioners. It is an open question, therefore, whether greater use of these services would have obviated the patients' use of the emergency department. The correlation analysis showed that mental illness, social dysfunction, and the occurrence of life events were all significantly related, but that while the occurrence of life events was significantly associated with the previous use of medical and social services, mental illness and social dysfunction by themselves were not. Therefore, it appears that the community resources are not being adequately used and that perhaps only a crisis, in the form of one or several life events, drives people to seek help. This raises the question of the definition of an emergency in terms of severity and urgency. Definitions of emergency refer to urgency or immediacy rather than clinical severity. A direct relation between clinical status and emergency admission has not, to our knowledge, been demonstrated and seems unlikely when factors such as patterns of practice, availability of beds, public attitudes, and availability of alternative forms of care are taken into account. The small proportion of people admitted as inpatients in this survey should not be taken as evidence that most of the cases were not emergencies. Nor can the scores on the tests be taken as quantitative measures of the clinical severity of the emergency; rather they are qualitative indices of the psychiatric or social impairment of the patient. In other words, the test scores were above the thresholds for normality or were comparable to those for other disturbed populations.

Criteria are needed to establish when immediate attention should be provided. In psychiatry there are cases that at first glance may not appear to be real emergencies but might become so if unattended. They might be called pre- or latent emergencies. A triage or screening procedure in the emergency department would permit immediate assessment for some patients and later, elective appointments for others. So, while there is no doubt that emergency patients constitute a disturbed group, the need for immediate help must be examined in each case. If the emergency department is staffed by a multidisciplinary team with appropriate techniques and knowledge of community resources, the triage procedure should be effective. Legally, emergency clinics are bound to offer help to all who seek it; so, to ensure that the problems are appropriate to the emergency clinic, better mechanisms of referral are needed. This is a highly complex educational exercise for primary care physicians, social agencies, and the public.

The high proportion of individuals in this survey with psychiatric and social dysfunction may seem surprising considering that elsewhere it was found that 25 percent of referred patients (i.e., those referred by a general practitioner) did not consider themselves ill and their expectations of psychiatric help were generally low (Kaesar and Cooper, 1971). It is not easy to compare our findings with those of other studies since the others have usually concentrated on attitudes and referral pathways rather than examining the clinical and social status of the patients. Too frequently emergency patients and outpatients have been studied to see whether they can fit into an existing hospital service rather than the converse. The aim of crisis intervention units is to be flexible in their therapeutic approach, and these units have been advocated for both general and psychiatric hospitals. Therefore, they need to develop the capability of managing emergencies with the use of multidisciplinary teams. A discussion of the development and evaluation of crisis intervention is beyond the scope of this chapter and has been described in detail elsewhere (Auerbach and Kilmann, 1977). For medicine to be effective and efficient the service–needs equation should balance. It appears that there should not be concern with the question of whether the patients suffer from psychopathologic or social difficulties, or both, but rather with the nature and urgency of the problems and whether the staff and techniques are appropriate to deal with them.

Finally, we make a plea for routine collection of information on emergency patients and booked outpatients, since this is not a requirement of the Ontario Ministry of Health. Any information on outpatients is arduously collected, and not frequently, despite the emphasis in psychiatry on outpatient community care. Such information is essential for the evaluation of psychiatric care and could prove an invaluable aid in the design of outpatient services.

REFERENCES

American Hospital Association (1976), *Roper Report.* New York: Roper Organization.

Auerbach, S. M., & Kilmann, P. R. (1977), Crisis intervention: A review of outcome research. *Psychol. Bull.,* 84:1189–1217.

Bartolucci, G., & Drayer, C. S. (1973), An overview of crisis intervention in the emergency rooms of general hospitals. *Amer. J. Psychiat.,* 130:953–960.

Brenner, M. H. (1973), *Mental Illness and the Economy.* Cambridge, MA: Harvard University Press, p. 36.

Eastwood, M. R., Mindham, R. H. S., & Tennant, T. G. (1970), The physical status of psychiatric emergencies. *Brit. J. Psychiat.,* 116:545–550.

Glasscote, R. M., Cumming, E., & Hammersly, W. D., et al. (1966), *The Psychiatric Emergency. A Study of Patterns of Service.* Washington, DC: Joint Information Service of the American Psychiatric Association and the National Association for Mental Health, p. 20.

Goldberg, D. P. (1972), *The Detection of Psychiatric Illness by Questionnaire: A Technique for the Identification and Assessment of Non-Psychotic Psychiatric Illness.* Maudsley monograph No. 22, London: Oxford University Press.

Holmes, T. H., & Rahe, R. H. (1967), The social readjustment rating scale. *J. Psychosom. Res.,* 11:213–215.

Kaeser, A. C., & Cooper, B. (1971), The psychiatric outpatient, the general practitioner and the outpatient clinic; an operational study and a review. *Psychol. Med.,* 1:312–325.

Krass, M. E. (1977), Non-urgent use of hospital emergency department. *Ont. Med. Rev.,* 44:181–184.

Morrice, J. K. W. (1968), Emergency psychiatry. *Brit. J. Psychiat.,* 114:484–491.

Ungerleider, J. T. (1960), The psychiatric emergency. Analysis of six months' experience of a university hospital's consultation service. *Arch. Gen. Psychiat.*, 3:593–601.

Watters, W. W., Goodman, A., & Molnar, J. G. (1972), Organization of a psychiatric ambulatory care service in a general hospital. *Can. Psychiat. Assn. J.*, 17:409–415.

Weissmen, M. M., & Bothwell, S. (1976), Assessment of social adjustment by patient self-report. *Arch. Gen. Psychiat.*, 33(suppl. 76):1111–1115.

Wilder, J. F., Plutchnik, R., & Conte, H. R. (1977), Compliance with psychiatric emergency room referrals. *Arch. Gen. Psychiat.*, 34:930–933.

Commentary

Ronald D. Stewart, M.D.

The past two decades have seen the hospital emergency department assume an increasingly important role in the provision of primary care to the community. It remains to be seen whether this is due to the decline of the house call and the scarcity of general practitioners, or the trend toward more and more specialization in medicine. Whatever the reason, the emergency department in a community assures the public of the availability of immediate care, whether the problem be of acute onset or whether it represents the exacerbation of a chronic complaint.

Eastwood and his colleagues attempt to describe the types of patients presenting as emergencies to an urban psychiatric institute, and to better define their problems and needs. In an effort to plan for the creation of a "crisis intervention unit" at the institute, the authors interviewed a random sample of emergency patients attending the outpatient department for an unscheduled appointment between 9 A.M. and 5 P.M. Each was assessed using a questionnaire designed to evaluate the psychiatric health of the patient (General Health Questionnaire), and a scale to determine the occurrence of significant life events during the previous year. Patients were interviewed to determine their use of medical and social services during the previous year.

In an attempt to develop a profile of the activity of an emergency unit, the authors report on the daily number of psychiatric emergencies, their distribution throughout the days and months of the year, and the characteristics of the patients themselves. Over 40 percent of patients had been seen previously at the same institute; 14 percent of the total seen over two years were admitted to the hospital. A peak in the number of patients occurred on Monday, with a decline during the week. August was the month with the highest number of patients seen, while significantly fewer were seen in May and December. Most emergencies occurred during the day (9 A.M.–5 P.M.).

Of the patients randomly selected for interview, most (59 percent) were males, with an average age of 33 years; over 50 percent were single, 22 percent were married, and one-half were employed. Over 80 percent of these patients had come to the emergency department voluntarily, of their own accord or on the advice of friends. Ninety percent of these patients scored above the threshold on the General Health Questionnaire, which is designed to indicate the probability of a psychiatric illness being present in the patient. Most (83 percent) scored high on a life events scale, indicating significant life-style changes during the previous year. On a social adjustment scale, patients' scores approximated those reported for a group of depressed outpatients, with evidence of significantly more problems with extended families.

To investigate whether greater access to and use of medical and social services might have obviated the need for emergency visits, the authors attempted to relate the presence and degree of mental illness, occurrence of life events, and the degree of social dysfunction to the extent of previous use of medical facilities. While the occurrence of significant life events was associated with the previous use of medical and social services, the degree of mental illness and social dysfunction was not.

In discussing the findings of their study, Eastwood and his group raise the question of the definition of an emergency, and urge that it be based on urgency or immediacy rather than on clinical severity. Although the profile shows that emergency patients constitute a disturbed group, the authors suggest that guidelines are needed as to when immediate attention should be given to the problem presented by the patient. A triage procedure is suggested for an emergency department, in which the immediate need for acute intervention could be assessed. The chapter concludes with a plea for directing our efforts toward determining the nature and urgency of the patients' problem and ensuring the staff and techniques to deal with them, rather than attempting to determine whether patients are impaired enough to warrant "emergency" treatment.

While this chapter is helpful in posing valid questions and correctly emphasizing immediacy rather than clinical severity as the chief element of that which constitutes an "emergency," there is serious question as to whether the authors' findings can be extrapolated and applied to most emergency department settings. The patient population studied was randomly selected from a large and well-known urban psychiatric institute, clearly identified in the eyes of the community as having special expertise in this aspect of health care. It is very likely that the patient mix presenting to such a facility would be somewhat selective and perhaps represent a more "impaired" population than might be present in a general emergency department. Simply put, the patient, his family, or friends would have perceived a need for psychiatric intervention, and would have "triaged" him to the proper facility (i.e., the psychiatric hospital). This would imply that the psychiatric illness was quite evident to the lay person and, by further implication, severe enough to be recognized as such. This is very different indeed from a patient with an underlying psychiatric illness manifesting itself as a medical condition presenting to a general emergency department.

The suggestion that patients be triaged for the nature and urgency of their complaint is an already standard procedure in the general emergency department. When all is said and done, the patient is the one who decides whether or not his condition represents an emergency. In most cases, our role is to ensure that the patient is promptly served by the medical resource appropriate to his needs. Patients requiring services specific to social or related problems can properly be triaged to the on-duty social worker or, if a medical condition is a priority, the social worker can become an integral part of the medical team treating the patient.

The plea by the authors to "cut the coat to fit the cloth" is well taken. That is, rather than fit patients with psychiatric problems into a rigid medical structure, we must design a system of care for psychiatric patients around their needs and ensure that staff and techniques are sufficient to care for them. That demands of the general hospital emergency department a concerned staff capable of dealing sensitively with both patients who have an overt psychiatric illness and those with a serious underlying emotional disturbance complicated or masked by a medical condition. A great emergency department, in planning for the care of such patients, should have a full complement of social service and psychiatric consultants who are part of the staff of the department. This crisis intervention team not only should conduct ongoing reviews and educational programs for other staff members, but also should have as part of their task the provision of group sessions during which the needs of the staff, as well as patients, are addressed. In turn, the psychiatric emergency unit must have in place a reliable service for medical consultation so that the physical needs of patients are determined and met.

The value of the review by Eastwood and his colleagues lies in the restatement of the importance of the role of the patient's perception of the urgency of his condition as the essential element in the definition of an "emergency" visit. In addition, the emphasis on the nature and immediacy of the patient's problem in the triage process underscores the key to the success of any emergency system; patients do not need to prove to us that they are sick—we need to prove they are, and if so, how seriously.

Annotated Bibliography

Ianzito, B. M., Fine, J., Sprague, B., & Pestana, J. (1978). Overnight admission for psychiatric emergencies. *Hosp. & Commun. Psychiat.*, 29:728–730.

A short paper discussing an alternative to psychiatric hospitalization. Patients identified as psychiatric cases on the emergency ward of a 1,036-bed teaching hospital were either released with outpatient referral, admitted to a psychiatric inpatient facility, or hospitalized in a general medical holding unit with a 24-hour stay. The authors review the demographic and diagnostic differences among the three groups, and comment on the advantages of overnight admissions as an alternative to regular psychiatric hospitalization and outpatient referral.

Bassuk, E. L., & Gerson, S. (1979). Into the breach: Emergency psychiatry in the general hospital. *Gen. Hosp. Psychiat.*, 1:31–45.

A general paper about the interface between the community and the general hospital that the emergency ward serves. The authors point out the increasing role that the emergency ward is serving in managing psychotic patients with chronic illness and psychosocial problems. Also discussed are various approaches to organization of services and evaluation of their effectiveness.

Comstock, B. S. (1983), Psychiatric emergency intensive care. *Psych. Clin. N. Amer.*, 6:305–316.

A discussion of the role of intensive short-term hospitalization units located in or near emergency settings. These units emphasize multidisciplinary approaches to a wide variety of psychiatric problems that are amendable to short-term care.

Lim, M. H. (1983), A psychiatric emergency clinic: A study of attendances over six months. *Brit. J. Psychiat.*, 143:460–466.

A paper from the United Kingdom which looks at 2,390 consecutive visits to a walk-in psychiatric emergency service. Only a third of the patients were from the catchment area. Psychotic patients and those admitted or kept overnight were more frequent after hours and among nonmedical referrals, especially family and police referrals; but suicidal patients often came from other hospitals. Attendance at follow-up appointments was poor and factors influencing attendance were examined. Keeping patients overnight avoided unnecessary regular admissions, and surprisingly, patients did not seem to abuse the service.

Slaby, A. E. (1981), Emergency psychiatry in the general hospital: Staffing, training, and leadership issues. *Gen. Hosp. Psychiat.*, 3:306–309.

A paper by a leader in the field examining some of the general issues of the increasing use of emergency care. Since emergency psychiatric care is time- and staff-intensive with unpredictable utilization, the adequate arrangement of staffing and training, and the need for creative leadership represent challenging issues.

Jacobs, D. (1983), The treatment capabilities of psychiatric emergency services. *Gen. Hosp. Psychiat.*, 5:171–177.

This paper reviews the treatment capabilities of the psychiatric emergency service of an urban and academically oriented hospital. The author discusses clinician features as well as the treatment goals of the unit which encompass symptomatic relief, maintenance of ongoing treatment, and referral and facilitation for definitive treatment. The treatment approach represents an integration of psychological, pharmacological, and physical management principles.

Appendix

Figure 4.1 First page of the Brief Evaluation Form (BEF).

UNIVERSITY OF PITTSBURGH
WESTERN PSYCHIATRIC INSTITUTE AND CLINIC

BRIEF EVALUATION FORM

(5/14/82)

Name: ______

WPIC Number ☐☐☐☐☐

Date: ____ M ____ D ____ Y

Evaluation Setting: ______

☐ Previous (latest) IEF completed at WPIC. Evaluation setting: Date: / /

IDENTIFYING INFORMATION, CHIEF COMPLAINT, AND SOURCES OF INFORMATION:

SUMMARY OF PRESENT ILLNESS *(Describe the history of present psychiatric illness, with focus on the most recent problems and events, and on changes in the patient's course of illness since the last Initial Evaluation Form was completed.)*

1. Number of weeks of psychiatric hospitalization during the past 12 months: ____________ ☐ Unknown

2. Modalities of mental health treatment received during the past 12 months (check all applicable):

☐ None	☐ Family psychotherapy	☐ Minor tranquilizers	☐ Stimulants	☐ Other/Unspecified medication
☐ Individual psychotherapy	☐ Specific behavioral techniques	☐ Antidepressants	☐ Anti-Parkinsonian medication	☐ ECT
☐ Group Therapy	☐ Neuroleptics	☐ Lithium	☐ Anticonvulsants	☐ Other/Unspecified modalities

3. ☐ Recent significant psychotropic medication change or discontinuation.

Figure 4.2 Inventory of current symptomatology on the BEF.

WPIC NUMBER ☐☐☐☐☐

CURRENT SYMPTOM INVENTORY

	CURRENT EPISODE N = Absent 1 = Mild 2 = Moderate 3 = Severe ? = Unknown	DURING INTERVIEW Y = Observed or reported as present
1. HYPOSOMNIA difficulty falling or staying asleep and/or early morning awakening	N 1 2 3 ?	Y
2. HYPERSOMNIA excessive amount of sleep	N 1 2 3 ?	Y
3. APPETITE DE-CREASED and food refusal	N 1 2 3 ?	Y
4. APPETITE IN-CREASED	N 1 2 3 ?	Y
5. WEIGHT DECREASED	N 1 2 3 ?	Y
6. WEIGHT INCREASED	N 1 2 3 ?	Y
7. DECREASED LIBIDO lack of sexual inter-est or activity	N 1 2 3 ?	Y
8. INCREASED LIBIDO	N 1 2 3 ?	Y
9. DISTURBED SEX-UAL PERFORMANCE impotence, inhibited orgasm, premature ejaculation, dispareunia	N 1 2 3 ?	Y
10. ABNORMAL SEXUAL OBJECT OR SITUA-TION paraphilias	N 1 2 3 ?	Y
11. SEXUAL IDENTITY PROBLEMS	N 1 2 3 ?	Y
12. ALCOHOL USE of concern to individ-ual or significant other	N 1 2 3 ?	Y
13. USE OF OTHER C.N.S. DEPRES-SANTS barbiturates, other hypnotics, minor tranquilizers	N 1 2 3 ?	Y
14. USE OF OTHER DRUGS stimulants, narcotic analgesics, marijuana, hallucin-ogens, cocaine	N 1 2 3 ?	Y

	CURRENT EPISODE N = Absent 1 = Mild 2 = Moderate 3 = Severe ? = Unknown	DURING INTERVIEW Y = Observed, or reported as present
31. BIZARRE BEHAVIOR idiosyncratic appear-ance and conduct, mannerisms and posturing	N 1 2 3 ?	Y
32. HOSTILITY belligerence, un-cooperativeness	N 1 2 3 ?	Y
33. DISSOCIATIVE SYMP-TOMS narrowing of consciousness	N 1 2 3 ?	Y
34. CONVERSION SYMP-TOMS functional paralysis, anesthesia, seizures, etc.	N 1 2 3 ?	Y
35. SLOWED SPEECH AND THOUGHT	N 1 2 3 ?	Y
36. SPEECH PRESSURE OR FLIGHT OF IDEAS rapidity & dominance or abrupt topic changes based on understandable asso-ciations, distracting stimuli or word plays	N 1 2 3 ?	Y
37. THOUGHT PROCESS DISORGANIZATION loose associations, incoherence, blocking	N 1 2 3 ?	Y
38. GENERAL ANXIETY motor tension, auto-nomic hyperactivity, apprehensive expecta-tion and scanning	N 1 2 3 ?	Y
39. PANIC ATTACKS discrete periods of sudden onset of intense apprehension or terror with autonomic symptoms	N 1 2 3 ?	Y
40. SITUATIONAL ANXIE-TY OR PHOBIAS persistent irrational fear of an object or situation	N 1 2 3 ?	Y

	CURRENT EPISODE N = Absent 1 = Mild 2 = Moderate 3 = Severe ? = Unknown	DURING INTERVIEW Y = Observed or reported as present
57. DELUSIONS OF REFERENCE, PERSE-CUTION, JEALOUSY OR GRANDIOSITY	N 1 2 3 ?	Y
58. DEPRESSIVE DELU-SIONS OR HALLUCIN-ATIONS nihilistic or derogatory content	N 1 2 3 ?	Y
59. OTHER DELUSIONS	N 1 2 3 ?	Y
60. IMPAIRED SENSOR-IUM AND ORIENTA-TION to time, place and person	N 1 2 3 ?	Y
61. ACQUIRED INTEL-LECTUAL IMPAIR-MENT deficit in mem-ory, calculation, knowledge	N 1 2 3 ?	Y
62. DEVELOPMENTAL INTELLECTUAL DEFICIT	N 1 2 3 ?	Y
63. POOR CONCEN-TRATION poor attention span distractibility	N 1 2 3 ?	Y
64. LACK OF INSIGHT about presence and nature of psychopathology	N 1 2 3 ?	Y

SUPPLEMENTARY INVENTORY FOR CHILDREN & ADOLESCENTS

65. FIRE SETTING	N 1 2 3 ?	Y
66. TRUANCY	N 1 2 3 ?	Y
67. RUNNING AWAY	N 1 2 3 ?	Y
68. DISOBEDIENCE persistent rule break-ing, defiance to authority	N 1 2 3 ?	Y

15. VIOLENT BEHAVIOR forceful aggressiveness, assaultiveness, destructiveness	N	1	2	3	?	Y
16. IMPULSIVITY poor impulse control	N	1	2	3	?	Y
17. OTHER ANTISOCIAL BEHAVIOR cheating, stealing, irresponsibility, lying	N	1	2	3	?	Y
18. HYPERSENSITIVITY TO CRITICISM or rejection	N	1	2	3	?	Y
19. EMOTIONAL DISTANCE OR COLDNESS limited capacity to form social relationships	N	1	2	3	?	Y
20. ECCENTRICITY oddities in thinking, perception, speech and behavior	N	1	2	3	?	Y
21. OVERLY DRAMATIC BEHAVIOR attention seeking and intensely expressed reactive behavior	N	1	2	3	?	Y
22. SELF-CENTEREDNESS grandiose sense and fantasies of self-importance and entitlement	N	1	2	3	?	Y
23. UNSTABLE AND INTENSE RELATIONSHIPS	N	1	2	3	?	Y
24. UNDUE DEPENDENCE ON OTHERS allowing others to assume responsibility for self	N	1	2	3	?	Y
25. UNDUE PERFECTIONISM overconcern with details and work, demandingness	N	1	2	3	?	Y
26. INTENTIONAL INEFFECTIVENESS indirect resistance to demands for performance	N	1	2	3	?	Y
27. DECREASED MOTOR ACTIVITY	N	1	2	3	?	Y
28. INCREASED MOTOR ACTIVITY restlessness, agitation	N	1	2	3	?	Y
29. SOCIAL WITHDRAWAL lack of spontaneous interaction, seclusiveness	N	1	2	3	?	Y
30. SELF-NEGLECT lack of attention to cleanliness and clothing	N	1	2	3	?	Y

41. DEPRESSED MOOD sadness, dejection, crying	N	1	2	3	?	Y
42. LOW SELF-ESTEEM	N	1	2	3	?	Y
43. LABILITY OF MOOD repeated, rapid shifts in mood	N	1	2	3	?	Y
44. ELATED MOOD euphoria, excitement, expansiveness	N	1	2	3	?	Y
45. FLAT or INCONGRUOUS AFFECT inappropriate for content of speech	N	1	2	3	?	Y
46. SUSPICIOUSNESS feelings that everything is not as it should be, inappropriate interpretiveness, hypervigilance, guardedness	N	1	2	3	?	Y
47. SOMATIC PREOCCUPATION hypochondriasis	N	1	2	3	?	Y
48. SUICIDAL INDICATORS death wishes, suicidal ideas or attempts	N	1	2	3	?	Y
49. HOMICIDAL IDEATION	N	1	2	3	?	Y
50. HOMICIDAL BEHAVIOR	N	1	2	3	?	Y
51. OBSESSIONS AND COMPULSIONS repetitive intrusive thoughts or behavior experienced against conscious resistance	N	1	2	3	?	Y
52. DEPERSONALIZATION experiencing self or surroundings as unreal	N	1	2	3	?	Y
53. SCHNEIDERIAN SYMPTOMS voices arguing or commenting on one's action or speaking thoughts aloud; somatic passivity; thought withdrawal; insertion or broadcasting "made" feelings, impulses or acts; primary delusional perception	N	1	2	3	?	Y
54. OTHER AUDITORY HALLUCINATIONS	N	1	2	3	?	Y
55. VISUAL HALLUCINATIONS	N	1	2	3	?	Y
56. OTHER HALLUCINATIONS smell, taste, touch	N	1	2	3	?	Y

69. TEMPER TANTRUMS screaming, breath-holding attacks	N	1	2	3	?	Y
70. SCHOOL REFUSAL	N	1	2	3	?	Y
71. ELECTIVE MUTISM refusal to speak in social situations	N	1	2	3	?	Y
72. DISTORTION OF BODY IMAGE	N	1	2	3	?	Y
73. FEAR OF OBESITY	N	1	2	3	?	Y
74. PICA persistent eating of non-nutritive substances	N	1	2	3	?	Y
75. TICS involuntary rapid movements or productions of noises or words	N	1	2	3	?	Y
76. STUTTERING	N	1	2	3	?	Y
77. ENURESIS	N	1	2	3	?	Y
78. ENCOPRESIS	N	1	2	3	?	Y
79. PARASOMNIAS e.g., sleepwalking, night terrors	N	1	2	3	?	Y
80. AUTISTIC WITHDRAWAL lack of responsiveness to other people	N	1	2	3	?	Y
81. RESISTANCE TO CHANGE IN THE ENVIRONMENT	N	1	2	3	?	Y
82. PECULIAR SPEECH PATTERN pronominal reversal, metaphoric language, echolalia, bizarre rhythm or intonation of speech	N	1	2	3	?	Y
83. SELF-ABUSIVE BEHAVIOR self-mutilation, biting or hitting self, head banging	N	1	2	3	?	Y
84. ODDITIES OF MOTOR BEHAVIOR peculiar posturing, peculiar hand or finger movements, abnormal repetitive movements, walking on tiptoe, etc.	N	1	2	3	?	Y
85. DELAYED LANGUAGE ACQUISITION difficulty in comprehending or expressing oral language	N	1	2	3	?	Y
86. DIFFICULTY IN ARTICULATION of speech sounds such as r, sh, th, f, z, l, or ch	N	1	2	3	?	Y

INSTRUCTIONS FOR DSM-III AXES I AND II

Axes I and II comprise the entire classification of mental disorders. Axis II includes Personality Disorders and Specific Developmental Disorders (listed within boxes on this page and on the back of page 7). All other disorders and conditions are included in Axis I.

On both Axes I and II multiple diagnoses may be made to describe the current psychiatric condition. Within each axis, diagnoses should be listed as primary, secondary and so forth, in order, with that being the focus of attention or treatment listed first.

The *Principal* diagnosis is that chiefly responsible for occasioning the evaluation or admission to clinical care. It will be assumed to be the first diagnosis on Axis I, unless the first diagnosis on Axis II is followed by "(Principal Diagnosis)".

The clinician may wish to indicate a significant degree of diagnostic uncertainty by writing "(Provisional)" following a given codable diagnosis in the main formulation section. Additionally, for each codable diagnosis, alternatives to be ruled out in a differential diagnosis process may be mentioned within the boxed sections of the diagnostic summary.

LIST OF AXES I AND II CATEGORIES AND CODES

LIST OF AXES I AND II CATEGORIES AND CODES

For most disorders, the DSM-III and ICD-9-CM codes are essentially the same. Whenever there is a substantial difference, the ICD-9-CM code is provided in parentheses after the diagnostic term. To ensure retrieval of DSM-III specificity, use always the codes to the left of the diagnostic terms. Data entry into the computer will include codes for both diagnostic systems.

The long dashes indicate the need for a fifth-digit subtype or other qualifying term.

DISORDERS USUALLY FIRST EVIDENT IN INFANCY, CHILDHOOD OR ADOLESCENCE

Other disorders with physical manifestations
307 00 Stuttering
307 60 Functional enuresis
307 70 Functional encopresis
307 46 Sleepwalking disorder
307 49 Sleep terror disorder (307 46)

Pervasive developmental disorders
Code in fifth digit 0 full syndrome present, 1 residual state
299 0x Infantile autism
299 9x Childhood onset pervasive developmental disorder

299 8x Atypical

327 01 withdrawal (292 00)
327 02 withdrawal delirium (292 00)
327 04 amnestic disorder (292 83)

Opioid
327 10 intoxication (305 50)
327 11 withdrawal (292 00)

Cocaine
327 20 intoxication (305 60)

Amphetamine or similarly acting sympathomimetic
327 30 intoxication (305 70)
327 32 delirium (292 81)
327 35 delusional disorder (292 11)

Mental Retardation
(Code in fifth digit: 1 = with other behavioral symptoms [requiring attention or treatment and that are not part of another disorder]. 0 = without other behavioral symptoms.)

317.0(x) Mild mental retardation, ______
318.0(x) Moderate mental retardation, ______
318.1(x) Severe mental retardation, ______
318.2(x) Profound mental retardation, ______
319.0(x) Unspecified mental retardation, ______

Attention deficit disorder
314.01 with hyperactivity
314.00 without hyperactivity
314.80 residual type

Conduct disorder
312.00 undersocialized, aggressive
312.10 undersocialized, nonaggressive
312.23 socialized, aggressive
312.21 socialized, nonaggressive
312.90 atypical

Anxiety disorders of childhood or adolescents
309.21 Separation anxiety disorder
313.21 Avoidant disorder of childhood or adolescence
313.00 Overanxious disorder

Other disorders of infancy, childhood or adolescence
313.89 Reactive attachment disorder of infancy
313.22 Schizoid disorder of childhood or adolescence
313.23 Elective mutism
313.81 Oppositional disorder
313.82 Identity disorder

Eating disorders
307.10 Anorexia nervosa
307.51 Bulimia
307.52 Pica
307.53 Rumination disorder of infancy
307.50 Atypical eating disorder

Stereotyped movement disorders
307.21 Transient tic disorder
307.22 Chronic motor tic disorder
307.23 Tourette's disorder
307.20 Atypical tic disorder
307.30 Atypical stereotyped movement disorder

Specific developmental disorders
Note: These are coded on Axis II.
315.00 Developmental reading disorder
315.10 Developmental arithmetic disorder
315.31 Developmental language disorder
315.39 Developmental articulation disorder
315.50 Mixed specific developmental disorder
315.90 Atypical specific developmental disorder

ORGANIC MENTAL DISORDERS
Section 1. Organic mental disorders whose etiology or pathophysiological process is listed below (taken from the mental disorders section of ICD-9—CM).

Dementias arising in the senium and presenium

Primary degenerative dementia, senile onset,
290.30 with delirium
290.20 with delusions
290.21 with depression
290.00 uncomplicated

code in fifth digit
1 = with delirium, 2 = with delusions, 3 = with depression
0 = uncomplicated
290.1x Primary degenerative dementia, presenile onset, ______
290.4x Multi-infarct dementia

Substance induced

Alcohol
303.00 intoxication
291.40 idiosyncratic intoxication
291.80 withdrawal
291.00 withdrawal delirium
291.30 hallucinations
291.10 amnestic disorder

Code severity of dementia in fifth digit
1 = mild; 2 = moderate; 3 = severe; 0 = unspecified
291.2x Dementia associated with alcoholism, ______

Barbiturate or similarly acting sedative or hypnotic
327.00 intoxication (305.40)
327.31 withdrawal (292.00)

Phencyclidine (PCP) or similarly acting arycyclohexylamine
327.40 intoxication (305.90)
327.42 delirium (292.81)
327.49 mixed organic mental disorder (292.90)

Hallucinogen
327.56 hallucinosis (305.30)
327.55 delusional disorder (292.11)
327.57 affective disorder (294.84)

Cannabis
327.60 intoxication (305.20)
327.65 delusional disorder (292.11)

Tobacco
327.71 withdrawal (292.00)

Caffeine
327.80 intoxication (305.90)

Other or unspecified substance
327.90 intoxication (305.90)
327.91 withdrawal (292.00)
327.92 delirium (292.81)
327.93 dementia (292.28)
327.94 amnestic disorder (292.83)
327.95 delusional disorder (292.11)
327.96 hallucinosis (292.12)
327.97 affective disorder (292.84)
327.98 personality disorder (292.89)
327.99 atypical or mixed organic mental disorder (292.90)

Section 2. Organic brain syndromes whose etiology or pathophysiological process is either noted as an additional diagnosis from outside the mental disorders section of ICD-9-CM or is unknown.
293.00 Delirium
294.10 Dementia
294.00 Amnestic syndrome
293.81 Organic delusional syndrome
293.82 Organic hallucinosis
293.83 Organic affective syndrome
310.10 Organic personality syndrome
294.80 Atypical or mixed organic brain syndrome

Figure 4.3 Mental status, medical history, and summary on the BEF.

WPIC NUMBER ☐☐☐☐☐

MENTAL STATUS REMARKS *(Comment on general appearance and behavior, speech and thought rate and pattern, mood and affect, thought content, perception, sensorium, orientation, intellectual functions and insight.)*

BRIEF MEDICAL HISTORY AND EXAMINATION *(Include current physical disorders, medications, allergies and a preliminary physical examination.)*

VITAL SIGNS: Pulse ________ B.P.: ______/______ Temp.: ________ Resp.: ________

NARRATIVE ASSESSMENT SUMMARY

PROBLEMS *(Psychopathological, physical and social)* **RECOMMENDATIONS** *(Diagnostic studies, treatment modalities, instructions to patient/family)*

LIST OF AXES I AND II CATEGORIES AND CODES (CONTINUATION)

SUBSTANCE USE DISORDERS

Code in fifth digit 1 = continuous, 2 = episodic, 3 = in remission, 0 = unspecified

305.0x Alcohol abuse, ______
303.9x Alcohol dependence (Alcoholism), ______
305.4x Barbiturate or similary acting sedative or hypnotic abuse, ______
304.1x Barbituate or similarly acting sedative or hypnotic dependence, ______
305.5x Opioid abuse, ______
304.0x Opioid dependence, ______
305.6x Cocaine abuse, ______
305.7x Amphetamine or similarly acting sympathomimetic abuse, ______
304.4x Amphetamine or similary acting sympathomimetic dependence, ______
305.9x Phencyclidine (PCP) or similarty acting arylcyclohexylamine abuse, ______ (328 4x)
305.3x Hallucinogen abuse, ______
305.2x Cannabis abuse, ______
304.3x Cannabis dependence, ______
305.1x Tobacco dependence, ______
305.9x Other, mixed or unspecified substance abuse, ______
304.6x Other specified substance dependence, ______
304.9x Unspecified substance dependence, ______
304.7x Dependence on combination of opioid and other non-alcoholic substance, ______
304.8x Dependence on combination of substances, excluding opioids and alcohol, ______

SCHIZOPHRENIC DISORDERS

Code in fifth digit 1 = subchronic, 2 = chronic, 3 = subchronic with acute exacerbation, 4 = chronic with acute exacerbation, 5 = in remission, 0 = unspecified.

Schizophrenia,
295.1x disorganized, ______
295.2x catatonic, ______
295.3x paranoid, ______
295.9x undifferentiated, ______
295.6x residual, ______

PARANOID DISORDERS

297.10 Paranoia

Other specific affective disorders
301.13 Cyclothymic disorder
300.40 Dysthymic disorder (or Depressive neurosis)

Atypical affective disorders
296.70 Atypical bipolar disorder
296.82 Atypical depression

ANXIETY DISORDERS

Phobic disorders (or Phobic neuroses)
300.21 Agoraphobia with panic attacks
300.22 Agoraphobia without panic attacks
300.23 Social phobia
300.29 Simple phobia

Anxiety states (or Anxiety neuroses)
300.01 Panic disorder
300.02 Generalized anxiety disorder
300.30 Obsessive compulsive disorder (or Obsessive compulsive neurosis)

Post-traumatic stress disorder
308.30 acute
309.81 chronic or delayed
300.00 Atypical anxiety disorder

SOMATOFORM DISORDERS

300.81 Somatization disorder
300.11 Conversion disorder (or Hysterical neurosis, conversion type)
307.80 Psychogenic pain disorder
300.70 Hypochrondriasis (or Hypochrondriacal neurosis)
300.71 Atypical somatoform disorder (300 70)

DISSOCIATIVE DISORDERS (OR HYSTERICAL NEUROSES, DISSOCIATIVE TYPE)

300.12 Psychogenic Anmesia
300.13 Psychogenic fugue
300.14 Multiple personality
300.60 Depersonalization disorder (or depersonalization neurosis)
300.15 Atypical dissociative disorder

PSYCHOSEXUAL DISORDERS

Gender identity disorders

FACTITIOUS DISORDERS

300.16 Factitious disorder with psychological symptoms
301.51 Chronic factitious disorder with physical symptoms
300.19 Atypical factitious disorder with physical symptoms

DISORDERS OF IMPULSE CONTROL NOT ELSEWHERE CLASSIFIED

312.31 Pathological gambing
312.32 Kleptomania
312.33 Pyromania
312.34 Intermittent explosive disorder
312.35 Isolated explosive disorder
312.39 Atypical impulse control disorder

ADJUSTMENT DISORDER

309.00 with depressed mood
309.24 with anxious mood
309.28 with mixed emotional features
309.30 with disturbance of conduct
309.40 with mixed disturbance of emotions and conduct
309.23 with work (or academic) inhibition
309.83 with withdrawal
309.90 with atypical features

PSYCHOLOGICAL FACTORS AFFECTING PHYSICAL CONDITION

Specify physical condition on Axis III.
316.00 Psychological factors affecting physical condition

PERSONALITY DISORDERS

Note: These are coded on Axis II

301.00 Paranoid
301.20 Schizoid
301.22 Schizotypal
301.50 Histrionic
301.81 Narcissistic
301.70 Antisocial
301.83 Borderline
301.82 Avoidant
301.60 Dependent
301.40 Compulsive
301.84 Passive-Aggressive
301.89 Atypical, mixed or other personality disorder

297.30 Shared paranoid disorder
298.30 Acute paranoid disorder
297.90 Atypical paranoid disorder

PSYCHOTIC DISORDERS NOT ELSEWHERE CLASSIFIED

295.40 Schizophreniform disorder
298.80 Brief reactive psychosis
295.70 Schizoaffective disorder
298.90 Atypical psychosis

AFFECTIVE DISORDERS

Major affective disorders

Code major depressive episode in fifth digit 6 = in remission, 4 = with psychotic features (the unofficial non-ICD-9-CM fifth digit 7 may be used instead to indicate that the psychotic features are mood-incongruent), 3 = with melancholia, 2 = without melancholia, 0 = unspecified.

Code manic episode in fifth digit: 6 = in remission, 4 = with psychotic features (the unofficial non-ICD-9-CM fifth digit 7 may be used instead to indicate that the psychotic features are mood-incongruent), 2 = without psychotic features, 0 = unspecified

Bipolar disorder,
296.6x mixed, ______
296.4x manic, ______
296.5x depressed, ______

Major depression,
296.2x single episode, ______
296.3x recurrent, ______

Indicate sexual history in the fifth digit of Transsexualism code:
1 = asexual, 2 = homosexual, 3 = heterosexual, 0 = unspecified.

302.5x Transsexualism, ______
302.60 Gender identity disorder of childhood
302.85 Atypical gender identity disorder

Paraphilias
302.81 Fetishism
302.30 Transvestism
302.10 Zoophilia
302.20 Pedophilia
302.40 Exhibitionism
302.82 Voyeurism
302.83 Sexual masochism
302.84 Sexual sadism
302.90 Atypical paraphilia

Psychosexual dysfunctions
302.71 Inhibited sexual desire
302.72 Inhibited sexual excitement
302.73 Inhibited female orgasm
302.74 Inhibited male orgasm
302.75 Premature ejaculation
302.76 Functional dyspareunia
306.51 Functional vaginismus
302.70 Atypical psychosexual dysfunction

Other psychosexual disorders
302.00 Ego-dystonic homosexuality
302.89 Psychosexual disorder not elsewhere classified

V CODES FOR CONDITIONS NOT ATTRIBUTABLE TO A MENTAL DISORDER THAT ARE A FOCUS OF ATTENTION OR TREATMENT

V65.20 Malingering
V62.89 Borderline Intellectual functioning (V62.88)
V71.01 Adult antisocial behavior
V71.02 Childhood or adolescent antisocial behavior
V62.30 Academic problem
V62.20 Occupational problem
V62.82 Uncomplicated bereavement
V15.81 Noncompliance with medical treatment
V62.89 Phase of life problem or other life circumstance problem
V61.10 Marital problem
V61.20 Parent-child problem
V61.80 Other specified family circumstances
V62.81 Other interpersonal problem

ADDITIONAL CODES

300.90 Unspecified mental disorder (nonpsychotic)
V71.09 No diagnosis or condition on Axis I
799.90 Diagnosis or condition deferred on Axis I

V71.09	No diagnosis on Axis II
799.90	Diagnosis deferred on Axis II

INSTRUCTIONS FOR DSM-III AXIS III: PHYSICAL DISORDERS

Axis III includes any current physical disorders or conditions relevant to the understanding or management of the individual. Such conditions are catalogued in the non-mental disorder sections of the International Classification of Diseases (ICD-9-CM). Physical conditions identified for an individual should be described in standard terms and will be coded later. Past disorders that are not currently active should be described in the Medical History but not listed in the diagnostic formulation.

Figure 4.4 Diagnostic summary and dispositional information on the BEF.

UNIVERSITY OF PITTSBURGH
WESTERN PSYCHIATRIC INSTITUTE AND CLINIC

BRIEF EVALUATION FORM

Name: ______________________

WPIC NUMBER | | | | | |

Date: ______ ______ ______
m d y

Evaluation Setting: ______________

DIAGNOSTIC SUMMARY

I. Clinical psychiatric syndromes *(Instructions and codes on back of pages 2 and 3)*

Main Formulation:	Codes	Alternatives to be ruled out	Codes
1.			
2.			
3.			
4.			

II Personality and specific developmental disorders *(Instructions and codes on back of pages 2 and 3)*

Main Formulation:	Codes	Alternatives to be ruled out:	Codes
1.			
2.			

III. Physical Disorders *(Instructions on back of page 3)*

Main Formulation:	Codes	Alternatives to be ruled out:	Codes
1.			
2.			
3.			
4.			

IV. Psychosocial stressors *(Instructions on back of this page)*

A. Ranked list:

	Codes
1.	
2.	
3.	
4.	

B. Overall stressor severity:

1	2	3	4	5	6	7	0
None	Minimal	Mild	Moderate	Severe	Extreme	Catastrophic	Unspecified

V. Highest level of adaptive functioning during the past year *(Instructions on back of this page)*

1	2	3	4	5	6	7	0
Superior	Very Good	Good	Fair	Poor	Very Poor	Grossly Impaired	Unspecified

VI. Current functioning: *(Instructions on back of this page)*

	Superior	Adequate	Slightly Impaired	Moderately Impaired	Markedly Impaired	Unspecified
A. Occupational	1	2	3	4	5	0
B. With family	1	2	3	4	5	0
C. With other indiv. & groups	1	2	3	4	5	0

DISPOSITION

A. Admission or Referrals

Name of program or facility	Date of admission or appointment (month/day/year)	Release of information signed (✓)

Remarks: ______

B. Were referrals and recommendations accepted by patient/family? ☐ Yes ☐ No If no, explain ______

C. Legal status after evaluation:

☐ Voluntary (regular) ☐ Voluntary-302 Commitment discontinued ☐ 302 Commitment in force ☐ 303 Commitment ☐ 304 Commitment ☐ Other involuntary

EVALUATORS *(Who interviewed the patient)*

1. ______ Signature of first clinician ______ Code ______ Date

2. ______ Signature of second clinician ______ Code ______ Date

3. ______ Signature of third clinician ______ Code ______ Date

INSTRUCTIONS FOR DSM-III AXIS IV: PSYCHOSOCIAL STRESSORS

Axis IV assesses psychological stressors (both discrete events and ongoing strains) judged to be significant in the development or exacerbation of the present disorder.

First, identify relevant stressors during the past 12 months as specifically as possible and list them (up to 4) in order of importance. To accomplish this, ask for a summary of events and strains from the patient, and then probe specifically to clarify the patient's initial report and to inquire about areas of the patient's life which may not have been mentioned spontaneously. Situations which mainly reflect the patient's symptomology or dysfunctions should be excluded.

Please consider the following categories of stressors:

1. **Health:** e.g. acute or chronic physical illness or injury either to the patient or to someone close to the patient, mental illness in significant others. A physical disorder, which is listed as such on Axis III, can also be a psychosocial stressor if it creates a considerable strain on the patient's life.
2. **Bereavement:** e.g., death of parent, extended family member, or significant other.
3. **Love and marriage:** e.g., separation, divorce, persistent marital discord.
4. **Parental:** e.g., pregnancy, birth of a child, loss of custody of child, behavior problems in children.
5. **Family stressors for children and adolescents:** e.g., cold or hostile relationship between parents, cold or hostile parental behavior towards child, stressful family situation.
6. **Other familial relationships:** e.g., acute or chronic serious family arguments other than with immediate relative, change in the frequency of family interaction.
7. **Other relationships outside the family:** e.g., terminating a close friendship, terminating organizational activities, serious disruptions in social relationships.
8. **Work:** e.g., demotion or promotion at work, significant changes in work conditions, having a difficult supervisor, becoming retired, lack of employment opportunities.
9. **School:** e.g., began or changed a school or training program, failed an important academic milestone, completing or failing a school or training program.
10. **Financial:** e.g., significant decrease in income, took a large loan or mortgage, foreclosure on a loan.
11. **Legal:** e.g., court appearances, major lawsuits, arrests, sentenced to (or served) a jail term.
12. **Housing/environmental:** e.g., change in residence, significant deterioration in living conditions, eviction or threat of eviction.
13. **Miscellanea:** e.g., being victim of a crime or assault, facing a new culture.

Next, rate the severity (from 1 to 7) of the summed effect of all the psycosocial stressors listed. This rating should be based on your assessment of the "objective" stress represented by the events or strains, not on the patient's "subjective" vulnerability to the stressors. The level of stress rated should be that likely to be experienced by an "average" person of similar socio-cultural circumstances as the patient and confronting the same events and strains. The following examples may be used as a guide in making your ratings:

Code	Term	Adult examples	Child or adolescent examples
1	None	No apparent psychosocial stressors	No apparent psychosocial stressors
2	Minimal	Minor violation of the law, small bank loan	Vacation with family
3	Mild	Argument with neighbor, change in work hours	Change in schoolteacher, new school year
4	Moderate	New career, death of close friend, pregnancy	Chronic parental fighting, change to new school, illness of close relative, birth of sibling
5	Severe	Serious illness in self or family, major financial loss, marital separation, birth of child	Death of peer, divorce of parents, arrest, hospitalization, persistent and harsh parental discipline
6	Extreme	Death of close relative, divorce	Death of parent or sibling, repeated physical or sexual abuse
7	Catastrophic	Concentration camp experience, devastating natural disaster	Multiple family deaths
0	Unspecified	No information, or not applicable	No information, or not applicable

In summing the effect of all stressors, it may be necessary to take into account both the number and the severity of stressors. For example, one moderate stressor would receive a rating of 4, while a combination of 3 moderate stressors might receive a rating of 5 or 6 (the same rating which a single more severe stressor would receive.)

INSTRUCTIONS FOR DSM-III AXIS V: HIGHEST LEVEL OF ADAPTIVE FUNCTIONING IN PAST YEAR

Axis V assesses an individual's highest level of adaptive occupational and social functioning (for at least a few months) during the past year.

Recommended rating steps:

1. Identify the best couple of months of adaptive functioning during the past 12 months and focus attention on that period for making the following assessments.
2. Separately judge the individual's performance and degree of impairment in the following two regards
   a) Occupational Functioning: This encompasses consistency and effectiveness of performance of expected role as worker, student, and/or homemaker. If an individual is unemployed, not primarily because of inability to hold a job but because of inavailability of employment, his occupational assessment should focus on alternative roles, e.g., homemaker.
   b) Social Relations: This encompasses frequency and quality of social interaction, i.e., meeting, communicating, and sharing common activities with family members and with other individuals and groups.
3. Combine the occupational functioning and social relations ratings using the scale below for obtaining the overall highest level of adaptive functioning in the past year. As noted, use of leisure time is considered only for the highest levels of functioning, and essential self-care only for the poorest.

Code	Term	Description
1	Superior	Unusually effective functioning in occupational functioning, social relations, and use of leisure time.
2	Very Good	Better than average functioning in occupational functioning, social relations, and use of leisure time.
3	Good	No more than slight impairment in either occupational or social functioning.
4	Fair	Moderate impairment in either occupational functioning or social relations, or some impairment in both.
5	Poor	Marked impairment in either occupational functioning or social relations, or moderate impairment in both.
6	Very Poor	Marked impairment in both occupational functioning and social relations.
7	Grossly Impaired	Gross impairment in virtually all areas of functioning, including essential self-care.
0	Unspecified	

INSTRUCTIONS FOR AXIS VI: CURRENT FUNCTIONING

Axis VI assesses current levels of functioning at work, school or homemaking, and relations with family, and with other individuals or groups.

Separately judge the individual's performance **during the past month** in the following three regards:

a) Occupational Functioning: This encompasses consistency and effectiveness of performance of expected role as worker, student, and/or homemaker. If an individual is unemployed, not primarily because of inability to hold a job, but because of inavailability of employment, his occupational assessment should focus on alternative roles, e.g., homemaker.

b) Functioning with Family: This encompasses frequency and quality of interaction with family members (i.e. meeting, communicating, and sharing common activities with them.)

c) Functioning with Other Individuals and Groups: This encompasses frequency and quality of interaction with non-family individuals and groups (i.e. meeting, communicating, and sharing common activities with them).

Determine the individual's current functioning level in each of these regards by using the scale given below.

Code	Functioning Level	Occupational Functioning	Functioning with Family and with Other Individuals and Groups
1	Superior	Highly regular and competent work	Very frequent and close personal contacts
2	Adequate	Acceptable work regularity and competence	Acceptable frequency and closeness of personal contacts
3	Slightly Impaired	Occasionally misses work and/or has some difficulty with competence	Rather restricted or irregular frequency and closeness of personal contacts
4	Moderately Impaired	Misses work frequently and/or shows moderate incompetence	Infrequent and superficial or troubled personal contacts
5	Markedly Impaired	Works rarely or not at all, and/or is grossly incompetent	Almost non-existent or grossly disturbed personal contacts
0	Unspecified		

Name Index

Subject Index